Lisha Simester

the natural health bible

stay well, live longer

quadrille

To Alan Dattelbaum with great love and admiration

This edition first published in 2007 by
Quadrille Publishing

Editor: Anne McDowall

Publishing Director: Anne Furniss
Creative Director: Mary Evans
Art Director: Françoise Dietrich
Editor & Project Manager: Lewis Esson
Art Editor: Rachel Gibson
Assistant Editor: Emma Noble
Production: Julie Hadingham

ISBN: 978 184400 5277

Printed in Singapore

Medical advisor:
Dr David Smallbone MB., ChB, LRCP, MRCS, MFHom, FCOH

Specialist consultants and contributors:
Patrick Holford BSc. Dip ION
Celia and Brian Wright
Pierre Jean Cousin MBACC, GCRCH
Eddie and Debbie Shapiro
Jennifer Dodd, ITEC, Dip. SPA
Caroline Turner RSA, ACE
Catharine Christof ITEC, ISTM
Dominique Radclyffe
Jerome Burne
Marci F. Murphy MS, ATC, CSCS
Christine Fletcher

contents

introduction

The fabulous scientific/medical and technological developments in recent centuries are awe inspiring. Yet, in spite of these, the world is neither safer nor healthier. While we can see stunning advances in medical, chemical, technological and surgical skills, they are not always without risks, side effects and failures. The frequency of errors and wrong calls make consulting a doctor, or a stay in hospital, a potentially dangerous process – a kind of roulette wheel. We know we can go into hospital with one thing and come out with another. There's no longer the old blind faith that doctors have all the answers and solutions to our health problems. We know they can't always give an accurate diagnosis, however brilliant their knowledge.

It would appear that God's medicine cabinet is not good enough, and unless we give it a chemical overhaul with double blind trials, costing huge sums of money, it is unworthy. Fortunately, modern medicine and the pharmaceutical and chemical industries are opening their eyes to the potency of nature in its natural state, showing respect for health systems with thousands, rather than hundreds, of years of history.

The discovery and regular use of antibiotics and vaccinations have wiped away many diseases that once ravaged the population with uncontrollable epidemics. But in their wake have emerged stronger and more deadly bacteria and viruses – 'superbugs' that can resist and overpower even the strongest drugs. At no other time in history have our immune systems been so challenged by changing environmental conditions and time zones: more people are travelling around the world than ever before and air travel circulates germs as well as people at sound-barrier-breaking speeds.

The information revolution ensures we are now much better educated about our minds and bodies. Yet many of us have lost touch with the simple folk knowledge about ourselves and the natural world that was second nature to our ancestors.

Today it is far easier to stay well as there are so many paths we can take to create and maintain optimum health. As more people wake up to the fact that there is a lot that can be done to prevent illness in the first place, it is up to each of us to discover a health regime that best fits our unique disposition, type and need. Each of us is in the front line when it comes to our own health: the way we treat our body and mind each day determines our state of health and well-being in the short- and the long-term.

Most of us in the developed world will live to a ripe age of 70 plus – a lot longer than our ancestors – and we can affect the quality of life we will experience in our advancing years. Will we spend our golden years struggling with degenerative diseases and ill health or will we live our days out in a state of wholeness and well-being, confident in our ability to adapt to the stresses of time, wear and tear and the normal aging process? If we learn to take better care of ourselves earlier we can prevent many of the illnesses so common today. We have the power – it is just a question of recognizing and using it, of really tuning into our bodies and minds and objectively assessing our condition, our type, and habits we have that might be contributing to negative lifestyle patterns that disturb the natural balance. It is possible to achieve a high level of well-being and vitality by creating an individual health programme tailored to our own needs and temperament. The choices we make play the largest role in the state of our health.

In this book we seek to explore the rich, varied and fascinating world of life-enhancing options from which we can choose to enhance the health of body, mind and spirit. We are not cataloguing health problems and cures in this volume, but rather emphasizing the joys of, and route to, positive natural good health. We are celebrating the many available paths to a more holistic, and therefore more vital, healthy life. Put simply, the purpose of *The Natural Health Bible* is to present many of the best options from which to choose and create a personal plan for positive well-being, increasing good health and improving quality of life. In calling this book a 'bible', I in no way mean to suggest this is the last word, or the most inclusive work on the vast subject of natural health. Rather, it is the reflection of a personal journey to wholeness which is, and will remain, ongoing as long as I live, and in that sense it is a personal bible. Each of the subjects within this volume could be a huge book on its own. I have been able to touch only briefly upon areas of natural health and well-being that warrant more in-depth exploration, but have set out to present the widest possible selection of options from which you may be stimulated to begin to create your own individual programme for lasting well-being.

the natural body

the healthy body

know your body type

Your body has more in common with that of everyone else than differences. But in spite of the fact that your physiological structure is the same as every other person's, the diverse expression of the human form seems infinite. Our physical differences are things like height, weight, coloring, size of features, and the finer, smaller details of our physiology. But we all have one head, one nose, two eyes, and so on.

As you look at the people around you and get past the small differences, huge variations, and many similarities, you notice that people seem to fall into specific "body types," like tall and thin or short and stocky. Students and teachers of physiology have attempted to identify and understand the major differences in body types, but different cultures have various approaches to classifying our diversity. For instance, Chinese and Indian medical systems have been filing types according to holistic elemental typing for thousands of years. Invariably, those attempting this sort of classification have found that there are strong links between body type and personality and emotional traits.

somatotypes

One of the systems we use in the Western world was developed in the 1940s by an American psychologist, W. H. Sheldon, although physicians from Hippocrates onward had attempted to classify "body types." Sheldon called his system, in which he observed very recognizable, distinct, identifiable body types, "somatotyping." Sheldon believed we have tendencies toward one type, but might also have some characteristics of one or both of the other types, that we are all an individual, unique mixture of the three somatotypes. Sheldon's body types are cast by body structure, not including height. You can be any combination of the three types, no matter what your height. You inherit your body type and basically there is not much you can do to alter the fact that you are seven feet tall and naturally lean or four feet six and naturally round.

Recognizing and accepting your body type is important to your wellbeing and, in some cases, your life direction: if you are a short endomorph, you would be smart to give up your dream of supermodel stardom and set your sights on a more realistic goal. However, it is important to remember that most of us are a rich mix of all three types.

Mesomorph

Muscular build, classic wide body and shoulders, small waist, narrow hips. Naturally athletic bodies. Aggressive, dynamic, competitive, courageous, and domineering personalities who need to win. Action men and women who like to take risks, have adventures, and participate in sports and exercise.

Endomorph

Large, round body, heavily built, possibly fat, short plump neck, thickly set legs and arms. Easygoing, tolerant, slow, relaxed, and sociable. A rather complacent personality.

Ectomorph

Tall and narrow, with a very thin angular body in which the muscle is lean rather than well developed. Nervous, sensitive individuals, smart and fussy, quick-witted, alert, and defensive.

the Ayurvedic types

THE DOSHAS

At the heart of Ayurvedic medicine (see pages 262–63) is the concept of seeking harmony by balancing the "doshas" or bodily humors. The three doshas are contained in every cell of the body, as they govern the three principles necessary to the maintenance of life: *Kapha* controls the physical structure and fluid balance of the body; *Vata* governs motion and movement throughout the body; *Pitta* manages digestion and metabolism.

All three are equally important to our mental and physical wellbeing, but all three are not present in equal proportions within us. It is our unique blend of doshas that creates our individual constitutional or body type (*prakriti*, the Ayurvedic term for body types, is the Sanskrit word for "nature"). We are a blend of all three doshas, but that blend is completely unique—a blueprint for our own innate characteristics and qualities. Knowing that blend can help us understand how to live appropriately for our particular nature and its needs.

For instance, what may feel natural in terms of diet and exercise for you is different from what feels "natural" for your partner, best friend, or sister. By exploring the three doshas and identifying your own dominant dosha, you can have a better idea of how to enhance, promote, and maintain your best health.

Vata

Vata governs motion and movement, so Vata types are full of vital energy and lead a creative and active life. Vatas usually have dry, coarse skin and hair and a fast metabolism; they are slim with little body fat. They are restless with lots of ideas and are very perceptive—Vatas are capable of intuitive leaps. They move quickly and their lifestyle can be variable and erratic; they strongly dislike routine.

A person strong in balanced Vata will sleep well, think clearly, and experience balanced and well-regulated bodily functions.

Unbalanced Vata

The Vata type becomes underweight. Their teeth decay easily and their skin tends to be overly rough and dry. They may have very bad circulation and often feel cold; they suffer from excess energy, which manifests itself in nail-biting, jumpiness, and occasional insomnia. Their thought patterns are erratic, they are sometimes impatient with friends, and their memory is poor. They have a tendency to be rash and to make hasty decisions. They are prone to nervous exhaustion.

Pitta

Pittas are of medium height and frame but slender. Their skin is soft and lustrous, but they may have freckles or birthmarks and should avoid too much sun. They have straight hair, tending toward oiliness, usually fair, and often prematurely gray. Pittas have strong teeth, good eyesight, and a highly developed sense of smell, and may even have a distinctive, but not unpleasant, smell themselves. Their appetite is good and they enjoy food.

A person strong in balanced pitta is intelligent, direct, ambitious and assertive, and an impassioned speaker.

Unbalanced Pitta

A tendency to overheat: they should stay out of the sun, away from explosive situations, and avoid spicy food. Fever and sweating may be a problem. Their hair may thin or gray easily. They can suffer poor digestion, possibly irritable bowel syndrome, and also inflammatory conditions—acid indigestion, gout, and skin disorders. Often poor vision.

Kapha

Kapha is the dependable force within you that builds cells, strengthens bones, and fights disease. Kapha people have well-developed bodies but tend to gain weight because of a slow metabolism. They have a vital, almost elemental, strength and a steady sexual appetite. They are good-looking: their hair is thick and lustrous and their eyes are big. They move slowly and calmly and see no reason to rush; they don't like change.

People strong in balanced Kapha are courageous, loyal, and caring. They should avoid cold, damp weather, oversleeping, and rich, heavy food.

Unbalanced Kapha
Unhealthy weight gain. They have a flabby physique and weak muscles. They may suffer a loss of sexual desire, perhaps frigidity or impotence. They are sluggish, constantly tired, and their digestion is poor. They are possessive and jealous. They may suffer from excess congestion, mucus, and fluid retention.

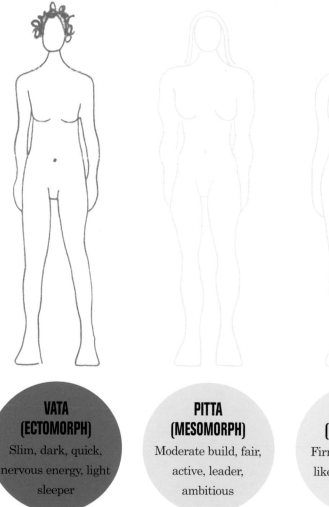

**VATA
(ECTOMORPH)**
Slim, dark, quick, nervous energy, light sleeper

**PITTA
(MESOMORPH)**
Moderate build, fair, active, leader, ambitious

**KAPHA
(ENDOMORPH)**
Firm, heavy-boned, likes routine, good appetite

which type are you?

To help you determine what your particular dosha mix might be, answer the three questionnaires that follow—one for each type. Score zero for "never" answers, 3 for "sometimes," and 6 for "often," then add up your total for each type. In most cases one dosha will have an obviously higher score—this will be your dominant dosha and you are a single-dosha type. If no single dosha dominates, you are probably a two-dosha type (most people are) and you must consider the traits of both. If all three scores are more or less equal, then you are that great rarity, a three-dosha type.

**No = 0
In between = 3
Yes = 6**

pitta

You have a medium build and strength.
You have red, blond, or light brown hair.
Your skin is fair or ruddy.
You have freckles or get them easily in the sun.
You get sharp hunger pangs and can't skip meals.
You get thirsty easily.
You can feel uncomfortable in hot weather.
You like to avoid the sun.
You tend to perspire easily.
Hot and spicy foods do not appeal to you.
You favor cold foods and cool refreshing drinks.
You have a strong appetite and can eat a lot at one time.
You tend to have regular bowel movements.
You see yourself as quite efficient.
You are very precise and orderly.
You tend to be a perfectionist.
You can be strong-minded and forceful in your manner.
You can lose your temper easily.
You tend to be impatient or easily irritable.
You are usually too hot rather than too cold.
You are considered stubborn by the people who know you well.
You can be very determined when you want something.
You can be highly critical of yourself and of other people.

kapha

You are well built, with a large, solid body.

You tend to gain weight easily.

You lose weight slowly.

You have good stamina with a steady level of energy.

You are a slow eater.

You can feel heavy after eating, especially after rich food.

You have a slow digestion.

You store fat easily and have a tendency to a full, plump body.

You are slow and deliberate in your movements.

You are naturally calm.

You are not quick-tempered or easily upset.

You have an easygoing, placid disposition.

You need at least eight hours of sleep a night.

You tend to oversleep and are slow to get going in the morning.

You are a very deep sleeper.

You are naturally relaxed and can't be rushed easily.

You are a slow learner, but once you learn something you really retain it.

You have a good memory.

You are methodical in your approach to learning.

You are methodical in your actions.

You don't like damp, cold weather.

You have a tendency toward sinus problems, mucus, and congestion.

vata

You have a thin build.

You don't gain weight easily.

Your hands and feet tend to be cold.

Your skin can be very dry, especially in winter.

Your eating and sleeping habits are irregular.

You often have difficulty falling asleep, and then sleep lightly.

You have a very active, restless mind.

You have a good imagination.

You learn quickly, but can forget equally quickly.

Your movements can be very quick.

You tend to walk quickly.

You worry easily and frequently become anxious.

You can find it difficult to make decisions.

You speak quickly.

Friends consider you talkative.

You are easily excited.

You are very active and your energy comes in bursts.

You have a tendency toward flatulence and constipation.

You are quite an emotional person and your moods change easily.

You are usually enthusiastic and positive.

You are the most uncomfortable in cold weather.

Since there are broad similarities between the somatotype and the Ayurvedic types, we have decided to use the Ayurvedic system to provide you with a quick guide that will help you find information appropriate to your body type in various parts of the book. Once you have established which Ayurvedic type(s) you are, you can go to the colored boxes appropriate to your type(s); for example, the Kapha box in the Healthy Eating chapter on page 49 to find broad guidelines on diet.

body basics

Of all our bodily functions, breathing is possibly the one we take for granted most. Without thinking about it, every moment of the day we are breathing in oxygen-rich air and, hopefully, breathing out wastes and toxins in the form of carbon dioxide. We are usually unaware of this basic instinct which is so necessary to our health and wellbeing—indeed, to our very survival!

Most people, particularly in the West, do not breathe deeply, undermining their chances for optimum health. Your body functions at its best when you are breathing to your full capacity. Your energy reserves may be lowered, and chronic fatigue, allergies, colds, and many more health problems may result from habitually breathing too shallowly, too fast, or too long.

breathing into being

"You can live two months without food and two weeks without water, but you can only live a few minutes without air."

HUNG YI-HSIANG, TAOIST MASTER

The supreme importance of breathing in maintaining true wellbeing is increasingly recognized by both health professionals and holistic practitioners. You might find it surprising to discover that good breathing stimulates the healing energies within the body. Paying more attention to your breathing patterns during times of physical illness or psychological stress can be completely empowering and supportive; conscious breathing and applied breathing exercises done at the right time can truly offer us help and hope during our greatest trials. For example, breathing exercises are among the most important ways in which a woman can take control over her labor and facilitate an easier, more pain-free, childbirth.

Learning how to breathe properly is an important part of health education. This is a long-accepted, fundamental technique in many Eastern traditions, particularly those of India and China. The increasing popularity of Indian yoga in the West is largely due to the practical health teachings of Pranayama, the art and science of breathing, traditionally practiced alongside physical postures.

According to yoga philosophy, this subtle energy or life force in the air is called *prana* and Pranayama is mastered by a series of breathing exercises that teach you how to be conscious of your breath. You can learn to use your breath properly in any good yoga class (see pages 168–81). Because we are not taught breathing techniques as part of our health education in the West, many people develop bad habits out of ignorance, combined with laziness. If we breathe too quickly, or the breath is shallow, then we retain too much stale air in our lungs. Then we begin to breathe in again before we have completed breathing out.

Research into breathing by Dr. Robin Monro, director of the Yoga Biomedical Trust, based at London's Royal Homeopathic Hospital, has shown that people who are very tense and suffering from stress problems tend to breathe too shallowly, using only the upper part of the chest and not using the diaphragm. Such shallow breathing can lead to rapid breathing and hyperventilation, from which many stressed people suffer and which only makes their condition worse.

To breathe correctly you must use your nose and not your mouth. The nose is designed to cleanse and warm the air before it reaches your lungs. Breathing through the mouth means an increase in the risk of infection. In correct breathing, when you breathe in, the lungs expand, the rib cage moves upward and outward and the diaphragm moves downward, pushing out the lower ribs and abdomen.

Deep breathing and using the respiratory system fully is particularly difficult for women who have been conditioned to "suck in those stomachs" since adolescence and have worn all sorts of attire like girdles, pantyhose, cinch belts, and Lycra ever since.

The habit of pulling in the stomach is difficult to reverse and is responsible for a lot of collective shallow breathing. Too many people use only the upper narrow part of the lungs, rather than the bottom part which has greater capacity.

Respiration begins when we breathe air through the nose and then the larynx, trachea, and bronchi, which clean, moisten, and warm the air to prepare it for absorption into the bloodstream through the lungs. The air is then pulled into a network of expanding and contracting air sacs. This is where blood and air meet. Blood enters the lungs through an artery and flows around the air sacs in capillaries. Here oxygen is taken in and carbon dioxide expelled. The blood then carries the oxygen through the pulmonary vein to the heart, and the respiratory system carries the carbon dioxide out of the body when we exhale.

Too much carbon dioxide is toxic, but we always need to have a little amount in the body to help regulate body chemistry and the function of the internal breathing mechanism. It is when the oxygen from the air meets and mixes with the glucose in the blood that vital energy is released and circulated.

Does the respiratory system have an important part to play in preventing illness in the first place, and if it does, what part does it play? Qigong (see page 183) is the Chinese equivalent of India's Pranayama. Meaning "energy control" and "breathing exercise," it has been a formal branch of Chinese medicine for over 2,000 years and is regarded as a science. The Chinese believe the body's supply of vital energy is created by correct breathing and that all our important functions, from blood pressure to hormone secretions, are regulated by our breathing, and that, therefore, the respiratory system plays the central role in our wellbeing and longevity.

Asthma

It is estimated around 16 million people in the United States suffer from the chronic lung condition, asthma. Although most common in children under the age of ten years old, people of any age can suffer from it. Too many people, including doctors, know too little about the condition, how to prevent it, and what to do in case of a serious attack.

Worldwide, asthma is on the increase and no one knows why or what causes it. Some people attribute their asthma to food allergies or a natural inclination to sinus problems, such as hayfever. Others connect their stressful life situations or challenging environmental conditions with the problem. Whatever the root cause of your asthma, this condition can be considerably helped by changing your lifestyle. Positive diet and exercise changes (including some regular relaxation and breathing exercises) are sometimes all that is needed to begin to turn the problem around.

Sufferers do not react to the same allergens in the same way. Many who suffer from asthma in childhood eventually grow out of it, but some people are affected throughout their whole lives. They can expect at any time—and often out of the blue—attacks of breathlessness and wheezing. A serious attack is very frightening. What starts out as an irritated cough can escalate to the muscles in the bronchial tubes contracting involuntarily and squeezing the tubes too tight, causing the sufferer, literally, to fight for breath.

If you are an asthma sufferer, you are probably under a doctor's care. Follow your doctor's instructions on using an inhaler. Try to work with the health professionals who manage your care to make the necessary adjustments to promote more balance and wellbeing in your life. Yoga is one of the best health programs for helping asthma conditions naturally. There are many simple things that asthma sufferers can do to help their own condition. The following is a list of a few natural hints for preventing or coping with asthma.

- Cut down on or, if necessary, completely cut out dairy and wheat products from your diet.
- Try to stay away from the food allergens or pollens and grasses that really irritate you.
- You could be sensitive to a number of airborne allergens including dust, animal hair, mites, mold, feathers, cigarette smoke or certain perfumes or petrochemicals. Try to keep your immediate environment clear of these kind of substances.
- Use natural fibers and floors rather than lots of heavy carpets, rugs, and curtains in your home.
- Keep your rooms well ventilated and your thermostat on low.

Exercise is an excellent and effective way to strengthen the lungs and the entire respiratory system, and also to increase confidence, which is important when fighting this condition. Breathing exercises are particularly effective, and slow, deep breathing is just one of many techniques that can help. Many asthma sufferers have reported tremendous benefits from yoga and from swimming, which also exercises the lungs. Some people believe yoga therapy has played an important part in curing their condition and there are many studies now in process.

SIMPLE BREATHING EXERCISE 1

Slowly inhale and exhale through the nose. With each breath, bring the air down to the diaphragm, allowing the abdomen to expand with each inhalation and contract with each exhalation, gently pulling in the abdomen.

SIMPLE BREATHING EXERCISE 2

To get in touch with the natural action of the diaphragm and abdomen in deep breathing, lie down on your back, relaxing your body, with your feet about a foot apart. Place your hands, palms down, on each side of your abdomen and follow your breath from your nose down through your chest to your abdomen and then back. As you inhale, allow the chest and then the abdomen to expand and as you exhale, allow the gentle contraction of first the abdomen and then the chest.

BREATHING FOR WEIGHT LOSS

Sounds too good to be true.... Most of us shallow-breathe into the upper chest, so the cells do not receive the full replenishment of oxygen. This can hamper attempts to lose weight and affect energy levels. Try breathing fully into the lungs using the diaphragm (see above). Oxygen depletion is common among many people, especially smokers and those who live in cities and polluted environments.

nurturing systems

We are consciously aware when eating that we are stimulating the digestive process but we often do not take that awareness to the next level and contemplate how what we digest can either nurture or harm us. Being conscious that what we eat nurtures us in the same way we nurture our children, or creatures in our care, is a way of keeping in mind the thought that what we eat can be either healthy or detrimental. Choosing what we eat and drink is a very self-empowering decision-making process that we go through many, many times every day. How conscious are we of the power we have to enhance our wellbeing by simply being aware of what we are putting into our mouths?

To feed and nourish your body and mind, the foods you eat and the liquids you drink journey through the entire digestive system before assimilation and nourishment can take place. Digestion begins in the mouth, where chewing food stimulates the production of saliva, which contains ptyalin, an enzyme that makes food easier to swallow, and begins to break down some starches into sugar. This is why you have teeth and why chewing your food well is so important. From the throat, food passes into a narrow channel about 25 cm (10 inches) long, called the oesophagus, which carries it into the stomach.

The stomach is an amazing muscular sac that releases hydrochloric acid to break down and dissolve food further, along with other digestive enzymes, such as pepsin, that are necessary for the digestion of protein. The stomach walls have a thick mucous lining that is constantly being renewed to protect it from the acid. Until about 25 years ago, gastroenterologists thought that the stomach's acid would kill off bacteria, but then an Australian scientist proved that most ulcers are linked to the presence of a bacterium called H. (Helicobacter) pylori and can be treated with simple antibiotics. This has been one of the biggest breakthroughs in the understanding and treatment of ulcers in years. The same bacteria is also now being linked to early stomach cancer.

Another cause of ulcers, some complementary practitioners believe, is excess acid, which in turn is the result of eating protein and carbohydrates together in large quantities. This is because hydrochloric acid is needed to digest protein but the stomach doesn't produce enough to do it properly when the protein comes with lots of carbohydrates. The result is that meat stays in the stomach longer than is either necessary or healthy.

This is one of the big food-combining secrets. Experts around the world are finding some agreement in the art and science of food combining (see page 83). It's probably quite difficult for you to believe that egg or hamburger and chips, or steak and baked potato, don't digest well together, but that is apparently the case. So it is far better to eat vegetables with your meat rather than starch, and avoid eating too much meat. Generally, food, with the exception of fruits and vegetables, remains in your stomach for 3–4 hours while it mixes with the digestive enzymes and is broken down further. Fruits and vegetables are digested in less than 2 hours, while proteins, starches and fats take considerably longer. Fatty red meat, for instance, can stay in the stomach for up to 6 hours.

This is why fruit is considered the healthiest food and the one that is easiest on your digestive system. Because of the high water content of most fruits, they also act as cleansers, as well as carrying easily absorbed nutrients. When toxins accumulate in your body and create too much acid, which can lead to a cycle of bloating and weight gain, fruit can help your body to retain the water needed to neutralize your acid level.

On leaving the stomach, food enters the duodenum, the first part of the small intestines, where partially digested food is further broken down by digestive juices released from the gallbladder and the pancreas. The pancreas, a gland behind the stomach, produces more enzymes, and the gallbladder in the liver produces bile, along with the intestine's own secretions, which are all alkaline and able to balance the stomach acids.

It is here that proteins are split into the building blocks of peptides and amino acids that can be made into new tissue, while carbohydrates become an energy source in the form of simple sugars, mainly glucose. The amino acid and sugars begin to be absorbed into the bloodstream through capillaries that run along the walls of the small intestine.

Your small intestine is about 6 metres (20 feet) long and its walls are covered by countless tiny soft hair-like projections called villi, which act as filters, separating nutrients from toxins and the rest of the mush that needs to pass further on for yet more processing. So it's important to reduce the risk of blockage and damage to your villi by cutting out of your diet, or at least reducing, substances that are known to irritate the stomach and intestines. These are:

- overeating
- gluten in wheat (bread and pasta)
- excess sugar
- fried foods
- alcohol
- tea and coffee
- carbonated drinks (sodas and colas)
- strong spices
- excess salt
- any overprocessed foods, junk foods and fast foods

OBESITY

Obesity is dramatically on the rise and contributes to heart disease, stroke, diabetes and many other diseases that can lead to premature death. The growing 'couch potato' syndrome, as TV and computers take up much more leisure time, and the huge increase in food portions are all contributing factors to this growing problem. In most fast-food chains, portions have tripled over the last 30 years. Eating little and often is much better than starving, which only encourages the body to store fat.

Obesity has also been linked to prolonged stress and to sleep deprivation – just a few nights of poor sleep significantly increases your body's ability to store fat.

Those proteins, carbohydrates and fats that the stomach and small intestines have failed to absorb may be stored in the heaviest organ of the body, the liver. This important organ is amazingly diverse and multi-talented. Perhaps because its functions are so numerous it is described in Chinese medicine as the 'minister of planning', organizing and storing nutrients for future use. The liver releases glucose into the blood and tissues in order to meet our energy needs and also stores vitamins, particularly some of the B vitamins that help red blood cells mature.

One of its other most important functions is to remove toxic waste substances from the blood. This is why too much alcohol places such stress on the liver. The accumulation of toxins from too much fermentation takes its toll over time. Only drink alcohol in moderation, or not at all, if you value your liver.

Bathed in digestive juices, chewed up and churned about, food takes a 4–8-hour journey through the small intestines, being pushed along by the waves of rippling muscular movements called peristalsis, while the villi stir up the materials, sorting nutrients out and absorbing them into the blood and lymph systems.

The last phase of the digestion process takes place in the large intestine over a period of 10–12 hours. And it is here that the biggest and most fascinating discoveries about the workings of the guts have been made recently. Even a few years ago, although we knew there was about a kilogram of bacteria living in the large intestines, nobody had more than the haziest idea about what they were doing or what role they played in our health. It is now becoming clear that the bacteria form an ecological system, known as the microbiome, that is as complex as a coral reef or a rain-forest. Not only is this system vital for extracting nutrients from the food that's passing through, but it is also involved in regulating such apparently separate functions as the effectiveness of our immune system, how much weight we put on and whether we develop inflammatory disorders such as asthma or eczema.

The link between the function of the large intestine and obesity is that 30 per cent of the calories we consume are made available by the action of gut bacteria. So just as people vary in how tall or how muscled they are, they almost certainly also vary enormously in the percentage of calories their microbiome can extract from a meal. One recent study involving mice found huge differences in the microbiome of fat and thin mice. As for immune disorders, another study, this time with humans, has recently discovered that newborn babies at high risk for eczema or asthma were 50 per cent less likely to develop these problems if they were fed probiotics in the womb and for several months after birth.

Just how sensitive this system is can be seen from the effect of camomile tea. What could be milder, yet in one study subjects who drunk a cup a day for two weeks were found to have a different pattern of chemicals being produced by the gut for two weeks after stopping the tea. In fact, it has been suggested that rather than being a collection of selfish genes we are nothing more than a mobile bacteria fementer.

Some simple guidelines for a healthy digestive system include:

- 'Graze don't gorge' is one of the health catch-phrases of the moment. Overeating places a lot of strain on the body systems.
- Remember that the digestive system needs the right foods at the right times to function efficiently.
- Through eating a wide and varied diet, high in fresh raw fruits, vegetables and whole grains, i.e. fibre, you can prevent many of the disabling diseases that are the result of poor diet, the root of an unhealthy lifestyle.
- Consult your doctor or a nutritionist if you believe you need to make major changes in your diet or if you have any chronic condition that you believe is linked to your digestive system.

Metabolic syndrome X

Dysfunctional metabolism appears to be one of the root causes of obesity, along with many other nasty illnesses. The evidence is mounting to support the direct relationship between bad metabolism, chronic stress and elevated cortisol levels. Excess cortisol over the long-term is dangerous: it weakens the immune system, leaving us vulnerable to infection and inflammation. Learning to deal effectively and safely, with the stresses of daily life appears to be one of our greatest challenges, one that we ignore at our peril.

Metabolic Syndrome X, a dangerous modern disorder, is considered a huge, increasing health problem in the USA and other Western countries. The name is given to the third stage of Potbelly Syndrome (PBS), a metabolic disorder manifesting itself in abdominal obesity, high blood pressure and, in its serious forms, type 2 diabetes. PBS is believed to affect about one-third of adults in industrialized societies.

In their groundbreaking book, *The Potbelly Syndrome, How Common Germs Cause Obesity, Diabetes and Heart Disease*, Russell Farris and Per Marin show that these conditions are caused not by bad habits but by chronic infections and inflammation. They quote an article, 'The Metabolic Syndrome X' by Dr. Barbara Hansen from the Obesity and Diabetes Research Center at the University of Maryland. She writes: 'The new millennium is likely to establish Metabolic Syndrome X as one of the most prevalent diseases of mankind, and one of the most costly in its contributions to morbidity and premature mortality,...by the year 2010, there may be some 50–75 million or more adults in the U.S. alone, with significant manifestation of this syndrome.'

FOODS TO SOOTHE AN IRRITATED STOMACH OR INTESTINE

Oatmeal
Milk
Rice pudding
White cabbage juice
Bananas
Melons
Camomile tea
Slippery elm powder
Aloe vera juice
Plain yogurt (necessary to eat if you are taking antibiotics to replace the healthy bacteria the antibiotics destroy along with the infection!)

COMFORT EATING

When we are unhappy or stressed, sweets and snacks provide momentary comfort. Replace unhealthy foods with seeds and nuts – particularly pumpkin and sesame seeds and almonds – lean meat and tofu. These all help keep up levels of serotonin, one of the feel-good brain chemicals.

the heart

In an average lifetime, the human heart beats around 2.5 billion times, about 100,000 times every day, and around 70 times every minute. It circulates about 7 litres (6 quarts) of blood through more than 96 thousand miles of blood vessels 3000–5000 times every day, bringing a constant supply of oxygen and nutrients to our tissues and removing waste and carbon dioxide.

And there are more impressive statistics. Every second, 7 million new blood cells are produced; by the end of an average lifetime your heart will have pumped 50 million gallons of blood. Most amazing of all is that the organ capable of all this is a muscle the size of a fist and weighing less than 500 g (1 pound)!

But the heart is also vulnerable and, by and large, our western life-style is not very good for it. More people die prematurely from diseases of the heart and arteries in the UK than anything else – 250,000 a year, half of this number from heart attacks and a quarter from strokes. A heart attack is caused by a blockage (known as a coronary) of one of the small arteries that lie on the surface of the heart; less and less blood gets to the heart until it can no longer do its job. A stroke may occur when a piece of plaque (gunge) building up on an artery wall breaks away and is carried in the blood stream to the brain, where it may block up a smaller artery. Yet both of these are largely preventable diseases with highly familiar risk factors, including poor diet, smoking, obesity and lack of exercise..

Until a few years ago a high-fat diet was seen as one of the main factors in encouraging the growth of plaque. As a result, since the 1980s, millions of people have been on low-fat diets, but no studies have linked a low-fat diet with longer life and people continue to get fatter. There seem to be two reasons for this: firstly, a low-fat diet generally includes more carbohydrates, often refined ones like sugar and white flour; secondly, it means low intake of omega-3, the essential fatty acids found in fish oils, nuts and seeds, which protect the heart. Basic healthy eating advice is now to consume more fresh fruit and vegetables, wholemeal flour and bean protein.

Diet can also help to bring down high blood pressure, one of the top markers for raised risk. Most people are aware that salt intake should be reduced, but that is only part of the story. The pressure in your blood vessels goes up when they are narrowed; this can happen because they are blocked with plaque or because the artery walls become tense. The stiffness is controlled by the flow of two pairs of minerals in and out of the cell walls of the arteries – sodium (salt) and potassium, calcium and magnesium. Too much of one of each pair – sodium or calcium – tenses them up. That's why you are advised to avoid salt and why one type of anti-hypertension drug – calcium channel blockers – blocks calcium.

FOR A HEALTHY HEART, CUT DOWN ON:

Animal fat
Dairy products
Sugar
Salt
Refined (white) flour
Fried food
Salty, processed food
Alcohol
Cigarettes

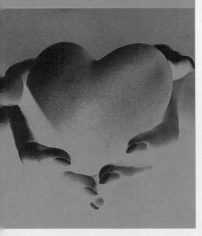

But what about the other two minerals? Nutritionists advise increasing your intake of potassium and magnesium to provide more of these relaxing minerals. And there is another dietary supplement your doctor probably won't suggest instead of drugs, an amino acid called homocysteine. This is a normal part of your metabolism but when levels get too high there is a raised risk of degenerative diseases, such as Alzheimer's, as well as heart disease. High levels are a sign you are not getting enough B vitamins, especially folic acid, B6 and B12, and the only way to lower it is by increasing your intake of them, possibly with a supplement if your levels are very high.

Everyone knows that raised cholesterol is a major factor in heart disease. Cholesterol, together with too much fat, forms the plaque that blocks the coronary arteries. But apart from taking statin drugs to lower cholesterol levels – and there is a big debate about how much it needs to be lowered – there are other ways in which you can make it safe. The first way is with antioxidants. Rancid butter is a good example of the oxidation of fat, and when considered on an internal level, this is something we want to minimize as much as posible. Vitamins C and E help to keep oxidation in check. Then there is the 'good' HDL cholesterol that clears 'bad' LDL cholesterol away. One of the most effective ways of raising HDL cholesterol is with the B vitamin niacin; 'good' cholesterol is also raised by omega-3 fatty acids.

Obesity is often linked with heart disease but being slightly overweight is probably not a problem so long as you stay generally healthy – and that means following familiar advice: don't smoke, avoid junk food and ideally take exercise every day, which stimulates all sorts of healthy repair processes. A brisk walk, swimming or dancing all provide an excellent full body workout (see pages 129-165).

Tips for a healthy heart

- Eat oily fish – e.g. salmon, herring, sardines, mackerel – at least three times a week. They contain the essential fatty acid EPA, which thins the blood and brings down cholesterol levels.
- Grill, steam or bake food instead of frying it. Don't add fat and avoid lots of saturated fat.
- Reduce your intake of sugar, salt, processed foods and alcohol.
- Increase your intake of fibre-rich foods, like wholemeal bread, oats and beans.
- Dramatically cut down on biscuits, cakes, crisps and all confectionery. Beware of trans fats found in some margarines and baked goods.
- Eat more fresh vegetables and fruit daily, especially dark green vegetables, which are rich in the vital minerals magnesium and potassium.
- Drink plenty of water. If your body is not getting enough it starts to store it in cells, which raises the amount of sodium in them, stiffening the arteries.
- Take more regular exercise.

FOODS TO REDUCE CHOLESTEROL WHICH SHOULD BE INCLUDED IN YOUR DIET REGULARLY:

Avocados
Olive oil
Oatmeal
Garlic and onions
Oily fish, sardines, salmon, mackerel
Dark green and orange vegetables
Sunflower seeds

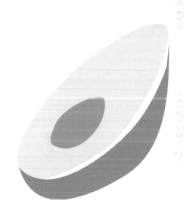

- Give up smoking! Smoking a packet of cigarettes a day gives you twice the risk of heart disease and 5 times the risk of a stroke.
- Reduce your stress levels – learn how to relax! Excessive stress increases the risk of high blood pressure and stroke.

Plant cholesterol busters

One of the ways of lowering cholesterol that has become increasingly popular is with hormone-like substances called plant sterols. Several large trials have shown that they can bring it down more effectively than statins. Sterols are relatively rare in the average Western diet so you may find yourself eating various foods you are probably not very familiar with such as soya – a particularly rich source – along with seeds, nuts, beans and lentils. They work by reducing the amount of cholesterol absorbed through the gut. But sterols aren't the only plant-based cholesterol busters. Others include oats, barley, aubergines and okra, all of which contain soluble fibre that does the job as well. A good daily combination would be 50 g (1 oz) of soya (a glass of soya milk, or a small serving of tofu, or a small soya burger), 35 g (1½ oz) of almonds (a small handful) and 25 g (1 oz) of soluble fibres from oats and vegetables (the equivalent of five oat cakes, plus a bowl of oats and three servings of vegetables).

12 aids for keeping your heart healthy

The following 12 nutrients, either obtained from foods or taken as supplements, will help reduce your risk of getting coronary heart disease or dangerously high cholesterol. If you are already suffering, the following can be beneficial in conjunction with your current treatment.

1 Omega-3 fatty acids A big study recently reported that fish oils decrease dangerous blood fats known as triglycerides by an average of 29 per cent and lower cholesterol by 12 per cent (lowering bad LDL cholesterol by 32 per cent and increasing HDL by 10 per cent). They also bring down inflammation, which is what can make plaque form in the first place. Linseeds (flax seeds) and their oils are also good. (See also pages 41–42.)

2 Vitamins A, C, E These highly beneficial antioxidant vitamins all have the ability to prevent deposits, including fats, sticking to artery walls and can help to prevent damage to the arterial lining caused by free radicals. Best sources of A are fish oil, egg yolk, liver; C is richest in citrus fruits, kiwis, strawberries, red peppers, peas; E in avocados, chickpeas, almonds, tuna, sunflower oil and muesli. (See also pages 94–98.)

Some people are naturally at risk because of hereditary factors, but most people exacerbate their potential for heart disease by unhealthy habits and lifestyle. A diet high in saturated fats, alcohol, salt, and sugar, and low in vegetables and fruits, will definitely increase your chances of developing heart disease. The simple lifestyle changes you could make to reduce your risk of heart disease considerably are:

- Reduce your intake of alcohol or give it up completely.
- Stop smoking.
- Eat a healthy diet.
- Exercise regularly.
- Lose weight if you are overweight.

3 Selenium Most of us are deficient in this valuable antioxidant mineral, which works with vitamin E to produce the prostaglandins that are needed for normal growth. It is found in lentils, wholemeal bread, sardines and Brazil nuts (see page 104).

4 Allicin The British Heart Foundation states that allicin, which is found most abundantly in garlic and also to a lesser degree in onions and leeks, may help in preventing blood clots from forming in coronary arteries. It is known to have blood-thinning properties.

5 Folic acid Folic acid helps reduce the risk of cardiovascular disease associated with high blood levels of homocysteine. Folic acid can be found predominantly in green leafy vegetables, mushrooms, pulses, nuts, fruits and root vegetables (see page 96).

6 Co-enzyme Q10 Co-enzyme Q10 is an antioxidant and is also a vital energy-releasing component and cardiac muscle strengthener. Levels of Co-Q10 in the system lessen due to old age, stress and illness; statin drugs reduce it further. Co-Q10 can be found in lean meat. See more on page 117.

7 Flavonoids Flavonoids inhibit the action of platelets, which are the blood cells that join to form blood clots. They are antioxidants that also help the absorption and action of vitamin C. Flavonoids can be found in fruit and vegetables, especially apples and onions.

8 Monounsaturated fatty acids These lower the levels of potentially harmful LDL cholesterol and maintain the necessary levels of beneficial HDL cholesterol (see pages 40–41). They can be found in rapeseed, walnut and groundnut oils, and avocados. Olive oil is another useful source and extra-virgin olive oil also contains protective antioxidants. See more on page 40.

9 Vitamin B6 This vitamin is essential for the production of healthy blood. B6 can be found in fish, pulses, nuts, chicken and potatoes (see pages 95–96).

10 Phytoestrogens These are currently under investigation as their health-giving properties seem prolific and include the ability to fight coronary heart disease. They reduce excess cholesterol, are rich in essential vitamins and minerals. They are found in soya, watermelon, onions, garlic, broccoli and even in tea.

11 Lycopene This is a carotenoid noted for its use in reducing the risk of coronary heart disease. It is fat-soluble and is therefore more efficiently absorbed when eaten with oil. It can be found in raw tomatoes and in any tomato product (see page 55).

12 Beta-carotene This is another carotenoid, which makes fruit brightly coloured. It helps to prevent the build-up of toxins in the arteries as well as having many other health-giving properties. It is found in spinach, tomatoes, cabbage, broccoli, peas, carrots and sweet potatoes (see page 94).

ASPIRIN

A report published in the *British Medical Journal*, on June 30, 2000, refutes the claim that a daily aspirin helps reduce strokes. It now appears there is a risk of developing bleeding in the stomach due to the blood-thinning properties of aspirin. More research is needed in this area, but it seems that those most likely to be prescribed aspirin (those with high blood pressure) are the ones most at risk of stomach bleeding. Even with low doses of aspirin, bleeding occurred in people with high blood pressure. Aspirin can be a more effective prescription for those with low blood pressure, but the risks could still outweigh the benefits, and other ways should be found of reducing high blood pressure.

the holistic back

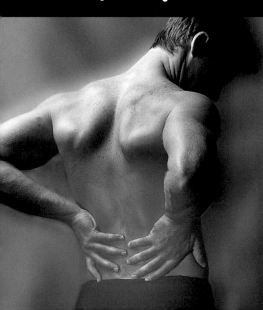

Research conducted by the American Academy of Orthopaedic Surgeons (AAOS) revealed that 80 percent of people will suffer at least one episode of back pain in their lifetime. The primary site for 85 percent of sufferers is the lower back area. To ensure that you do not join the unhappy throng of sufferers, treat your back respectfully and try to maintain strength and suppleness throughout life.

Back problems can affect anyone. Although back pain is most prevalent in 45 to 64 year-olds, back injuries are the leading cause of disability in the United States in those under 45. According to the Bureau of Labor Statistics, back pain is the second leading cause of absenteeism from work, after the common cold, with back injuries accounting for 100 million lost days of work annually.

Manual workers are at higher risk than white collar workers. Any job that involves heavy physical work, lifting and forceful movements, bending and twisting, standing, or static work positions is putting the employee at risk of back pain. Some of the occupations that can cause back pain without involving injury are: farm labor, driving a truck, work involving intensive use of telephones without headsets, and stationary computer work.

Back pain is rarely "cured" by surgery or treatment of the spine itself. Dr. Art Brownstein, in his book *Healing Back Pain Naturally*, suggests that most back pain is caused by problems in the muscles. When the back muscles are in a state of imbalance, they may be tense, tight, weak, and untoned, and therefore unable to support the spine. As they influence almost every major muscle group in the body, injured back muscles can cause a knock-on effect of pain throughout the whole body, and this can create dramatic problems—not just in the back. There may be other causes of back pain, such as a structural injury because of accidents or habitual poor posture, but it is the muscles that transmit pain messages to the brain because they are directly connected to nerves.

Many people do not recognize how damaging stress and tension can be to the back. Tension causes muscles to stiffen. Even if you are undergoing treatment for back injuries, the back will not heal if you are emotionally distraught and tense. Healing just cannot take place in tight muscles. If you have had a diagnosis of pinched nerves, disc problems, or any other condition, you can be sure, according to Dr. Brownstein, that the problem began in the muscles and not the spinal column.

The only way to a back problem-free existence is to reclaim full use and mobility of the back by keeping the muscles toned and healthy, and by avoiding excessive stresses. Shutting out the powerful message of pain by using painkillers and pain relievers denies you the wisdom of the message. Ways to release endorphins and encephalins, which are the body's natural painkillers, include exercise, laughter, deep relaxation, and stress management techniques. Learn stretching techniques that work the back muscles and relax the muscles with breathing exercises and general exercise.

Stretching is a very important and powerful way of relieving muscular pain. The muscles can be retrained to be resilient and elastic and loose, as they should be. Stretching is probably the single most important physical activity you can do to make sure that your back will be healthy for years to come. When you stretch, you release stored-up tension in your muscles, releasing knots, tightness, spasms, and pain.

Any negative, angry, distressing thoughts you have travel via powerful electrical impulses through the nerves to every part of your body, especially the muscles of the back. Learn ways of relaxing that are powerful enough to really induce a feeling of long-lasting ease and peace. Practice makes perfect, and retraining will take time and patience. However, the effects of stretching, stress management, and deep breathing will be felt immediately. With repetition and retraining, the muscles will "learn" to remain relaxed and to not tense up unnaturally, even if this has been habitual for many years. You need to practice the techniques for only a few minutes every day to help your back and, for that matter, your whole body and mind.

A well balanced, whole diet, along with regular exercise, is vital for keeping your back healthy. Other parts of the body need to be well maintained, too, in order to take stress out of the back. For example, weak leg muscles place stress on the back when walking. Walking, jogging, and bicycling are all simple exercises that develop muscular strength in the legs.

Abdominal muscles are essential because the abdomen holds up the body and supports the back. Sit-ups are a good way to build strength in these muscles. Start by doing just five a day. Don't do fast, jerky repetitions; always keep movements slow to enhance the action of the abdominal muscles. Build to no more than 50 per day. Crunches, which are done with bent knees, place less stress on the back and are often recommended when there are back problems.

INFLAMMATION

A new understanding of the root cause of all physical pain, and almost every disease, is now possible. Many of our most debilitating diseases can be traced to an inflammatory cause. Asthma, arthritis, chronic back pain, diabetes, obesity, heart disease, Alzheimer's disease and many forms of cancer have inflammation as one of the underlining causes.

In his groundbreaking book, *The Inflammation Syndrome*, published by Wiley in the U.S., Jack Challem identifies the reasons for chronic inflammation and, more importantly, what we can do about it. He provides a new, drug-free, approach to healing inflammation-related problems through a simple nutrition and supplement programme.

Challem's research shows how, far more than genes, poor eating habits are at the core of most modern degenerative disorders, including chronic inflammation. *The Inflammation Syndrome* is supported by hundreds of scientific studies.

The book provides a brilliant understanding of this universal problem, and a plan for you to empower yourself to safely prevent and overcome inflammatory disorders.

bones of the matter

Osteoporosis is a common medical condition linked to the aging process, where the level of bone density begins to fall as the rate of bone loss accelerates. Osteoporosis is a thinning of the bones, which makes the bones more fragile and vulnerable to breaks and fractures. More women develop this degenerative condition earlier than men: 80 percent of sufferers are women. An even more alarming statistic, reported in Great Britain by Dr. Margaret Rees in *Medicine & You*, shows "that more women die from hip fracture than from cancers of the cervix, womb, and breast combined."

Unless you take steps to prevent this debilitating and life-threatening condition, osteoporosis could gradually affect you. Women become much more vulnerable to bone loss after the menopause because the ovaries are no longer producing the hormones that help the body maintain the balance of bone loss with new bone formation.

Throughout life, your bones replace lost bone with new bone formation, although unfortunately this process does slow down as we age. Good bone formation in childhood and puberty is crucial for bone health in later life; calcium intake in the first ten years of life affects the peak bone mass in adulthood and about 45 percent of adult skeletal mass is formed in adolescence. There are two main types of cells in your bone: osteoblasts, which make new bone, and osteoclasts, which eat away areas of old bone. When their activity is equal and balanced, you are in the healthy state of homeostasis. However, when nutrients, hormones, enzymes, pH factor, and other elements in the body's internal balance get upset, the osteoclasts are more active, so more bone is lost than is replaced. Sometimes intense bone loss is the result of a sedentary lifestyle or immobility, which will greatly accelerate bone loss at any age in either the weight-bearing kind, is also important in maintaining the state of homeostasis, or "balance."

How to prevent osteoporosis

1 Make sure that you eat good-quality fresh produce every day, concentrating on fruit and vegetables as the main components of your diet. Your vitamin and mineral balance is essential in preventing osteoporosis. For example, it is not only your bones that need calcium—your blood does, too. If you have too little calcium in your body, your blood takes it from your bones to keep the level normal.

2 Maintaining or increasing bone density is encouraged by a regular weight-bearing exercise program. Exercise helps keep the bones strong

SQUATTING

Squatting is excellent for the pelvic, sacral, and lower spine, and also for strengthening your leg and hip muscles. This is a natural pose to adopt and is one that many Eastern peoples can attain with ease. Children find squatting effortless and easy. Anthropologically, when humans gathered from the land, they almost certainly worked in this pose. In some countries birthing is undertaken in the squat pose.

and improves tone. Weight-bearing exercises are essential for building strong bones and to improve tone, strength, flexibility, stability, and balance in the musculature. This gives your skeleton the best and strongest support, while helping to prevent the falls which can lead to more serious bone problems if osteoporosis does start to develop. Over the last 50 years, as cars, labor-saving devices, computers, and home entertainment have taken over, normal everyday exercise has been neglected. Making exercise a routine part of your day will help prevent problems in later life.

3   Reduce the stress and anxiety in your life! When you are stressed or distressed, your adrenal glands produce adrenaline, the "fight or flight" hormone. Too much stress stimulates too much adrenaline, which can be a disaster for your skeletal system because adrenaline is capable of dissolving bone! Give up or reduce your intake of coffee, since it stimulates the adrenal glands to secrete adrenaline. Also, stress increases the need for magnesium and vitamin C, both of which are required for good bone structure.

4   Avoid fast food and drugs that upset the body's chemistry and natural state of balance. Refined processed foods, coffee, tea, carbonated drinks, sugar, salt, alcohol, antacids, and drugs all upset the delicate balance in the body, affecting your body's ability to absorb and use the nutrients it needs when it needs them.

5   Osteoporosis is known to occur more frequently in very thin women, who have a lower bone mass and less fat tissue. At the menopause, fuller-figured women have more estrogen in their systems because the natural steroids in fat also produce estrogen. Even though the ovaries may stop functioning, a fatter body keeps the estrogen flowing much longer.

6   Keep your endocrine system in balance. The parathyroid gland naturally produces a hormone called calcitonin, which plays an important role in normal bone function by slowing down the cells that eat away at old bone. Salmon is a good food source for stimulating calcitonin levels.

Dr. Nancy Appleton, in her book Healthy Bones, places the endocrine system balance high on the list of preventative approaches to osteoporosis. She writes, "The endocrine glands, which are scattered throughout the body, secrete hormones into the bloodstream that help regulate the body chemistry. Each of these glands—the adrenals, pancreas, thyroid, parathyroid, pituitary, and gonads—plays an important part in maintaining homeostasis. Whenever we upset our body chemistries, a chain reaction occurs among these guardians of homeostasis. As they try to bring balance back to the bloodstream, they often pull calcium and other minerals from the bones. When this happens repeatedly over years of upset bone chemistry, osteoporosis is a likely result."

the endocrine system

If you've ever had butterflies in your stomach, felt hungry or had an orgasm, you've experienced the power of hormones. These are the chemical messengers that are produced by glands all over the body and carried by the blood stream to regulate hundreds of vital functions – the release of milk in breast feeding, how much water your body loses, how fast you grow, when you ovulate and so on. When you are alarmed or anxious, for instance, hormones flow from the hypothalamus to the pituitary in the brain and then to the adrenal glands on top of the liver, which produce the stress hormone cortisol – the one you feel in your stomach. Producing extra cortisol day after day in a very stressful job can lower your immune system and make you more prone to infections.

Some hormones have very precise effects, for example the parathyroid hormone (PTH), which maintains your calcium balance – vital for proper muscles and brain functioning. Too little and PTH stimulates the 'osteoclasts' to start mining bones to release calcium. A diet that makes your blood slightly too acidic can start calcium release too, which can lead to osteoporosis.

Other hormones, such as oestrogen, have much wider functions. At puberty, rising levels contribute to the development of women's fuller lips and a smaller chin as well as breasts and less body hair. During the menopause its decline dries out the skin, reduces vaginal lubrication and triggers mood swings.

The huge range of effects hormones can have make them a favourite target of drug companies, who can manufacture synthetic versions to increase or reduce hunger or regulate sexuality, for example. However, synthetic hormones very often don't work in quite the same way: HRT (hormone replacement therapy), can reduce the symptom of hot flushes and keep the skin plumped up, but it also raises the risk of cancer and heart disease. The action of any one hormone is carefully balanced by another, so taking a synthetic version regularly almost always has unwanted side effects.

The wrong balance of hormones can lie behind all sorts of disorders, from constant and extreme fatigue to lack of libido. Problems with the effectiveness of the hormone insulin makes for an unbalanced blood sugar level, for instance, which can lead to type 2 diabetes. Hormone therapy is very individual and should be undertaken only with the guidance of an expert.

AN ALTERNATIVE TO HRT

A possible replacement for HRT is what are known as 'bioidentical' hormones. HRT contains slightly altered molecules of oestrogen and progesterone; otherwise they couldn't be patented.

Treatment with bioidenticals not only involves exact copies of the ones your body makes, but also replaces all the hormones that decline with the menopause: three types of oestrogen, progesterone, testosterone and DHEA.

Testosterone levels, which are linked with female libido, drop more than oestrogen levels do and DHEA is used to make all the others. Care is taken to find the amounts that work best for you. Proper nutrition and supplements can sort out some hormone imbalances but long-term effects are still uncertain.

the immune system

Why do some people seem never to catch infections, while others fall ill when anyone sneezes? The secret is your immune system, an awe-inspiring network of chemicals, cells and fluids that recognize and destroy the millions of bacteria, viruses and pathogens that pass through us every minute. We all know about the arteries and veins that carry blood around the body; less familiar is the equally vital and complex lymph system that winds around it and removes waste and debris.

Cruising both the blood and the lymph systems is an army of immune cells (lymphocytes) whose job it is to seek out and destroy any foreign particles. Like an army, it's made up of many divisions and brigades, each with specialized tasks. The two main classes of 'soldier' are known as B cells, which are made in the bone marrow, and T cells, made in the thymus, an organ in the centre of your chest.

The T cell units have names like natural killer (NK) cells and T-helper cells, while the B cell units are divided into 'immunoglobulins' with names like IgE, IgA and IgG. Too few NK cells is a sign your immune response is weak, while an overactive IgE response is what triggers an allergy like hay fever. The command posts of the lymph system are the lymph nodes, which are found in places like the groin, armpits and neck. Here B cells are stored ready to swarm out on the attack when they get an alarm signal from the T cells. This is why you can get a painful swelling in those areas when you've got an infection.

A major difference between mainstream and complementary medicine is in the way each handles the immune response; drugs that target it tend to damp it down, like steroids, while the complementary approach is usually to strengthen it. When you're fighting an infection and producing billions of B cells you use up a lot of resources, so for peak effectiveness you may need to supplement certain vitamins: A, the B vitamins (especially B6), C and E – and the minerals zinc and selenium in particular. And you can get a lot more specific: thymus extract, for instance, can normalize the relationship between suppresser T cells and helper T cells; royal jelly enhances the functioning of the lymph nodes; while Reishi mushrooms restore the helper T cells knocked out by radiation therapy. Balance is vital: too little response allows infection; too much brings allergies and auto-immune disorders.

The mainstream is now accepting that your mental and emotional state has an impact on your immune system. Students worried by exams or people who have lost a loved one often show up with a dramatically reduced immune response, for example. Meditation and relaxation can improve this response, as too can laughter and an optimistic outlook, so keep your sense of humour in shape for optimum health. (See Laughter and Chocolate, page 206.)

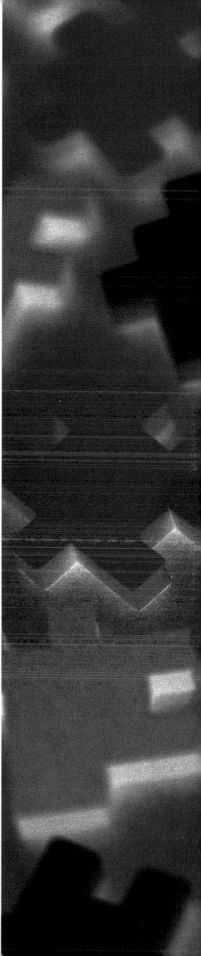

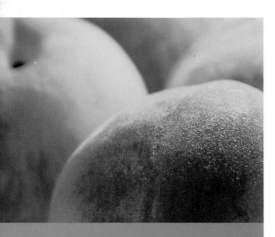

skin

The skin is an incredible organ of the body, and the largest. In addition to protecting us and helping to regulate our fluid levels and temperature, it also breathes in air and excretes unwanted material. The skin is covered in tiny pores which open and close to allow such processes to take place. It contains nerve endings which carry the direct messages about the joys and pains of the outer world inside to our internal one. The skin is the conduit of delicious sensual sensations that promote all sorts of feel-good actions in our mind and body.

Skin consists of layers. The outer layer that you can see, the epidermis, has different layers: the top, horny level that sheds dead cells which constantly flake and fall off; and the bottom basal level, which produces new cells that push upward as they divide, moving toward the skin's surface. If this layer of skin gets damaged, it will heal without scarring. The inner layer, or dermis, is rich in blood vessels, sweat glands, nerves, elastic fibers, and layers of collagen, which provide support, keeping the skin firm and supple. The deepest layer, the subcutaneous, consists mostly of fat cells and fibrous tissues.

Not only does the body breathe through the respiratory system—the nose, mouth, and lungs—but also through the skin. The skin is covered in countless tiny pores, which take in from the atmosphere around and eliminate anything unwanted. If the pores are clogged with creams that do not allow the skin to breathe, then the natural shedding process can be inhibited. Dead skin cells will then build up on the top layer and the skin will become dull and lifeless.

Notice the silky smoothness of a baby's skin. Over time, your skin is bound to suffer from some of the effects of stress and the pressures of environmental pollution, cigarette smoke, alcohol, candy and other junk food, and lack of exercise, sleep, or just plain tender loving care. To minimize negative effects on your skin, follow a few simple rules.

1 Keep your skin clean. Make skin cleansing a regular part of your morning and evening health rituals. Although not easily seen by the naked eye, your skin easily accumulates dirt, grime, old make-up, sweat, dead cells, and oil, which will lead to a bacteria build-up and potential skin problems. Clean skin is not a good host to poor skin conditions.

SKIN FACTS

- Our skin covers between 17 and 21 square feet and weighs up to 7 pounds.

- One square inch of skin has about 645 sweat glands, 65 hairs, 95 sebaceous glands and 20 feet of blood vessels.

- Each day we get rid of about 4 percent of our entire quantity of skin cells.

- The thickness of our skin varies in different parts of the body, with the face being the thinnest. On the palms and soles it can be more than ⅛ inch thick.

- Skin reflects health habits. Clear, glowing skin indicates a healthy lifestyle. Sallow, dull skin indicates lack of self-care and an unhealthy lifestyle.

2 Protect and nourish your skin with regular applications of moisturizing cream. To help conserve the skin's own natural moisture, it is essential to moisturize your skin regularly. Daily lubrication helps protect skin against inclement weather and environmental hazards, prevents the deterioration of the skin's layers, and helps keep it soft and smooth.

3 Gentle exfoliation, about once a week, can help to alleviate a build-up of dead skin cells. Pimples and acne can often be attributed to dead skin cell build-up. Weekly full-body exfoliation will help alleviate this and give you smoother, clearer, and unblemished skin. Exfoliation also has great health-giving benefits since it leaves the skin free to breathe.

4 Try to buy body products, bath and shower products, and skin creams that are natural and not overloaded with chemicals. Not only will you be helping your skin and your whole body, but you will also be helping the environment. Everything that you flush down the sink goes toward potentially damaging the environment. Your skin deserves the best, and natural products will help keep you looking and feeling healthy.

Using deodorants

Antiperspirants and deodorants, although seemingly essential in our society, are potentially damaging to the body. Because the armpits are full of lymph nodes, it is important to keep them clean and clear of chemicals. The chemicals and alcohol used in many deodorizing products travel directly into the blood system through the lymph nodes and capillaries in the armpits. The fact that some also inhibit sweating makes them doubly harmful, since sweating is an essential part of the elimination process. Sweating is the body's way of keeping cool in the heat and of eliminating toxins; when sweating is suppressed, toxins remain in the body and travel back into the system through the lymph and blood stream.

Try using mineral deodorant stones instead. These include salt water, or rock salt, do not inhibit sweating, last for six months, and are cheaper in the long run. Check your diet. If you suffer from body odor, you are probably eating a diet rich in unhealthy foods or strong, spicy foods, drinking too much alcohol, stressed, or even possibly ill. Toxins need to come out. Try switching a coffee or two a day for just plain water. Plenty of water will help detox the body and soon you will find you need deodorizing less often! Eating nutritious food also helps in the general elimination of toxins, as well as in keeping you healthy.

HEALTHY SKIN GUIDELINES

- The number one tip is never to go out without sunscreen. Even winter sun in the Northern hemisphere can be damaging to the skin, not just those hot days of summer. Use creams with UVB and UVA protection at all times of the year.

- Clean thoroughly but not excessively. Overcleaning can remove natural oils from the skin that are essential to keep it looking and feeling fresh, and can also lead to premature aging.

- Read the labels on products. Different areas of your face, neck, and body have different needs. The skin around the eyes, for example, is much thinner than that on the cheeks and it also has no oil glands. It may be wise to use different lotions in different areas.

- Avoid products that are heavily perfumed, riddled with chemicals, or contain a lot of alcohol. Always try to use the most natural products you can find. For example, using products with high-quality pure essential oils will work much more favorably for your skin than heavily perfumed alternatives. Take time to seek out what feels right for you.

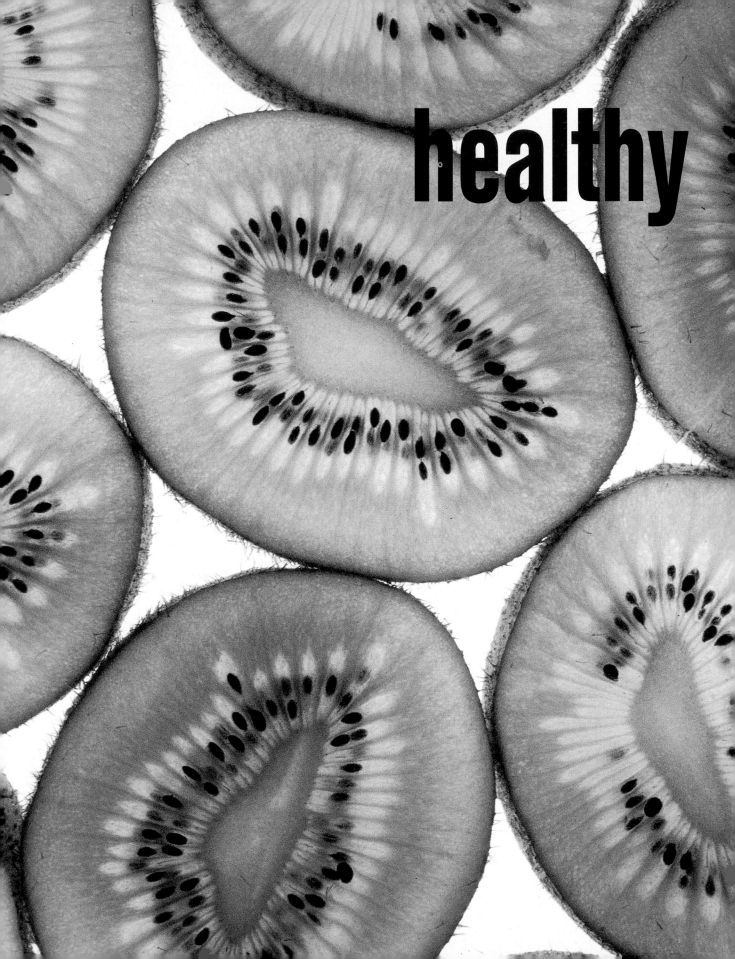

healthy

eating

In addition to being one of life's greatest pleasures, eating well is the most important contribution that we can make to our ongoing health and wellbeing. Taking our eating habits for granted is easy; our tastes have been with us for a long time. At some point, though, it dawns on most of us that our chosen diet and lifestyle hold the key to the state of our body and mind. We need to realize that the front line in the battle for the health of our whole being lies in our diet—in what we choose to put in our bodies and, just as importantly, what we choose *not* to eat or drink.

Most people would agree a well body is one that is free of serious imbalances, excesses, toxins, and dysfunction, and certainly free from degenerative disease. To reach a level of whole health and wellbeing, you need simply to realize that you have the ability to achieve a balanced body and mind. By reviewing your dietary habits and lifestyle honestly and implementing a few simple changes, you can redress the balance.

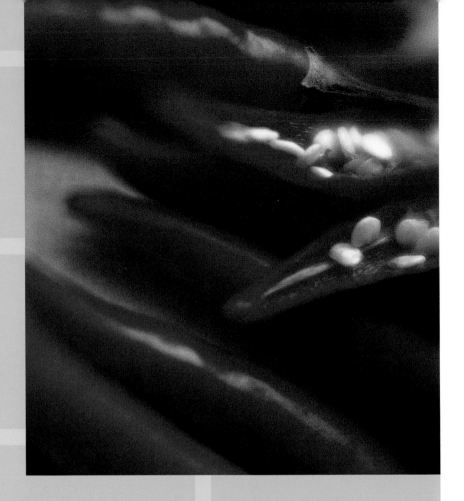

laying the
foundation

The consensus of medical and nutritional experts around the world is that we should eat more fresh fruits and vegetables, more whole-grain bread, pasta and cereals, lean meat and oily fish and drink more water. All the nutrients we need are to be found in a balanced diet like this. We should eat much less red meat and fatty foods, refined flour and sugar products like cakes and cookies, less white bread, junk food, salt, carbonated and caffeine drinks and alcohol. Golden rules for good nutrition.

OUR BODIES' BASIC NEEDS:

Carbohydrates

These provide energy and other nutrients. There are two kinds: simple carbohydrates, which are sugars, and complex carbohydrates, which are the starchy foods like grains and vegetables. Although sugars are an excellent source of quick energy, it is much healthier to get most of our energy from complex carbohydrates, since they have few health drawbacks and come in forms that bring lots of other nutrients and benefits.

Fats

These are another good source of energy and fat-soluble vitamins A, D, E, and K (see pages 94–98). Some fat in the body is essential for maintaining body heat, protecting vital organs, and providing cell wall structure (see also The Fat Crisis, page 40).

Proteins

Necessary for the growth, maintenance, and repair of body tissue, proteins help the building of cells, hormones, and enzymes by providing the amino acids that are the "building blocks" of life. Among meat-eaters and lacto-vegetarians, most proteins in the diet come from animal products, but vegetables contain adequate proteins, too. However, most vegetable proteins don't contain a full share of the essential amino acids the body needs. (Only eggs contain all eight essential amino acids.) In a good balanced diet, rich in a wide variety of vegetables and whole grains, this is not a problem because each type of food contains a different range of amino acids.

Proteins are an important energy source, but you may need less than you think. Most Americans consume over the recommended level. Too much protein can break down muscle and can create a toxic reaction over time. Serious illnesses may be linked to consuming too much meat—particularly red meat.

Fiber

As well as providing the bulk that facilitates the passage of foods through the system, fiber in sufficient quantities may also help prevent several intestinal problems, including bowel cancer. Derived from plant cell walls, fiber is classified as "insoluble fiber," which is cellulose, and "soluble fiber," mainly pectin, which is important in helping reduce blood cholesterol levels and stabilizing blood sugar. A diet rich in fruit, vegetables, and grains will ensure you get adequate fiber.

Vitamins and minerals

These are the substances, required in fairly small amounts (apart from the bone- and tooth-building minerals such as calcium), that are essential for the body's processes to function correctly (for a full discussion, see pages 91–105).

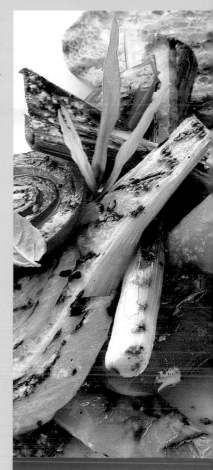

THE IDEAL BALANCE OF NUTRIENTS IN THE DIET

Nutritionists recommend that we get a minimum of 55 percent of our calories from carbohydrates, up to 15 percent from proteins, and a maximum of 30 percent in the form of fat.

Perhaps because of its obvious correlation with body weight, the one message about healthy diet that has now entered into public consciousness is that high fat intake is bad. Unfortunately, all too often this message has produced a general fear of fat that is not only unnecessary but dangerous. There are several different types of fat and only two are really harmful, while others are not just highly beneficial in moderate quantities, but are also essential for our wellbeing.

THE DIFFERENT TYPES OF FAT

All the fats and oils we eat are a combination of what are termed "saturated" and "unsaturated" fats. The fat in most foods is a mix, but usually either saturates or unsaturates predominate.

Saturated fats

These are the fats that naturally go hard when left at room temperature. Most animal fats, including those in poultry and dairy products, are predominantly saturated. Saturates are implicated in high blood cholesterol levels, atherosclerosis, and coronary heart disease. They are considered the type of fat you need to keep firmly in check and even reduce in your diet.

Unsaturated fats

These are generally the fats that are naturally liquid at room temperature. The oils from vegetables, nuts, and seeds are predominantly unsaturated. Unsaturated fats have the effect of reducing the bad (LDL) cholesterol in the blood (see below).

There are two main categories of unsaturated fats: monounsaturated fats, at their highest level in olive, peanut, and canola oils; and polyunsaturated fats, at their highest in corn, sunflower, safflower, and fish oils. Monounsaturates seem doubly health in that they not only help reduce bad cholesterol, but can also help maintain or even boost levels of good (HDL) cholesterol.

Cholesterol

This white, crystalline, organic compound is found in most animal and vegetable tissue and is essential for many metabolic functions. The body makes its own cholesterol and normally regulates levels in the blood, no matter how much we consume. However, it has been established that when the diet is high in both damaged cholesterol and saturated fats, then blood cholesterol levels rise.

the fat crisis

Cholesterol is a constituent of lipoproteins, which carry fats in the blood. Low-density lipoprotein cholesterol (LDL cholesterol), in excess, forms deposits on the artery walls, leading to cardiovascular disease. On the other hand, high-density lipoprotein cholesterol (HDL cholesterol) acts as a scavenger, helping clean the blood of fats and cholesterol. Sex and stress hormones are made from cholesterol.

Trans fats

For decades, people all over the world have been replacing butter with margarine, believing they were making a healthier choice. Experts still maintain it is essential to keep a tight rein on the intake of saturated fatty acids to avoid the risk of heart disease, and that favoring cooking oils and spreads that are high in monounsaturates and polyunsaturates is much healthier. To complicate matters somewhat, recent research has shown that not all fats, margarines, and spreads made from vegetable oils are necessarily healthier. The reason for this is the presence of trans fatty acids (often called trans fats), which consist of unsaturated fats, the normal molecular shape of which has been altered by hydrogenation, the chemical process that makes oils solid at normal room temperatures. They are called trans fats because they are "transformed" fats.

Many studies have demonstrated that trans fats have the same effect on blood cholesterol levels as saturated fats; they raise the level of LDL cholesterol—the bad cholesterol—and reduce the blood levels of good cholesterol—the HDL cholesterol. Some trans fats do actually occur naturally in dairy products, but these do not have the same potentially harmful properties as the trans fats in hydrogenated oils, and they are not as potentially damaging to your health. Trans fats are found in many packaged foods, such as cookies, crackers, and pastries.

The effects of trans fats are now considered so detrimental to our health that most food manufacturers are seriously reducing or eliminating them. Indeed, now an ever-increasing number of brands and products are carrying labels: "no trans fats".

The essential fatty acids

As we have seen, there are fats that are bad for us and fats that are good for us, but some fats are actually vital for the correct functioning of our metabolism. Recent reports from Boston University Medical Center in America claim that a diet very low in fat is not good for your heart. Such diets may lack essential fatty acids (EFAs). Research indicates that those with low levels of EFAs in their blood are also deficient in HDL cholesterol, the good cholesterol that protects against heart disease (see above).

The essential fatty acids are almost all to be found in vegetable oils, such as olive and sunflower oils, as well as in the omega-3 oils in oily fish like salmon, mackerel, and sardines. These are necessary for a healthy heart and a healthy body. Some of

GUIDELINES ON FAT INTAKE

Dietary guidelines released in October, 2000, by the American Heart Association recommends:

- Cut fat in the diet to less than 30 percent of total calories.
- Cholesterol intake should be under 300 milligrams a day.
- Use more oils high in monounsaturated fatty acids, such as olive and canola oils.
- Limit foods high in saturated fats, trans fats and/or cholesterol.
- Eat less than 6 grams of salt daily.

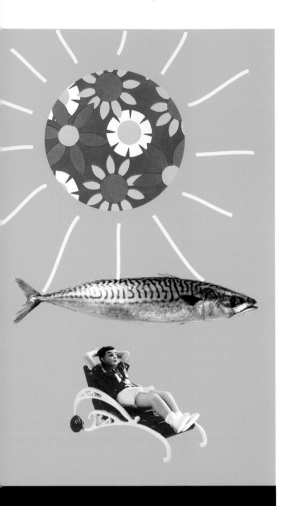

FISH OILS AND SKIN CANCER

Fish oils may be as powerful a sunscreen as commonly used SPF creams and also may help prevent skin cancer. Eating a meal of fish rich in omega-3 fatty acids every day may boost your immunity to skin cancers and reduce the risk of burning through overexposure to the sun.

us get most of the omega-6 we need from vegetable oils. However, we are nearly all deficient in omega-3, which is mainly found in oily fish and flaxseed oil.

A deficiency of omega-3 oils has been strongly implicated as a principal contributor to heart disease, cancer, immune dysfunction, and many other modern illnesses. Such conditions as allergy, asthma, alcoholism, arthritis, dry skin, eczema, inflammatory conditions, learning difficulties, poor memory, schizophrenia, and a great many others, all relate to fatty acid deficiencies or imbalances.

The huge change to our diet this century means that almost everyone has a deficiency of these essential nutrients, or at least an unbalanced consumption of them, which can also cause chaos in our chemistry. Understanding how to correct these imbalances could be life-saving. It could also help to heal long-standing symptoms and delay the progress of degenerative disease. There is evidence that we are already lowering the collective IQ by feeding babies formulas that are deficient in essential fatty acids. Many breastfeeding mothers are deficient, too.

In 1992, in his book *Nutrition and Evolution*, Dr. Michael Crawford, director of the Institute of Brain Chemistry at the University of North London, England, put forward the revolutionary theory that nutrition was the true driving force in evolution. The development of the human brain appears to have been dependent on the people living in locations with unlimited access to seafoods and fish, high in the omega fatty acids.

Dr. Lesley Rhodes, a consultant dermatologist at the Royal Liverpool University Hospital, says: "There is a big link between the effect of fish oil in preventing sunburn and what we suspect will prove to be its effect in helping prevent skin cancer, because the same wavelengths of light are responsible for both. What we also know is that the process which triggers sunburn and the process involved in the development of skin cancer over a period of time are the same"

Dr. Rhodes goes on to explain that sunburn is the result of tissue damage, which is, in turn, part of the process that leads to skin cancer. Through trials conducted, the tolerance to sunlight increased with the more fish or flax oils consumed—in fact, the threshold for sunburn doubled! In the U.S., the results of a recent laboratory experiment, released by researchers at the New York Medical College and the American Health Foundation, show that a main component of fish oil, called DHA, is effective in inhibiting the growth of human melanoma cells, suppressing cell and tumor growth.

Everyone needs fat in their diet

Although most people may still eat too high a level of saturated fat from fatty meat, butter, or cheese, or too much trans fats—the kind found in most margarines and such processed foods as cookies, cakes, and pastries (see page 41)—others are cutting out too much of the right kind of fats from their diet.

In addition to being aware of the problems that high fat intake may produce, we must never forget that fat is essential to good health. Fat is:

- An important energy and heat source; the body burns off fat calories when active.
- Vital in providing a protective cushion around the organs and in insulating the body against heat loss. Obviously fat is even more important in cold climates, and you need more in winter than in summer.
- A source of the fat-soluble vitamins A, D, E, and K.
- Important in the diet of women to help them make the hormone estrogen.
- A source of the essential fatty acids, linoleic acid (omega-6 oils) and alpha-linolenic acid (omega-3 oils), that are essential to health and which help the body make other polyunsaturated fatty acids necessary to wellbeing. They also help your body metabolize cholesterol.

THE GLYCEMIC INDEX

The glycemic index measures the effect of eating a particular food on your blood sugar levels against a pure glucose standard, which rates 100 on the index. Foods with a low glycemic index (GI) rating are absorbed more slowly than foods with a higher rating, therefore affecting blood sugar levels less radically. You should try to include plenty of these foods in your diet because they provide long-term, sustained energy with fewer highs and lows. High-GI foods, on the other hand, provide quick-release, short-term bursts of energy, which is useful for athletes; for the rest of us, however, these foods should only be eaten in moderation.

The index rates only high-carbohydrate foods, because high-protein foods and fats do not have much of an effect on blood sugar. However, both types of food eaten in small amounts with a carbohydrate help to lower its GI rating, so it does help to have a little protein and fat with your carbohydrates (for example, salad dressing or parmesan on pasta).

Some common foods and their glycemic index:

Apple	39
Banana	62
Beans, kidney	29
Beans, lima	36
Beets	64
Brown rice	66
Carrots	92
Cherries	23
Chickpeas	36
Corn	59
Cornflakes	80
Glucose	100
Grapefruit	26
Grapes	45
Honey	87
Lentils	29
Milk, whole	34
Milk, skim	32
Oatmeal	49
Oranges	40
Peanuts	13
Pears	34
Peas	51
Plums	25
Potatoes, baked	98
Potatoes, new	70
Raisins	64
Shredded wheat	67
Spaghetti	50
Sweet potato	51
Tomatoes	38
White bread	69
White rice	72
Wholewheat bread	72
Yogurt	36

LIQUID REFRESHMENT

Water

It is a fascinating fact that water makes up about 70 to 75 percent of the body. Without this "elixir of life," we would burn up or dry out; our core temperature is regulated by drinking water and we couldn't survive without it. In fact, dehydration is a very serious —and potentially fatal—condition, which must be remedied immediately if it occurs.

Some people seem to function quite normally by unknowingly walking around in a state of semidehydration. One of the first symptoms of dehydration is that the skin becomes dull and dry. Not only does water help regulate our temperature but, just as importantly, it is a powerful internal cleanser, dissolving waste material for elimination to prevent toxic build-up, and essential to the absorption of nutrients we need to live.

For these reasons it is recommended that we drink six to eight 8-ounce glasses of water a day to replace what is lost. This may not be easy for those brought up in a coffee-, juice-, cola-, and alcohol-drinking culture like our own! People on high-fiber diets, especially, must drink at least the recommended minimum in order to avoid intestinal problems, particularly constipation.

Because the recognition of water's important role in our health has widened, there has been an enormous rise in concern over the level of pollutants in the drinking water supply. Unfortunately, this has been matched by an increase in reports of contamination in the last decade. Threats from man-made compounds, detergents, pesticides, and industrial by-products can seep into the water supply. Other chemicals have been added to our drinking water as a matter of course for various reasons, although some occur naturally.

Ammonia and chlorine are added to drinking water as disinfectants, but they can also cause skin problems. Chlorine is also known to react with other chemicals in water to produce trihalomethanes, certain ones of which can cause cancer. Many water companies also add fluoride to help prevent tooth decay, but this may not be good for the skin or bones. Pesticides get into the water system, too, via rainwater in the fields moving into the rivers and streams. Some pesticides contain chemicals that mimic the action of the hormone estrogen, and fertility researchers are linking the rise in male infertility to the increase in pesticide residues in the water supply.

The Safe Drinking Water Act of 1974 requires the Environmental Protection Agency to set standards for quality, but the responsibility to monitor contaminant levels falls to the local water utilities. For advice on the drinking water in your area, contact your local water supplier and public health department.

Although millions have since been spent to clean up tap water, and there are some real improvements, we still cannot assume it is always perfectly pure; in fact, its safety may be questionable. Is it any surprise that sales of water filters and bottled water has increased so dramatically over the past two decades?

EMOTIONS EFFECT WATER

A pioneer Japanese researcher, Dr. Masaru Emoto, believes that water has the ability to absorb, hold and even transmit human feelings. He has discovered, and documented photographically, how thoughts and emotions can impact the molecular structure of water.

Using high-speed photography, he found that crystals formed in frozen water reveal changes when specific, concentrated thoughts or emotions are directed toward them. Water exposed to loving words shows brilliant, colourful snowflake patterns, while water exposed to negative words forms incomplete patterns with dull colours. Taking this look at energy medicine a step further, music, visual images and the written word were also seen to have an impact on the structure of the crystal.

Dr. Emoto believes his work can further the cause of peace. As the Earth, along with its peoples is made of 70 per cent water, we can affect the planet and each other by consciously expressing love and good will.

Water filters generally work on the principle of passing the water through activated carbon and ion exchange resins to remove impurities such as lead, nitrates, pesticides, and herbicides, and to improve taste and odor. The carbon-filter cartridges need to be changed frequently to avoid creating a breeding ground for bacteria. Some people opt for filters that are installed directly in the plumbing of their home; these are much more expensive, but very convenient, and can be more effective if reverse osmosis filters are used. Whichever filter system you choose, follow the manufacturer's instructions exactly or you could make the quality of your water worse.

- Keep your filter reservoir and water container clean.
- Change the filter cartridge regularly, as directed by the manufacturer.
- It is safer to keep filtered water in the refrigerator, and the water will taste better.
- Boil water for babies' food or drink.

If you can't find bottled water when traveling and you are unsure of local water quality, always boil your water before drinking it or cooking with it. In the U.S., the Food and Drug Administration regulates bottled waters, although sparkling waters are not regulated in the same way. Water labeled as spring water comes from a natural spring. Buy from an approved source, as some spring water may contain dangerous levels of pesticides and nitrates, for example.

Alcohol

The question of whether or not alcohol is good for you continues to spark a lot of debate in medical and non-medical circles alike. Most experts are agreed, however, that there is nothing harmful about drinking in moderation, but excessive drinking is very damaging to your health and well-being, and will dramatically affect you and your family. Alcohol tolerance is a very individual thing and can greatly vary depending on your age, sex and other physical and psychological considerations.

Moderate intake of red wine is reputed to be beneficial and may even protect the heart and lungs. In countries where moderate amounts of red wine are frequently drunk with meals, the incidence of heart attacks is much lower than it is in the UK, for example. One or two small glasses per day, with water to accompany the wine, would be considered a moderate amount.

the medicine cabinet in your food

"Superfoods" is a recent term for some fairly everyday foods of all types, which are highly nutritious, possess powerful properties for promoting wellbeing, and help to prevent or fight illnesses. Most of the superfoods are common vegetables, fruits, seeds, or herbs. It is the quality, quantity, and regularity with which you eat the superfoods that count. A wide selection, eaten regularly, is a good way of getting all the nutritional and medicinal benefits they offer.

Almond

A very concentrated, highly nutritious food, full of protein (a third more than eggs), almonds are rich in some B vitamins and minerals like potassium, zinc, calcium, magnesium, and phosphorus. The body absorbs these nutrients best when eaten with foods rich in vitamin C. Almond milk is an ancient natural remedy for respiratory and digestive problems. The soothing properties of almond oil have been widely recognized for centuries.

Apple

The power of the apple has been documented at least since biblical times. Modern day nutritionists support what our great-grandmothers and the ancients already knew: an apple a day does keep the doctor away. Apples are full of the antioxidant vitamin C and rich in pectin, which helps protect from the ravages of pollution by binding to toxic heavy metals in the body, such as mercury and lead, and carrying them out. This delicious, highly nutritious fruit is a natural aid to healthy digestion, and its tartaric and malic acid content helps the body cope with rich foods or excessive protein. People with rheumatic pain often experience relief from their symptoms after adding apples to their daily diet.

Apricot

This small but powerful fruit is packed with beta-carotene and iron, which combat free radical activity and help fight respiratory and other infections. Some researchers claim they help in the prevention of cancer. Dried apricots are a good source of iron.

Avocado

This delicious and nutritious fruit is an amazing, almost complete food, rich in antioxidant vitamins A, C, and E, some B complex, potassium, a little protein, starch, and monounsaturated fats. Make avocado a regular part of your diet to help lower LDL cholesterol levels (see pages 40–41). Avocados are reputed to be good for your heart, digestion, skin, and sex life. Researchers have also found a unique antibacterial and antifungal in the flesh.

Banana

This sweet, soothing, easy-to-eat, easy-to-digest fruit has calming and restorative qualities, perhaps the reason it is one of the very earliest solid foods introduced to babies. Bananas are a good source of potassium, which is so important to the healthy function of every cell in the body. They are a rich source of many other nutrients, including vitamin B6, calcium, folate, iron, and zinc, as well as a source of the valuable fiber, pectin, which helps in the elimination of toxic wastes.

Barley

People have been growing this soothing, strengthening, highly nutritious, and easily digested, grain for thousands of years—Roman gladiators ate it for strength. Used to relieve inflammation, constipation and diarrhoaea, to improve digestion, respiratory and liver function, it is also reputed to help fatigue and stress, and to strengthen the nervous system. Rich in the B and E vitamins, calcium, and potassium, barley is a good restorative for invalids and improves brain function and mental alertness. Barley water helps to relieve a sore chest or throat and to soothe cystitis.

Basil

This popular herb is reputed to be a natural tranquilizer, helping to calm the nervous system and aid sleep!

Beans

Beans of all types, fresh and dried, are high in fiber and protein and low in fat. Rich in soluble fiber, they slow down the rate of digestion, reduce blood cholesterol, steady blood sugar, and combat anemia. Their high levels of iron and folate rival those of meat and fish, and they are rich in potassium.

Young, green barley shoots and wheatgrass juice are among the new superfood stars and are used in many natural health spas for cures and fasts. They are rich in proteins, vitamins, and minerals, and form the basis for many fasting programs to cleanse and regenerate the body.

Berries

Berries, particularly blackberries and blueberries, are renowned for their high vitamin C content and antioxidant properties. Strawberries are also known as protectors against free radicals.

Beet

For many centuries this sweet vegetable has been known for its positive effect on the entire digestive system, but most particularly the liver. Eastern Europeans have particularly valued the healing and tonic qualities of this plant, with the fresh, raw juice used to cleanse and "build" the blood and to treat people recovering from serious illness by strengthening their immune system. Beets are best eaten raw for the full power of their healing properties.

Black cumin seed

The Prophet Mohammed said, "black cumin heals every disease—except death," and it has become known as "the medicine of the Prophet." Containing nigellin, which stimulates digestion, it has many other qualities, including as a heart-protector and an antibacterial. Used externally, it can treat skin diseases and many allergies. It is a valuable source of the essential fatty acids.

Black currant

Best known for their high vitamin C content, black currants' dark purple color comes from flavonoids, which are known to strengthen the walls of the small blood vessels. Black currants are also rich in vitamin E and carotenes, making them a valuable source of antioxidants. Also a good source of potassium and a diuretic, their health-giving properties include helping to relieve inflammation and lowering the risk of heart disease, stroke, cataracts, and cancer. They are rich in anthocyanins, flavonoids which counter the common bacteria that can cause food poisoning and urinary tract infections, and their high pectin levels can help relieve diarrhea. The seeds also contain the fatty acid, gamma-linolenic acid (GLA) used to treat the inflammation associated with rheumatism, skin conditions, eczema, and psoriasis.

Brazil nut

This is one of the richest vegetable sources of the antioxidant mineral selenium, which is so important for fertility and hormone metabolism. It also helps the function of the thyroid.

Broccoli

Part of the crucifer family, which includes cauliflower, kale, Brussels sprouts, cabbage, and radishes, this iron-rich vegetable is stocked with beta-carotene and vitamin C, antioxidants reputed to have the power to inhibit free radical activity, help prevent certain cancers and heart disease, and treat joint problems and fatigue. They are also the best source of anticarcinogenic glucosinolates.

Brown rice

This complete food is high in fiber, which soothes, cleanses, and protects the intestinal tract. It is also rich in the B vitamins, which keep the nervous system healthy and in the antioxidant vitamin E. Brown rice is a good source of methionine, needed to make enzymes that combat free radicals, and pangamic acid, which is said to lower cholesterol.

Cabbage

A member of the brassica or crucifer family, cabbage has healing qualities that have been known for centuries. Cabbage is a tonic and disinfectant in respiratory infections, and its raw juice treats ulcers successfully. It is a notable cleanser, particularly of the liver, blood, and skin. Anemics benefit from eating lots of cabbage, since it is rich in both iron and chlorophyll, chemically very similar to human blood hemoglobin. Cabbage is also rich in vitamins A, B, C, and E, as well as iron, sulphur, silica, magnesium, and calcium. It boosts the immune system and helps protect against stress and in treating cancer (see also Sauerkraut, page 54).

Camomile

Camomile is renowned for its relaxing properties and has been widely used since at least the 17th century in Europe by those seeking restful sleep. Its uses are varied and it is valuable in treating stomach upsets, irritable bowel syndrome, period pain, headaches, migraines, and muscle spasms (see also page 107).

Cardamom

Cardamom is an excellent digestive tonic and is also used to treat some respiratory disorders. The seeds contain volatile oils, including borneol, camphor, and pinene. Chewing the seeds releases the oils, giving a comforting, not-too-fiery warmth that eases indigestion and flatulence.

Carrot

These sweet brightly colored vegetables are rich in vitamins A, B, and C, minerals like calcium, iron, and potassium, and other antioxidants. They are good sources of beta-carotene; you can get your full RDA of vitamin A in just one carrot, hence the vegetable's reputed efficacy in eye and skin disorders, as well as respiratory infections. The mighty carrot is also high up on the list of foods that protect against cancer. Raw carrot juice makes a wonderful tonic and is often recommended for supporting the liver and for preventing wrinkles, making it a popular antiaging food.

Cauliflower

Cauliflower is another member of the nutritious crucifer family (see also Brussels sprout, opposite) and a good source of folate, antioxidant vitamin C, and the cancer-fighting glucosinolates.

Celery

Celery is a good substitute for sea salt because it is higher in sodium than most vegetables. It is also a good source of potassium, which counterbalances sodium in the body to help prevent raised blood pressure. It contains a phytochemical which lowers blood pressure and blood cholesterol. Celery juice can help reduce acidity levels, making it an excellent preventative food for osteoarthritis.

Celery, taken as a juice or eaten raw, or used liberally in vegetable soups, is also an excellent natural diuretic. Celery is also known to act synergistically with cabbage, for example, in breaking down fat cells, so it is a useful food for those wishing to lose weight in a healthy way.

Cinnamon

Latest research indicates that cinnamon can inhibit the growth of *E. coli* bacteria. This comes as little surprise to herbalists, who have known of its antibacterial, antifungal, and antiviral effects for many years. It can treat stomach upsets and vomiting, and reduce cold and flu symptoms. A dash of ground cinnamon in a honey and lemon drink can soothe a sore throat. In the form of a tea, cinnamon is also an antispasmodic and eases menstrual cramps.

Chilies

Chili peppers are, in fact, a fruit and they provide three times more vitamin C than oranges. Moderate amounts of any type of fresh or powdered chili will induce sweating—a cooling mechanism that could explain the seemingly perverse popularity of chilies in hot climates. The unique chili pepper heat comes from a component called capsaicin, concentrated in the internal pale rib membranes and seeds. Capsaicin can relieve nerve pain and is used in a medically prescribed cream to ease the pain of shingles. Herbalists advocate chili to warm the body, improve the circulation and stimulate metabolism. However, chilies may be

contraindicated in certain "hot" conditions, such as acne rosacea, which causes abnormal facial flushing.

Cloves

Cloves are a well-known toothache remedy. Simply apply clove oil to the affected area or clamp a whole clove between your teeth; the clove is thought to act as a mild anesthetic. Cloves have strong antiseptic and germicidal qualities.

Cranberries

The juice is excellent for the treatment of cystitis and for preventing urinary tract infections because it helps flush out the bacteria that are known to cause these conditions.

Fenugreek

High in ingredients that soothe and heal, freshly ground fenugreek seeds can be used in cooking or as an infusion to ease inflammatory conditions of the stomach and intestines. They can be sprouted, and the green parts eaten, together with the seeds. Fenugreek can be used in a soothing poultice for abscesses and boils. It should not be used medicinally in pregnancy but increases breastmilk after.

Garlic

A member of the onion family, along with chives and shallots, this plant is now widely recognized as one of the most potent medicinal plants. It is a natural diuretic, increasing kidney function, and is traditionally used to clean and treat wounds and bites. It is a natural expectorant, helping the expulsion of mucus from the lungs and throat.

In ancient times a remedy for most pains and disease, garlic is now highly recognized for its natural antiseptic and antibiotic qualities. Recently published research claims that garlic powder can kill bacteria known to cause stomach ulcers. Another recent study showed that natural chemicals found in garlic can suppress tumors and that these may even help to prevent cancer.

Garlic is renowned for lowering the risk of heart disease and strokes, helping to reduce cholesterol and improving the circulation. It also has a powerful effect on blood clotting mechanisms by "thinning" the blood.

The sulphur in garlic is responsible for its pungent aroma; garlic contains hundreds of components, with sulphur involved in most of them. Allicin is the most notable of these, and on crushing garlic, the allicin is released. Allicin is believed to be responsible in helping to reduce cancer risk. Recent research has shown that regular consumption of garlic reduced the risk of stomach cancer by 25 to 50 percent.

A research team from the Chelsea and Westminster Hospital in London, England, has shown that taking garlic during pregnancy reduces the risk of pre-eclampsia (raised blood pressure and protein retained in the urine).

Everyone can benefit from regular consumption of raw and cooked garlic to fight common colds, flu, coughs, and bronchitis, as well as other respiratory and digestive infections. Garlic is highly effective as a liver cleanser and can help reduce blood sugar.

Ginger

Ginger root is valued for its cleansing, warming, and stimulating qualities. It aids digestion, helps remove gases from the stomach and intestines, has antiseptic qualities, and helps loosen mucus. It is widely used to alleviate the symptoms or colds and flu. Ginger helps improve circulation and, with its warming qualities, can be useful in the treatment of rheumatism and arthritis.

Grape

This cleansing and strengthening fruit is best eaten fresh or as a juice; eat it on its own, because it ferments in the gut quickly. One of the most popular and effective cleansing fasts practiced is a grape fast. Grapes seem to have the effect of stimulating the body's regenerative powers and are highly effective for combating stress and fatigue; they are often included in the diet during convalescence.

Horseradish

Horseradish acts as a digestive aid, stimulates blood circulation, and increases urinary flow. An infusion made from the root, with some crushed mustard seeds added, can help disperse excess fluid and reduce water retention.

Lemon balm

This plant, also called balm, is native to Southern Europe and grows in some areas of the U.S. It can help treat anxiety and tension, or even mild depression.

Lentils

Lentils are a nutritious source of protein, cholesterol, and fiber, as well as iron, magnesium, potassium, and B vitamins. They are also rich in lignans, which fight hormone-dependent cancers.

Mango

In its raw state, this delicious tropical fruit is a useful source of vitamin E, iron, and vitamin C. It is also a rich source of beta-carotene, giving it valuable antioxidant properties.

Manuka honey

The healing and antiseptic qualities of honey have long been acknowledged, but a senior lecturer in biochemistry at the Waikato University in New Zealand, Dr. Molan, has found that Manuka honey, which comes from the flower of the famous, healing New Zealand Tea Tree Bush has medicinal qualities not found in other honeys. It is purported to strengthen the immune system, help heal wounds and fight all kinds of infections, and is particularly effective for colds, sore throats, skin eruptions and cuts, burns and fever blisters. It is also used for acid reflux, heartburn and stomach ulcers.

Melon

Cleansing and mildly stimulating to kidneys and bladder, melons are gently laxative—perfect for a summer fast.

Mushrooms

The Chinese have understood the usefulness of mushrooms in medicine for centuries, and the Japanese in a recent study showed that eating only 3¼ ounces of shiitake mushrooms every day caused blood cholesterol levels to plummet after

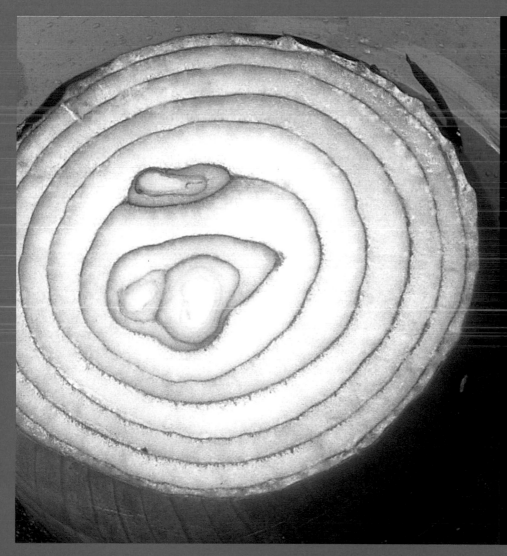

THE TOP 20 ANTIOXIDANT VEGETABLES

Bean, green
Beet
Broccoli
Brussels sprouts
Cabbage
Carrot
Cauliflower
Celery
Corn
Eggplant
Garlic
Kale
Lettuce, Iceberg
Lettuce, leaf
Onion
Pepper, red
Potato
Potato, sweet
Spinach
Squash, yellow

only one week. Mushrooms contain vitamin B, potassium, iron, and protein, as well as beneficial chemicals called polysaccharides, which are known to stimulate the immune system because they are so similar to bacteria cell walls.

Nutmeg

"Traditionally added to milky drinks given to convalescents, nutmeg contains myristin, a substance that, in small amounts, can cause drowsiness and a sense of wellbeing," says diet consultant Joanna Hall. Just a pinch of the finely grated spice can also treat flatulence, nausea, and vomiting. Grated nutmeg in a suitable carrier ointment is reputedly excellent for hemorrhoids. However, too much nutmeg taken internally is highly dangerous—as little as two whole nutmegs could be fatal.

Oats

This staple food is perhaps the most important grain after brown rice and should hold a regular place in the diet. Oats are highly stabilizing to blood sugar levels, making them excellent for diabetics. Oats have been shown to help lower blood cholesterol levels, one of the reasons people with heart or circulatory problems are advised to eat oats, especially as oatmeal and oat bran. Many digestive disorders, including constipation, respond to regular eating of oats and its demulcent quality soothes the stomach and intestines. Oats are traditionally known for their qualities as a sedative and nerve restorative, which is not surprising when you consider how nutritious they are, and rich in the B complex vitamins and vitamin E, calcium, magnesium, potassium and silicon.

Oily fish

Fish like herring, mackerel, salmon, and halibut are rich in the important omega-3 fatty acids, which help lower blood cholesterol, protecting against heart disease, stroke, cognitive decline, and skin conditions.

Olive oil

This delicious, healthy, and popular oil is rich in cholesterol-neutralizing monounsaturated fats and vitamin E, and is a free-radical inhibitor. It encourages the digestive system and regular bowel movement, and is good for easing rheumatic conditions.

Onion

High in the B vitamins and potassium, onions are considered to be in the food front line when helping to reduce heart disease, stroke, and cancer risk. They also help process fatty foods, preventing the blood-clotting rise in cholesterol after a fatty meal. People who eat raw onions regularly have more balanced, healthier cholesterol levels. Onions are a popular folk remedy for colds, arthritis, asthma, bronchitis, gastric and urinary infections, early aging, rheumatism, and gout.

Orange

Oranges are renowned for their infection-fighting qualities. With their high content of vitamin C, beta-carotene, and bioflavonoids,they help

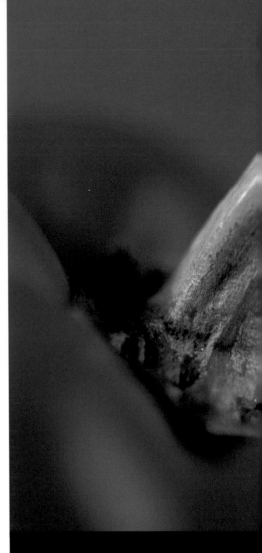

HOW TO GET ENOUGH!

The best sources of each of the major antioxidants should be:

VITAMIN C: Red and green bell peppers, oranges and their juice, black currants, kiwifruit, broccoli, and leafy green vegetables.
VITAMIN E: Nuts, seeds, vegetable oils, avocados, and whole grains.
SELENIUM: Brazil nuts and seafood.
CAROTENOIDS: Red bell peppers, cantaloupe, spinach, mangoes, and oranges.

the body's defenses. Bioflavonoids aid the support of the immune system by strengthening vitamin C's antioxidant powers, helping to enhance the strength of the blood capillary walls. Eaten fresh, oranges provide pectin, which helps reduce blood cholesterol.

Parsley

This popular herb is so widely used that we take it for granted and forget how much it can help improve our health, as well as the taste of the dishes we prepare. It is an excellent source of potassium and calcium, and is particularly rich in the antioxidants, carotenes, and vitamin C. Recognized as a special herb, since at least Roman times, parsley also has expectorant and diuretic powers. It is considered an emmenagogue—with the power to stimulate the menstrual process. Pregnant women must not eat medicinal doses of parsley, and take it only lightly and occasionally, if at all.

Peppers

The sweet bell pepper, or capsicum, has very high levels of vitamin C, especially the riper yellow and red varieties. They are an excellent source of beta-carotene, iron, and potassium. Red and yellow bell peppers rank high in the antioxidant army's war against cancer and heart disease. As with most plant foods, it is best to eat them raw and fresh to get the maximum nutritive value you can.

Peppermint

This plant is noted for its usefulness in a wide range of digestive disorders. It

apparently works by reducing the time food spends in the stomach by stimulating the gastric lining and also relaxing the stomach muscles. It is also a useful antispasmodic (see also page 108).

Pineapple

Hundreds of research studies have shown the positive action of the powerful bromelain enzyme found in the fresh, raw juice or full fruit of the pineapple. This enzyme can digest many times its own weight of protein in a few minutes. Pineapple is a delicious cure for all types of digestive ailments, and it is also prized for its anti-inflammatory action and for speeding up the healing process.

Prune

These contain twice as much antioxidants as any other fruit or vegetable. They also have a high fiber content, which is why they are so popular as a natural laxative.

Pumpkin seed

In Eastern Europe, pumpkin seeds are said to protect the prostate gland and to be a good tonic for men generally. These tasty seeds are good for everyone and a valuable source of B complex vitamins, calcium, iron, magnesium, and zinc.

Radish

An important member of the crucifer family, radishes are hot and astringent in their action. They should be eaten fresh, and regularly but not in excess. Their powerful juice stimulates the discharge of bile from the gallbladder, but too much

can irritate both the gallbladder and the liver. A good source of calcium, potassium, and sulphur, radishes have long been recognized for their detoxifying liver-toning qualities.

Raspberry leaves

For centuries a tea made from raspberry leaves has been taken by women during late pregnancy. The leaves are now known to help relax the uterine muscles for labor. Raspberry tea also soothes throat irritations and mouth ulcers.

Rosemary

This astringent herb has a deserved reputation for its strengthening and toning effect on everything from muscles to hair. Rosemary increases perspiration and has a calming action on the stomach, showing a nervine or sedative quality. It can help psychological tension, head colds, lethargy, and flatulence, and is used to relieve many varied symptoms, such as bad menstrual cramps and circulation problems. It has natural antibacterial, antifungal, antiseptic, and relaxant powers, and is a good brain and memory tonic (see also page 108).

Sage

In traditional folk medicine, this pungent herb has been regarded as an aid to memory and to fight the symptoms of aging, especially failing eyesight. It has strong antiseptic, antispasmodic, and astringent properties, fighting infection and boosting the immune system. Sage tea or infusions are excellent for asthma, catarrh, colds, flu, sore throats, swollen

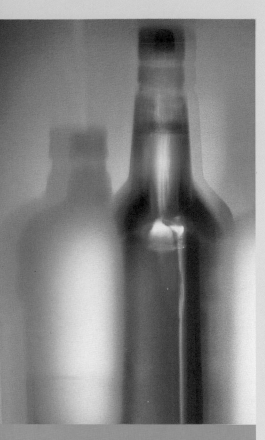

glands, and respiratory infections. Sage is an excellent remedy if you are suffering from stress, anxiety, or exhaustion, or if you are convalescing after illness. However, pregnant women and epileptics should avoid it.

Sauerkraut

This amazing medicinal food is made by fermenting slices of raw cabbage layered with sea salt and a few spices or juniper berries. The cabbage ferments in its own juices over the three to four weeks it takes to create this nutritious food. It is packed with important enzymes and high in calcium and vitamin C. It helps eliminate toxins in the gut and arrests autointoxication, regulates digestion, and helps cultivate intestinal flora. Because it promotes a healthy colon, some say that it helps prolong youth.

Sesame seed

Rich in protein, antioxidant vitamin E, iron, magnesium, calcium, zinc, essential fatty acids, and important amino acids, these tasty little seeds are excellent for toning up the kidneys and liver, stimulating circulation and fertility, treating fatigue, and enhancing your sex life and your sense of vitality. You can mix the seeds, whole or ground, with other foods, or use tahini (sesame seed paste) instead of butter. Halvah is a Middle Eastern confection made from ground sesame seeds and a little honey.

Soybean

Soybeans and most soy products, like tofu and soy milk, are nutritious foods, rich in the B complex vitamins, calcium, iron, and lecithin. They are known for their positive effect on the nervous system, especially when eaten in moderation and, as in the Japanese diet, fermented and combined with sea greens and rice. Recent research has shown that soybeans contain materials that, on digestion or fermentation, release genistein and daidzein, which help prevent breast and prostate cancer and form a natural hormone-replacement therapy for those in the menopause. They are referred to as "plant estrogens," and in fact, are a type of flavonoid which is a good estrogen balancer.

Spinach

To maximize the nutritious value of this dark green leafy food, it is best to eat it fresh and raw or very lightly cooked. Spinach is very rich in iron and potassium, and antioxidant. Eaten raw, a couple of times a week, it increases antioxidant protection and may help reduce the risk of cancer and eye degeneration in later years.

Sprouted seeds

Sprouted seeds are a storehouse of food energy and have a regenerative effect on the body. Generally eaten raw, they are packed with vitamins and minerals, and rich in enzymes and complete proteins. A seed's nutrient value increases many times over when sprouted. The vitamin E content of wheat, for instance, increases 300 percent after just four days of sprouting. Sprouts are an excellent source of the B complex vitamins and the

DIET GUIDELINES FOR VATA TYPES
(see pages 11–15)

Warm, well-cooked oily foods are the best choices. Vatas prefer sweet, salty, and sour tastes. The majority of their diet should be foods that are warming and grounding: brown rice, oats, couscous, lentils, root vegetables, all nuts and seeds, tofu, honey, plain yogurt, bananas, berries, cherries, grapes, pineapples, apricots, lemons, and limes. Vatas should favor foods that are orange, red, and yellow in color, as well as warming spices.

antioxidant vitamins A, C, and E. They are one of the main foods of the Hunzas of the Western Himalayas, who are renowned for their longevity and vitality. Their rich enzyme concentration stimulates a heightened enzyme activity in the metabolism, leading to the regeneration of many of the body's processes, particularly those in the digestive and circulatory systems (For more detail on how to sprout your own seeds, see page 82).

Sunflower seed

Rich in B vitamins and polyunsaturated fats, protein and minerals, sunflower seeds are a concentrated nourishing food that provides energy and helps keep in check irritability, fatigue, and depression when eaten regularly.

Sweet potato

This delicious low-fat food is not related to the ordinary potato and possesses a much higher content of vitamins, minerals, and antioxidants. It has a particularly high level of vitamin E, which can help lower the risk of many degenerative conditions, and it is also a good source of iron and potassium.

Thyme

This herb has many medicinal uses because it is astringent, antimicrobial, and expectorant. It can be used for digestive and respiratory infections, helping to ease the symptoms of asthma, bronchitis, and whooping cough; as a gargle it soothes irritable coughs and sore throats (see also page 108).

Tomato

People all over the world, but especially in the Mediterranean countries, enjoy this juicy, sumptuous fruit regularly in their diet. In addition to being the vegetable most commonly eaten raw, it is used in countless cooked dishes and made into a wealth of different sauces, especially for pasta and other vegetables.

Long regarded as imbued with the power to enhance your love life, tomatoes are filled with nutrients, including the minerals iron and potassium and the antioxidant vitamins C and E, as well as beta-carotene. Lycopene, the main form of carotenes found in tomatoes (and the reason for their vivid red color), works in a unique way with vitamin C to make it an even more powerfully protectant antioxidant.

People who eat large quantities of tomatoes are known to be less likely to suffer from heart disease and cancer, particularly of the prostate, lung, and stomach. Worldwide studies recently carried out on women who consume high levels of tomatoes and tomato products showed that they are also less likely to suffer from breast, cervical, and ovarian cancers.

The quantity of lycopene in a tomato depends more on the fruit's degree of ripeness than on type of tomato, and does not seem to be much affected by cooking, which means that sauces, soups, purees, concentrates, and even ketchup are as valuable in this respect as fresh tomatoes. Of course, some of these products contain high percentages of salt and sugar, so be

careful of this. Children usually love tomato ketchup on everything, so do let them eat this product. Try buying an organic brand without additives.

Recent studies also suggest that lycopene might slow down the onset of age-related macular degeneration (AMD), perhaps the most common cause of poor vision and blindness in old age.

Turmeric

Turmeric contains liver-protectant compounds. Herbalists use extracts to treat conditions such as hepatitis, cirrhosis, and jaundice. It is antiseptic, calms the digestive system, and . stimulates the gallbladder to release bile, improving the digestion of fats. Adding turmeric to beans can help reduce flatulence and bloating. Curcumin, an active component, is thought to have anti-inflammatory and antitumor effects. A University of Miami School of Medicine study suggests that curcumin causes breast cancer cells to self-destruct.

Watercress

This is an excellent, nutritious source of vitamins A and C, with some good amounts of B vitamins, together with iodine, calcium, iron, potassium, and zinc. This reputed illness preventative helps treat and prevent anemia, all kinds of infections, catarrh, eczema, and countless other more serious degenerative diseases. Rich in antioxidants, especially when eaten raw, this leaf is purported to offer some protection against various cancers, particularly of the lungs and intestines.

superfood recipes

Stuffed flounder Italian-style *serves 2*

2 fresh, skinless flounder fillets

1 tablespoon melted butter

2 tablespoons lemon juice

a few sprigs of parsley, to garnish

lemon wedges, to serve

for the stuffing:

about 1½ ounce fresh breadcrumbs

1½ ounce Parmesan cheese, grated

1 tablespoon chopped parsley

1 teaspoon chopped basil

½ small beaten egg

Preheat the oven to 350°F. Make the stuffing by mixing the breadcrumbs, Parmesan cheese, parsley, and basil with the egg in a small bowl.

Halve each flounder fillet lengthwise. Spread the stuffing evenly over each fillet. Roll up each fillet, starting from one end, and secure with wooden skewers.

Place the fillets on a foil-covered, buttered broiling pan. Mix together the butter and lemon juice and pour over the fillets.

Bake for 20 to 30 minutes until the fish is cooked and flakes easily when tested with a fork. Carefully remove the fillets from the broiling pan and serve immediately, garnished with the parsley sprigs and lemon wedges.

Rainbow vegetables *serves 2*

You can substitute bell peppers, broccoli, or cauliflower florets for any of the vegetables listed below.

6–8 cherry tomatoes, cut in half

2 celery sticks, sliced at an angle

2 inch cucumber, thickly sliced

6–8 baby carrots

a few sprigs of flat-leaf parsley

for the avocado dressing:

½ large avocado, peeled and pitted

½ small garlic clove, crushed

juice of ½ lemon

2 tablespoons low-fat plain yogurt

sea salt and freshly ground
        black pepper

Make the dressing: place all the ingredients in a blender with 2 tablespoons of water and process until smooth. Add a little more water if the mixture is too thick. Arrange the vegetables in a colorful pattern on two serving plates. Spoon over the dressing and decorate with the sprigs of parsley. Serve immediately.

Teriyaki salmon with tossed steam-fried vegetable noodles *serves 2*

2 fresh salmon fillets, each about
   5½–6 ounces
2 tablespoons grated fresh ginger
2 green onions, finely chopped
2 tablespoons teriyaki or soy sauce
2 tablespoons white wine
parsley, chervil, or dill, to garnish

for the noodles:
2 celery sticks
1 small red bell pepper, deseeded
16–20 snow peas
6–8 green onions
1 teaspoon extra-virgin olive oil
3½–5½ ounces Asian noodles

Prepare the noodles: bring a large pan of water to a boil. Cut the vegetables into thin sticks. Steam-fry in the oil and a little water for about 3 minutes until cooked to taste. Meanwhile, add the noodles to the boiling water and cook for about 3 minutes, or as directed on the pack. Drain the noodles and add to the vegetables.

Place the salmon fillets, skin-side down, on two serving plates and spread with the ginger. Sprinkle over the green onions, teriyaki or soy sauce, and wine. Fill two large saucepans with water and bring to a boil. Reduce the heat and place a plate on each pan. Cover the fish with another plate and steam for 7 minutes. Carefully turn the salmon over and steam for 5 to 7 minutes more, depending on their thickness, until cooked; try to avoid overcooking. Drain the juice into the noodles. Pile the noodles onto two serving plates and arrange the salmon on top. Garnish with herbs and serve.

Date and orange tart *serves 2*

3 ounces dried dates, pitted and chopped
2 ounces ground almonds
1 tablespoon honey
4 tablespoons plain yogurt
2 oranges, peeled and with zest removed and sliced separately

If possible, chop the dates even more in a food processor. Mix in the almonds and honey and press the mixture into the bottom of a 6-inch shallow tart pan. Place in the refrigerator and chill for at least an hour, or until required.

Remove the tart from the pan. Mix the yogurt with the grated zest of ½ an orange and spread over the base. Arrange the orange slices on the top and serve.

Recipes from *The Optimum Nutrition Cookbook*, Patrick Holford and Judy Ridgway.

the Mediterranean diet

The benefits of a diet similar in content to that eaten by the people of the Mediterranean region has been proven to be much lower in cholesterol than the average American diet. The Mediterranean diet is a rich blend of colorful and enticing foods, with a very high fruit and fresh, raw vegetable content. It is also high in oily fish, known to provide the essential fatty acids and omega-3 and -6 oils, as well as in olive oil. In Italy, for example, the benefits of olive oil are widely acknowledged by doctors and the oil is revered as virtually an elixir of life.

Today foods produced in the area, and enjoyed by most people all over the world, include complex carbohydrates, such as pasta, legumes, and rice. The region is abundant in vegetables, particularly those that are known to have protective properties, such as dark green leafy vegetables like broccoli. Yellow, orange, and other brightly colored vegetables, such as peppers of all kinds, carrots, pumpkins, salads, and many of the orange-colored fruits, such as melons, apricots, peaches, nectarines, and oranges, all help boost the immune system and fight off infections.

Dairy products are kept to a minimum in the Mediterranean diet. Cooking is achieved primarily with olive oil, which has many health-giving properties (see page 52). Protein is eaten in small amounts and is mainly in the form of oily fish, such as mullet, mackerel, tuna, sardines, and salmon, which contain essential and valuable quantities of omega-3 oils. Those who live in the region receive their fiber quotient from complex carbohydrates, like pasta and rice, which are known to lower blood cholesterol and reduce the risk of some cancers.

The Mediterranean diet also includes plenty of garlic, which contains an active ingredient, allicin, now proved highly effective in reducing blood pressure and preventing blood clots. It is also antibiotic, antiviral, and antifungal, in addition to being a general tonic for the body when eaten regularly in small amounts, preferably raw or lightly cooked, or in a salad dressing (for more on garlic, see page 50).

FOODS IN THE MEDITERRANEAN DIET WITH PROTECTIVE PROPERTIES

Complex carbohydrates

Pasta, rice, and other grains; beans, lentils, and other legumes; fruits and vegetables; nuts and seeds.
Protective constituent: fiber and a wide range of vitamins, minerals, and phytochemicals.
Beneficial effect: lower cholesterol; may protect against heart disease and some cancers.

Fruits and vegetables

Brightly colored vegetables, such as bell peppers, carrots, and tomatoes.
Protective constituent: as above, especially antioxidants and phytochemicals.
Beneficial effect: protect against the damaging effect of free radicals (see page 26).

Dark green vegetables

Broccoli, peas, and asparagus, collard greens, spinach, watercress, and cabbage.

Protective constituent: as for complex carbohydrates, especially antioxidant vitamins C and E, and beta-carotene, which converts to antioxidant vitamin A.

Beneficial effect: combat damaging free radicals; reduce cancers of colon, breast, and lung; delay and reduce the effects of aging.

Fats

Olive oil and oily fish, such as tuna, sardines, and anchovies.

Protective constituent: essential fatty acids, omega-3 oils.

Beneficial effect: reduce harmful LDL cholesterol levels and increase good HDL cholesterol; stimulate the pancreas to reduce risk of stomach ulcers.

Garlic

Protective constituent: allicin, sulphides, antioxidants.

Beneficial effect: antiseptic/antifungal and possibly antiviral; prevents blood clots, destroys free radicals, and lowers blood pressure and blood cholesterol levels.

The variety of foods available from which to choose makes this a delicious, interesting, and exciting way to enjoy food so vibrant in color, flavor, and texture.

the Mediterranean way

The following is a week's eating plan that will stimulate your appetite and tempt you to try the Mediterranean way to health!

Every day

Breakfast   Plain yogurt with a little honey
Fresh fruit chosen from the following: apricots, cherries, grapefruit, grapes, melon, nectarines, peaches, plums, oranges, raspberries, and strawberries

Day One

Lunch   Taramasalata with pita bread
Greek salad of tomato, red onion, and feta cheese

Dinner   Seafood risotto
Plate of assorted fruit sorbets

Day Two

Lunch   Eggplant dip with a selection of crudités

Dinner   Pasta with garlic and chilies
Grilled bell pepper salad with lemon dressing

Day Three

Lunch   Grilled or broiled mackerel with fresh tomato sauce
Fresh fruit salad

Dinner   Braised lamb shanks with lemons
Mashed potatoes with olive oil and shredded basil leaves
Baked figs

Day Four

Lunch Salad niçoise with green beans, watercress, and potatoes
Small baguette

Dinner Tarragon roast chicken with grapes
Pears poached in red wine

Day Five

Lunch Baked potatoes dressed with hummus and olive oil

Dinner Spicy steamed seafood
Broccoli and cauliflower florets with pine nuts
Chilled melon balls and cherries

Day Six

Lunch Broiled tomato, mozzarella, and anchovy bruschetta

Dinner Shrimp and mushroom lasagne
Arugula salad
Fruity panettone

Day Seven

Lunch Frittata
Tomato and red onion salad

Dinner Seared lemon-marinated chicken breasts
Spinach and walnut salad
Mixed fruit compote with gingered mascarpone

DIET GUIDELINES FOR PITTA TYPES
(see pages 11–15)

Pittas favor bitter, sweet, and astringent tastes. It is good for them to start and end meals with sweet-tasting foods. They should avoid very hot or spicy foods, like chilies and peppers. Pittas do better with cooling foods, such as salads and seafood. They should favor lots of green vegetables, melons, grapes, and other fruits with a high water content, sweet fruit juices, mint, peppermint, and alfalfa teas, and plain cool water.

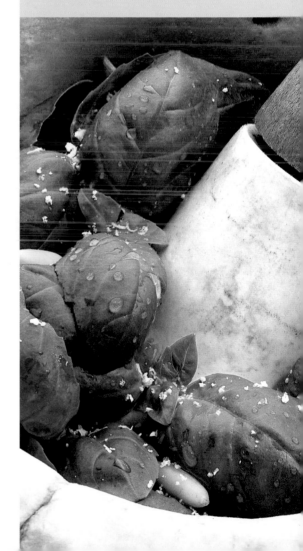

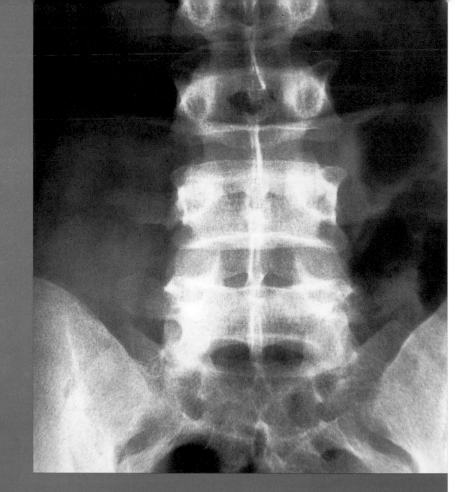

diets for your needs

Obviously what constitutes a good balanced diet varies considerably according to all kinds of factors, such as age, gender, activity level, time of year, climate, stress levels, and even your genetic make-up. In this section, we look at some of these topics in detail and try to make suggestions as to how you can adjust your eating habits to best suit your own personal needs. This is an opportunity to make your life fit your mind/body and reap untold benefits in terms of health and wellbeing.

A growing interest in genetics has researchers considering that your blood type might determine the conditions to which you may be prone. Eating foods and taking supplements that support your genetic makeup might be the key to optimum health. Dr. Peter D'Adamo with Catherine Whitney, in their book *The Eat Right Diet,* have made this link between food and disease and blood types. There has been much literature in the area, but D'Adamo amd Whitney are the first to research it in great depth. The blood group links have historical and anthropological origins. For example, originally there was only one group among the peoples of Europe—the Type O—and this is still the most common group there, whereas Type B began among the Mongols.

TYPE O

Type O's were the hunter-gatherers who lived on meat, fish, vegetables, and fruit. As this was pre-agriculture, going back over 200,000 years, farmed grains and dairy products just weren't available. Type O's cannot effectively digest these foodstuffs even today.

Health problems O's may experience: low thyroid activity, leading to fatigue and weight gain; ulcers because of high stomach acids (for digesting animal protein); allergies, arthritis, and blood-clotting problems.

Sensitivities: "new" foods; farmed foods, such as wheat and milk, can lead to arthritis and allergies.

Positive attributes: strong defenses against infection; hardy digestive system; with sufficient exercise and the right diet, they metabolize food well and stay lean and strong.

Type O Diet

Eat freely: fish, meat, vegetables, and fruit (except oranges).

Restrict intake of: oranges, dairy products, corn, and wheat.

Ideal supplements: iodine (kelp), vitamin B, vitamin K, and calcium.

Ideal exercise (energetic): aerobics, running, and martial arts.

TYPE A

Descended from the first farmers, these were the earliest vegetarians, going back a mere 10,000 years. They thrive on vegetable proteins, grains, and beans, and were the first to cultivate wheat, but should restrict their intake because their muscles may develop acidity. They are not genetically disposed toward dairy foods, since these can cause them blood sugar problems.

Health problems A's may experience: cancer, anemia, liver/gallbladder problems, diabetes (type 1), and heart disease.

Positive attributes: these are not as specific as for O's, since this group did not have as many demands made on them. They make good followers and community members.

THE GREAT MILK DEBATE

After suffering five bouts of breast cancer, geochemist Professor Jane Plant decided to treat herself by diet. Her researches, outlined in her book, *Your Life In Your Hands,* showed that incidence of breast and prostate cancer is much less in China and Japan than in the West. She put this down to our "unnatural" reliance on dairy foods and eliminated them from her diet. Her tumor shrank and she is convinced that her diet saved her life. She also eliminated or reduced levels of harmful chemical additives in her food by eating organic whole food and cutting out refined, preserved, and overcooked foods, at the same time including as many foods known to combat cancer as she could.

Type A Diet:

Eat freely: tofu, grains (except wheat), beans and other legumes (except kidney and lima beans), fruit, soy foods, and seafood.

Restrict intake of: dairy products, kidney and lima beans, wheat, and meat.

Ideal supplements: folic acid, vitamin B12, vitamin C, and vitamin E.

Ideal exercise (calming): yoga and t'ai chi.

TYPE B

Type B's evolved after A's, and originated in the Himalayan highlands, as Caucasian and Mongolian tribes mingled. Mongols then brought the Type B blood group to Europe. Many Jewish people from Eastern Europe are Type B. They are sturdy and can often resist most killer diseases, like cancer and heart disease.

Health problems B's may experience: immune disorders; multiple sclerosis; lupus; chronic fatigue syndrome, and diabetes (type 1).

Positive attributes: with correct diet they can live long and healthy lives. Type B's can eat the widest variety of foods, including dairy products, lamb, and venison.

Type B Diet:

Eat freely: dairy products, beans and other legumes (except lentils), vegetables, fruit, and meat (but not poultry).

Restrict: poultry, lentils, peanuts, sesame, buckwheat, wheat, and corn.

Ideal supplements: magnesium.

Ideal exercise (moderate): hiking, cycling, tennis, and swimming.

TYPE AB

This, the rarest of all major groups, is found in less than 5 percent of the world's population and is only 1,000 years old. It is a blend of Type A Caucasians with Type B Mongolians.

Health problems AB's may experience: certain cancers, anemia, and heart disease.

Positive attributes: they combine the best of all worlds and are resistant to allergies, arthritis, and other autoimmune diseases.

Type AB Diet:

Eat freely: seafood, dairy products, tofu, beans and other legumes (except kidney and lima beans), fruit, grains (except buckwheat), meat, and vegetables (except corn).

Restrict: kidney and lima beans, corn, seeds, red meat, and buckwheat.

Ideal supplements: vitamin C.

Ideal exercise (calming/moderate): hiking, cycling, tennis, yoga, and t'ai chi.

the circadian diet

A book published in the U.S., *The Circadian Prescription*, by Dr. Sidney MacDonald Baker and Karen Baar (published by G. P. Putnam's Sons, 2000) assures us that the smooth functioning of the body is reliant on the types of food we give it at specific times of the day. Getting your eating habits in tune with your body clock is a powerful disease deterrent.

Our body clock, or circadian rhythm, goes through many stages in a 24-hour period. We cannot affect the natural pace at which our personal body clock progresses, but we can make the processes it goes through more effective; for example, by eating the right foods at the right times of day for us. It is obvious that our bodies utilize less energy at night, when we are resting and sleeping, than they do during the day, when energy is expended to enable us to function at work and play. Why is it then that so many of us eat huge meals at the end of the day, when we don't actually *need* the energy that the food provides? What goes into those meals is also important.

Often we load up on carbohydrates in the mornings and during the day. Whether in the form of sandwiches, croissants, muffins, cereal, or even fruit juice, all are high in carbohydrates. Dinner can often be high in protein, such as chicken, fish, or red meat. In fact, it is during the "day shift" that protein is actually needed. At this time it creates the correct chemical reactions in the body that enable us to stay mentally alert and physically active. If we are low on protein during the day, we suffer from poor attention span, confusion, and low energy—even apathy. The "night shift" is the time for carbohydrates, which are essential then because they enable the body to perform crucial repair work to damaged cells and produce new ones, detoxifying our systems and ensuring we get adequate rest and healthy, beneficial sleep.

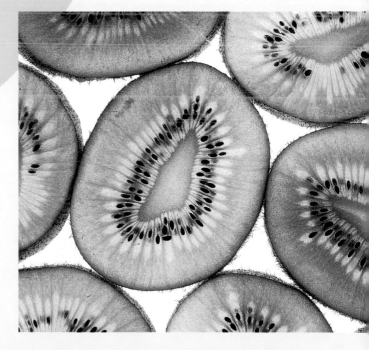

Following such a regime is a tall order for most people, whose normal habits will literally need to be turned head over heels. However, the general indication is that great health benefits can be achieved if the majority of protein is eaten in the morning and at lunchtime, and the majority of carbohydrate in the evening. It is believed that adopting this eating pattern could be instrumental in alleviating or even curing a variety of recurring health problems.

Our cultural habit is to eat too much carbohydrate, in the form of starchy and sugary food, too frequently. This is a fairly recent occurrence, historically, and we just have not evolved as quickly as our eating habits have changed. Problems with processing carbohydrates in the body, and specifically a disorder called insulin resistance or carbohydrate poisoning, are responsible for many conditions blamed on high cholesterol, such as weight gain and some cardiovascular disease. Generally too much carbohydrate causes overly high insulin levels, which can lead to insulin resistance, which in turn can contribute to heart disease, diabetes, and chronic inflammatory problems. The circadian diet addresses this common problem by reducing the number of times a day that carbohydrates are eaten to one, as would have been the common practice of our ancestors.

Conditions that are known to respond to the circadian diet include asthma, arthritis, premenstrual problems, infertility, and menopause and prostate problems, to name but a few.

CIRCADIAN MEALS

10 POWER BREAKFASTS:
Sliced fruit, cottage cheese
Herb omelet
Ham omelet
Crème fraîche over slices of melon and strawberries
Peanut butter thickly spread on a thin slice of toast
Nut protein bar
2 eggs and ham fried in olive oil
Broiled tomatoes with broiled fish
Chopped bacon and scrambled eggs
Honey and nuts in plain yogurt

10 PROTEIN LUNCHES:
Green salad, lamb and onion kabob
Salad with egg mayonnaise
Salad with clam chowder/fish soup
Green salad with cauliflower and cheese
Green vegetables with broiled pork chops and applesauce
Salad with salmon or lox
Beef stew
Salad niçoise
Chicken casserole
Chicken salad

10 CARBOHYDRATE DINNERS:
Green salad with vegetable bake
Wholewheat pasta salad with bell peppers
Vegetable burger in seeded bun with salad
Thick vegetable soup, green salad, and warm bread
Potato and mushroom bake
Dolmades (grape leaves with rice) with hummus and pita bread
Tomato macaroni, herb sauce, and green salad
Warm focaccia bread, large potato, onion and chive salad, carrot and raisin salad, and watercress salad
Vegetable casserole with wholewheat bun
Vegetable lasagne

seasonal diet

Seasonal eating

Your dietary needs, and even your lifestyle habits, naturally change with the season. The changes seem obvious when we look at them, but how often do you really think about the way you eat in the summer as opposed to the winter? Or your different sleeping patterns in winter and summer? We respond quite instinctively to the natural cycles, the seasonal patterns within which we live. For example, in winter you need more than extra layers of clothing; you also feel the need for extra inner padding; consequently, you begin to hunger for more warming soups, stews, and hot food in general. In summer, on the other hand, you hanker for more fruits, salads, and cold drinks.

Here we look at some of the simple healthy foods you can eat to help avoid the winter blues.

Warming food and drink for the winter blues

Brown Rice An excellent winter food, rice is a healthy, balanced grain, which makes a good replacement starch for potatoes or pasta.

Garlic Eating raw garlic may not be the easiest thing to do, but you do get the most benefit from its potent healing and antiseptic qualities. There are other ways you can ingest garlic: you can take garlic capsules or cook it lightly in food. In its natural state, garlic is reputed to be a food that gives you strength. What could be better? That's just the thing you need in winter. When you are feeling low, with little energy, fighting off yet another invading germ, garlic can help pick you up and fight off infection.

Ginger To reap its full warming benefit, ginger root is best ingested in the form of a tea or infusion. It helps fight colds and flu, aids digestive problems, improves a sluggish circulation, and is excellent for aches and pains, particularly those brought on by damp weather.

Oats On top of all its health-giving, cholesterol-lowering qualities, oatmeal is essentially one of the best comfort foods there is. Warming and filling, it meets the most important criteria for a winter food.

Mustard This spicy condiment is great for sustaining warmth. Good for preventing or treating muscular pain, you can eat mustard or mix mustard powder with warm water to use as a poultice for treating rheumatic or arthritic conditions.

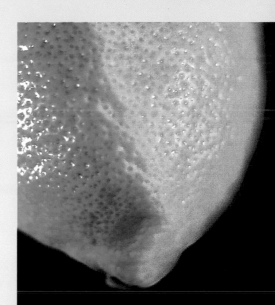

SOME SURPRISING WARMING FOODS:

APPLES This healthy fruit helps with rheumatic pain, so it can be quite useful in a winter diet. Apples also have a calming and relaxing effect on the digestive system.

LEMONS An excellent food for inner cleansing, lemons are really effective for purifying the liver and kidneys, and are also very good for treating colds, flu, and circulation problems.

ONIONS These can help prevent or ease rheumatic pain, respiratory problems, and ear disorders. This vegetable is also good for your sex drive.

SPINACH An excellent leafy vegetable to eat in plentiful amounts. Longer nights in winter mean we need brighter eyes! Spinach helps prevent nightblindness because it is so rich in the "eye" vitamin, A.

eating through the ages

We need to eat well at every stage of life. To live life to the full and prevent illness and degenerative conditions, eat a diet rich in fresh foods, fruit, salads, and vegetables throughout life. Get plenty of physical activity (according to your needs and condition) during the different stages of life, and you can be assured of continued good health into old age. Eating well and exercising regularly will also help prevent stress and provide satisfying and nourishing sleep, the third and equally important component of becoming a healthy individual.

There are general rules of thumb which traverse time and age.

- Fruit and vegetables must play a significant role in everyone's diet, making up the main component of your daily diet.
- Limiting your fat intake and opting for essential fats (see The Fat Crisis, page 40) in correct quantities will help prevent conditions associated with high-fat and wrong-fat intake.
- Protein is an integral part of everyone's diet, but not in the high proportions to which so many of us are now accustomed.
- Complex carbohydrates, found in vegetables and some seeds and grains, are essential for energy and a well-balanced diet.

There are many schools of thought regarding the order of intake, quantities, and how often to eat. "Little and often" is a good guide and philosophy to adopt. Do not overeat and strain the digestive system, especially if you are sedentary. It is a good idea to try foods that appeal to you and find the overall "diet plan" that works well for you and your lifestyle.

Parents can play an important role in their children's lives by "training"them into healthy eating habits from the beginning! So many of us are unlearning the bad habits passed onto us: those habits formed such an important part of our early years that they are often hard to shake off, even if we know they are bad for us. Children learn quickly and well, and seeing you eating nutritious food will encourage them to do the same.

As it is important for children to eat well, so it is for all of us. The middle years are perhaps the most significant in terms of our health to come in the later "golden" years. This is the time when the metabolism begins to slow down, we no longer have the unlimited energy supplies we had in our youth, and we are now realizing that we really do need to take care of ourselves at this stage to ensure good health and fitness in later life.

The following categories offer nutritional guidelines for the stages of life, which should be adjusted as you go through the different phases.

PREGNANT WOMEN

Throughout life, women have a daily requirement of about 2,000 calories. During the last three months of pregnancy, this increases to 2,300 calories per day, and while breastfeeding to 2,400 to 2,600 calories. It is important that the diet remains healthy during both pregnancy and breastfeeding to ensure good health for both mother and baby.

Tips for a healthy pregnancy for mother and baby

- Green vegetables and fruit are musts during pregnancy, to provide sufficient intake of vitamins, folic acid, iron, and fiber. Always buy the best quality available, preferably organic.
- The need for dairy products increases because of the extra calcium requirement. For those eating dairy products, try skim or low-fat milk, low-fat cheese and yogurt, preferably organic. For those on a dairy-free diet, calcium-enriched soy milk is a good alternative, as are almonds and sesame seeds.
- Eat small amounts regularly to maintain constant energy levels.
- Protein needs are high. Fish provides high amounts, together with essential fatty acids. Avocados are a useful alternative for vegetarians, vegans, or allergy sufferers. Eggs are full of protein.

Avoid

- Refined or processed foods and fast food.
- Excess salt and sugar in foods.
- Vitamin A can be harmful in very high quantities, so liver and any products that contain liver (which is very high in Vitamin A) should be avoided.
- Alcohol should be excluded.
- Smoking.

Trying to conceive?

- Try to take folic acid supplements for three months before aiming to become pregnant and during the first three months of pregnancy to prevent neural tube defects, such as spina bifida.
- Limit or exclude alcohol.

PREADOLESCENCE (UP TO 14)

Preadolescent children grow rapidly. They need plenty of starchy carbohydrates, like rice and pasta, and calcium-rich foods to create healthy bones. At this stage children need some saturated fats. The American Academy of Pediatrics recommends a 30 to 40 percent of total fats in a normal child's diet. Introduce nuts and seeds, or at least peanut butter, into the child's diet—they are an excellent source of calcium and essential fats.

Although many preadolescents would love to live on junk food alone, they can be encouraged to eat a diet full of fresh fruits and vegetables, essential to good health. Growing uses a lot of energy and you may marvel at the amount of food a child can put away in a day. They usually know instinctively just how much they need. Encourage them to use their judgement and to enjoy food! Children's instincts are usually good and they will carry them into later life. Sitting them at the table with huge plates of food to be tackled, with constant probings from parents or carers, may not be appropriate. In other cultures, for example, a small bowl is offered to each at the table and appropriate quantities of each food item taken from a large serving dish and placed in the bowl. This way what is needed and desired will be eaten, not what is forced.

The habit for overindulging on food comes, perhaps, from historical times of hunger, particularly in Western culture. Feeding children well was a status symbol, and it was important for families to show that they could. Today we have more money and choice where food is concerned. Listen to your child's needs and let them decide, while encouraging them in healthy habits and directing them as needed.

Tips for diet in childhood

- Limit candy. Try introducing a "candy day" (or days)—special days when children are allowed to eat a limited number of these items. This should help to avoid candy becoming a daily necessity.
- Satisfy their need for sugar with fresh or dried fruit. For example, children often love grapes because they are sweet and very juicy.
- Encourage children to drink plenty of water – without anything added. This is a wonderful habit to set up in their early years and will help to reduce the risk of sugar addiction that sweet, carbonated drinks can create. Even fruit juices may have added sugars.

- Salty, fatty snacks, like potato chips and french fries, should be limited to indulgent treats, not part of their daily diet.
- Helping children to understand food (get them involved in its preparation) can be fun for them and will help to increase their awareness about nutrition.
- If their schools provide meals, make yourself aware of the weekly menu. If they have to have school meals, make sure that whatever is missing gets provided for in the evening meal or at breakfast, where appropriate. If possible, give them packed lunches.

ADOLESCENCE (15–18)

Calcium still plays an important role in the diet during this period, as adolescents' bones are still growing. A healthy balance of foods, with as much variety as possible, is highly recommended. The calorie requirement at this time of life is higher than at any other time, due to the amount of energy expended just by living an adolescent life. On average, males need 2,755 calories and females 2,100 per day. They will amaze you with the quantity of food they can eat and the extent of their appetites. They need calories because they are still growing, going through puberty, studying hard, and playing hard, and going through the often troublesome process of transforming from child to young adult.

Emotions can often run high and will need sensitive and intelligent nurturing. Emotional energy can burn up a lot of calories. Make sure your adolescents continue eating well, especially when they have the blues, are preparing for tests or sport activities, and generally going through the ups and downs of puberty. They are still instinctive at this age and, as much as they use energy, they require sleep—sleeping in to noon and beyond is not unusual.

During this time it is important to encourage them to eat foods that supply energy without causing damage. Continue with the vegetable and fruit theme, making sure that adequate quantities of all food types are eaten.

Tips for diet in adolescence

- Adolescents often start experimenting with alcohol at this time. Your own habits in this area will come into play now: if you are a moderate drinker, your children will probably follow your lead to some extent. Peer pressure—and just the desire for *fun*—will potentially increase the desire for alcohol and experimentation. Talk to them about this and advise them of the safe limits and possible side-effects.
- Their hunger levels will be at an all-time high: encourage them to eat foods that include starchy carbohydrates so they get enough energy, and limit or cut out junk food.

ADULTHOOD

All the general recommendations of healthy eating apply throughout adulthood, and healthy patterns established in early adulthood will prove their worth in middle age and later life. Ideal calorie intake depends on many factors, such as metabolism and height. Throughout adult life, the average man has a consistent calorie requirement of about 2,550. A man who exercises frequently, or has a very physically active lifestyle, should increase his intake under guidance. Women, however, tend to need fewer calories from around the age of 50, although the same recommendation applies regarding exercise and physical activity. Pregnant or breastfeeding women require higher calorie levels (see page 69).

Tips for diet in adulthood

- During this period, taking care of your health will help to avert problems in later life. Exercising regularly and eating well will help you maintain good, consistent, and appropriate energy levels.
- Get your energy requirements met by eating starchy carbohydrates found in fruit, vegetables, and grains.
- Limit the amount of fat in your diet.

Establishing healthy patterns for prevention of disease

- Bowel problems, such as colon cancer, can be minimized by eating plenty of fiber-rich complex starchy carbohydrates.
- The benefits of moderate drinking (no more than two glasses of red wine per day) are now common knowledge. It is advised, of course, not to go over this amount and certainly not to binge drink, as this can be more harmful than regular drinking. The reputed benefits, to men in particular, include reduced blood cholesterol and lowered risk of heart disease.
- To encourage a healthy heart, salt levels should be restricted. Even better, don't add *any* salt to food in cooking or when raw. This will help prevent high blood pressure and other heart-related problems.
- Keep to your calorie levels between ages 40 and 50. This is the time of "middle-age spread," often caused by lack of activity and more indulgence in food. Of course, food can—and should still be—a source of pleasure and socialization. With potentially increased earnings, you can also afford to indulge yourself in luxury foods that are good for your health. It is important to continue to keep physically active to maintain flexibility and mobility. If you have not been an avid enthusiast at the gym, start now! At the very least, try walking more and further, and at a faster pace. You will enjoy the exercise and appreciate it now and definitely in the future.

THE GOLDEN YEARS (50+)

As men and women mature, their calorie requirement changes—earlier for women than for men. From the ages of 50 to 75 years, the average woman needs about 1,900 calories per day, and about 1,800 from then on. Men, on the other hand, have a consistent need for 2.500 per day up to about age 60, with a gradual decline to 2,100 per day by the age of 75.

Tips for diet in old age

- As you become less and less active, you need less energy from food. Reduce your intake, sensibly maintaining a healthy balance. Exercise to retain flexibility, mobility, and good health, and to avoid weight gain and any of the degenerative diseases which seem to be the modern-day plague in Western culture.
- Everyone should eat a cooked meal every day—but especially after retirement. Cooked food is easier to digest. Always eat a varied and well-balanced diet, rich in fruit and vegetables.

Antiaging foods

As the population continues to grow worldwide, with more people living longer than 85, and with one-fifth of the world population destined to be over 65 by the year 2020, the issue of defying age-related conditions becomes ever more relevant to us all. We want to live longer and stay healthy at the same time. Age-related disease is not inevitable.

Research consistently bears out the theory that eating right not only promotes longevity but defies the age-related diseases that we may have come to accept as almost inevitable. The theories behind why we age seem to rest in two main courts: one holding that cells are lost due to oxidative stress (when cells are attacked by free radicals) and two that aging involves "glucation," a process by which damage is caused to the body's tissues by excess sugar in the blood.

PREMATURE AGING

New research from the USA identifies the biggest reasons for premature aging as being overweight and leading a sedentary lifestyle. People are eating much larger portions of food than they were even just 20 years ago – approximately three times the amount in any serving, in fact. The electronic age means we sit much more than ever before, and hence are exercising the body less. We need a wake-up call. It is estimated around 67 per cent of Americans are overweight and the figure is rising.

ten foods that can help you live longer

1 DARK FRUITS

Red or purple fruits, black grapes, blueberries, black cherries, and blackberries contain a lot of vitamin C and flavonoids.

2 WHOLE GRAINS

They include brown rice, wholewheat bread, and oatmeal, all keeping bowels regular and efficient to prevent toxins, which have been processed by the liver and sent to the intestines, from re-entering the blood. Whole grains are also rich in vitamins E and B, which keep your nervous system healthy. Brown rice contains methionine, which forms enzymes that fight free radicals.

3 CABBAGE FAMILY

All members of the cabbage family, especially broccoli, Brussels sprouts, and greens are rich in chemicals that help the liver break down cancer-causing toxins and pollutants. They are also rich in carotenes, more agents against free radicals. The cabbage family helps prevent osteoporosis, since it is an excellent source of vitamin K, which is needed for bone formation and repair.

4 OILY FISH

The omega-3 oils found in oily fish, particularly mackerel, herrings, and halibut, may help prevent red blood cells from clumping and blocking blood vessels. Oily fish are also rich in zinc, which helps prevent prostate problems in older men.

5 SOYBEANS

Recent research has shown that soybeans contain materials that can be converted by digestion and fermentation to genistein and daidzein, which help prevent breast cancer and prostate cancer and also form a natural hormone-replacement therapy for those in the menopause. Referred to as "plant estrogens," they are, in fact, a type of flavonoid which is a good estrogen balancer. To receive all the benefits soy has to offer, eat tofu, soy yogurt, soy flour, and soy milk, but more especially fermented soy products such as miso and tempeh.

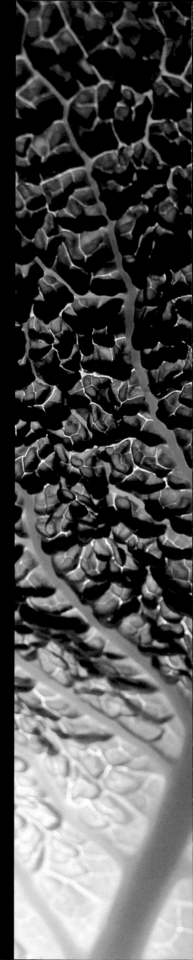

6   BRAZIL NUTS

Selenium is found in Brazil nuts, which are actually one of the very few good sources of this mineral, needed in the body to make the antioxidant enzyme called glutathione peroxidase, which helps prevent free-radical damage to your cells. Studies continue to show that people who eat selenium-rich food greatly reduce their risk of developing cancer and heart disease. Research also indicates that selenium helps the kidneys to clean toxins from the body more efficiently. Other sources include whole-grain cereals, seafood, and seaweed.

7   CELERY JUICE

Meat eating can cause overacidity, which can lead to illnesses such as osteoarthritis. Celery juice, made with an extractor or juicer, will help reduce acidity. It is credited with being one of the best treatments for the prevention of osteoarthritis. Drink one to two glasses daily, even more if it seems to help.

8   SESAME SEEDS

Although bones obviously need calcium to remain strong and healthy in later life, they also need the osteoporosis-fighting nutrients magnesium and zinc. Sesame seeds are rich in both and contain high levels of calcium. Mix them with other foods or use tahini (sesame seed paste) instead of butter.

9   ORGANIC LIVER

Liver is rich in vitamin A and zinc, which are both high in the antiaging nutrient list and help prevent hormone deficiencies. Liver also contains folic acid and other B vitamins, which could help prevent heart attacks and Alzheimer's. In addition, it contains chromium, which helps keep blood sugar levels down. Not everyone likes to eat liver; those who dislike it but who are happy to eat meat can buy desiccated liver tablets, although they are quite difficult to find in organic form. Vegetarians need to eat a varied diet and take vitamin A, or safer beta-carotene, which is converted to vitamin A (but not readily in diabetics), and mineral supplements. It is not advisable for pregnant women to eat nonorganic liver because it has a high retinol content.

10   WATER

A fluid loss of just 2 percent can result in the first signs of dehydration. Stimulants, such as tea, coffee, and alcohol, increase our need for water because they cause dehydration, increasing the potential for kidney problems. The average adult should drink between six and eight glasses of water daily to flush out toxins and maintain adequate hydration. Athletes need to drink more.

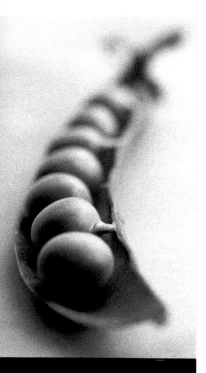

the de-stress diet

Your body/mind needs the appropriate and best-quality fuel to run at optimum performance levels. A poor diet destroys more than our physical health—our mental health and wellbeing may be totally undermined. Most of the symptoms of nutrient deficiency show up first in the brain and central nervous system. Your moods, memory, and ability to concentrate and make decisions are all affected by what you eat and drink.

You can also help control and cope with the symptoms of stress by regularly eating a varied, balanced, and nourishing diet. In fact, this can do more than de-stress; it can improve your memory and overall mental performance, enhancing your mind and improving your behavior and moods.

When you are under prolonged stress, your immune system can become depressed along with your mood. You are more prone to digestive problems because the autonomic nervous system, which governs stomach action, is stimulated by anxiety. This triggers the secretion of excess stomach acid juices, which can eat away at the stomach's coating and, over time, lead to inflammation and ulcers.

Stress also doubles your risk of catching a cold and other viral infections. It triggers all sorts of other health problems, from asthma and eczema to high blood pressure, heart disease, and even possibly cancer. You can counteract many of the unhealthy effects of excessive stress by choosing nutritious meals and snacks to calm your nerves and increase your vitality.

It is not only what you eat, but how you eat that matters when looking at your diet and how to reduce stress levels. Eating little and often is better than having large meals that may overtax an already stressed system, or large spaces between meals, when your blood sugar levels can fall dramatically. Avoid skipping meals, even if you feel you are too stressed and/or overworked to eat; take time for at least a piece of fruit and a yogurt. A nutritious diet is the best defense against the destructive effects of stress in a healthy body. Although it is generally considered good advice to avoid eating when you are very angry or rushing around in a stressed state, it is obviously not practical or healthy to diet or eat irregularly when you are under prolonged stress or pressure. During these times, it is especially important to stop what you are doing and allow yourself to relax before eating. Eating wholesome foods that are easy on the digestive system will help you cope with stressful situations while maintaining your health.

Here are some guidelines for stress-free eating habits:

- Give yourself time off to eat. Acknowledge the importance of nurturing your body and mind by allowing enough time to enjoy each meal.
- Take time to eat, and put some thought into what you eat and the environment in which you eat.
- Don't eat if you are very anxious or angry; wait for the moment to pass.
- Don't eat your food quickly or eat on the run.
- Eat breakfast. During stressful times it is important to keep your blood sugar level steady to sustain your mental as well as physical energy. Breakfast is an essential high-carbohydrate meal that will set you up for the day and keep you going for hours. If you starve yourself in the morning, it can play havoc with your blood sugar levels as the day progresses.
- Chew food slowly and well—the mouth is where digestion begins. Good chewing and saliva production help break down and process the food you eat.
- Choose fresh food, preferably home-cooked.
- Eat plenty of whole unprocessed foods, like oats, barley, rice, whole-grain breads and cereals, fresh fruit and vegetables, nuts, seeds, sprouts, dried beans, and peas.
- Eat fresh fruit and vegetables every day. Some experts recommend at least five servings a day.
- Don't eat too many high-sugar or fatty manufactured snacks. They have practically no nutritional value and can alter your moods and clog your digestive system.
- Don't add salt to your food. It can stimulate a state of high blood pressure.
- Replace unhealthy salty or sugary snacks, like potato chips, candy, cookies, and cakes, with healthy snacks, such as sunflower and pumpkin seeds or trail mixes. Mixed seeds provide concentrated nourishment, and are packed with B-complex vitamins, calcium, iron, zinc, and protein. They are ideal for countering irritability, depression, and lack of energy. This healthy snack contains important nutrients to help maintain you under pressure. Bananas are another delicious, nutritious, and filling snack. Whole and nourishing, they are packed with minerals.

The following are considered excellent for protecting you against the ravages of stress:

Apples
Apricots
Asparagus
Avocado
Bananas
Barley
Beet
Bell pepper
Broccoli
Cabbage
Carrots
Celery
Figs
Grapes
Kiwifruit
Lettuce
Oats
Oranges
Peaches
Raspberries
Spinach
Strawberries
Watercress

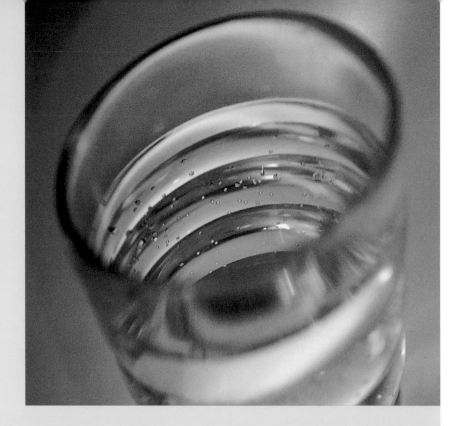

is a good diet enough?

it's not just what you eat

It's not just what you eat that matters for health, but how you eat it. Grabbing snacks at work in a standing position or on the move, or sitting in front of the TV, can all lead to a build-up of toxins in the body and malabsorption in the digestive system. You may be eating the healthiest diet possible, but your body may just not be assimilating it correctly. Poor assimilation of food could be the root of many minor and more serious illnesses from headaches, lethargy, fatigue, and weight gain to irritable bowel syndrome. Sitting down to eat a meal (even if you are alone) and making sure you chew slowly, aid correct absorption.

Good health can be attained by reducing toxicity and can be maintained by keeping the body free of impurities. Clear systems can have a profound effect on the mind, emotions, and spirit—you will lose weight, have glowing skin and more energy, and be calmer and more able to concentrate. The following simple steps will encourage you to eat well:

1   Don't eat too much at any one sitting. Eat regularly to avoid getting overly hungry and being tempted to indulge in unhealthy snacks or junk food.

2   Chew food well. Saliva contains predigestive juices—these start the breaking down of starchy food before it even reaches the stomach. Gulping food means that it fails to break up sufficiently, is harder to digest, and will not be absorbed well.

3   Drink plenty of water (not with meals, since it dilutes the digestive juices). About six to eight glasses per day is recommended. Fruit juices and herbal teas are also advised, to dilute toxins and expel them through the kidneys more easily.

4   Eat at least three times as much vegetables as starch or protein.

5   Never eat in a rush, or when angry or upset. Eat calmly.

6   Avoid processed or convenience foods at all costs.

7   If you are taking antibiotics, make sure you also take acidophilus tablets at the same time. Antibiotics kill off the benevolent stomach bacteria which aid digestion.

8   Try to listen to your body. Keeping your blood sugar level on an even keel throughout the day will ensure your energy levels are consistent. Are you very tired after eating lunch? If this is the case, you may have a plummeting blood sugar level. Many people find that eating as many as five small meals throughout the day maintains a consistent energy level without causing the familiar after-lunch siesta!

9   Breakfast is an important meal. The old adage, "breakfast like a king, lunch like a prince, dine like a pauper," is appropriate. You utilize energy gained from food throughout the day, so it makes sense to eat more at breakfast than in the evening, especially if you expect to expend little or no energy after eating. Eating breakfast will kick-start the metabolism into action; otherwise, your body will react and go into "starvation emergency mode" and start to store food rather than process it, encouraging weight gain.

10 Make food exciting with herbs and spices instead of salt and heavy sauces.

TEN GOOD REASONS TO BUY ORGANIC

1 Foods are nutritious and flavorful.
2 No chemicals in the foods.
3 Buying organic saves energy and reduces global warming.
4 Helps to restore biodiversity.
5 Ensures water quality.
6 Protects future generations.
7 Prevents soil erosion.
8 Protects farm workers' health.
9 Helps small farmers.
10 You pay real money for real food.

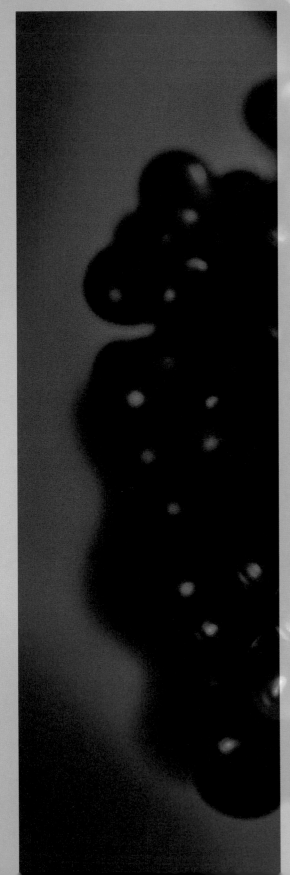

Fasting and cleansing

Fasting is one of the most natural and effective methods of stimulating and regenerating your body's own dynamic healing power. It can help you fight many minor and major ailments and has been employed as a therapeutic treatment for over 2,000 years. Some natural therapy practitioners recommend one 24-hour fast once a month, or every other month, as well as at least one longer fast every year. Only liquids, preferably pure water or freshly pressed vegetable or fruit juice, or a gentle cleansing herb tea, should be ingested in the fast.

If your diet is rich in meat and processed or packaged food, you should seriously consider a regular fasting program. Short-term fasting allows the body to concentrate on cleansing and detoxifying. It can help with obesity, high blood pressure, arthritis, rheumatism, food allergies, eczema, and even psychiatric problems like schizophrenia and depression. Short-term fasting is perfectly safe if properly undertaken, but longer-term fasting should be done under professional supervision and at the most appropriate times of the year (not high summer or deep winter).

Cooked foods and protein foods, especially meats, produce more waste matter than raw food and tend to cause a build-up of waste material in the digestive system, particularly the bowel. This can inhibit intestinal absorption of nutrients. If you regularly eat meat, you might consider a longer fast annually or even biannually.

A water fast is not for everyone. If you are suffering from any debilitating illness, then a more nourishing fast would be more appropriate. Seek professional advice.

A popular three-to-five day fast is the green grape fast. Just replace your normal three meals a day with a filling portion of grapes and only drink water. For best results (and least discomfort during the fast), this fast should be preceded and followed by a one-to-two week cleansing diet.

A cleansing diet is made up predominantly of fresh, raw foods and juices—vegetables, fruit, salads, seeds, and some cooked vegetables—cutting out all fats, meats, sugar, and starches. This annual "spring clean" is best done in summer, when we might expect to need less food to keep warm there is plenty of fresh local food, and we are more relaxed and likely to be outdoors taking in the fresh air and sun, as well as gentle exercise.

Prepare for fasting by eating organically grown vegetables, fruits, seeds, sprouts, and legumes for two or more weeks preceeding, and do the same after you fast to minimize the discomfort and maximize the healing effect. Some people experience headaches, nausea, irritability, fatigue, and aching muscles while fasting. You may feel cold and lethargic, and alternate from a state of euphoria to exhaustion. Certainly, toward the end of your fast, you will experience light-headedness. This is because the body quickly starts to release and eliminate stored toxins that have accumulated over time, which irritate muscles, tissues, and nerves.

These reactions should pass after a few hours and it is generally a good idea to rest and drink some water while symptoms persist. Be sure to rest a lot when you are fasting, taking only mild, regular exercise. Never undergo a fast during a busy or demanding period.

Some experts recommend starting a fast by taking a heaped teaspoon of Epsom salts in 1¼ cup of hot water and then drinking a hot cup of herbal tea. This helps purge the bowels and can be repeated at the start of the second day of your fast, together with a 2 ¾ cup warm-water enema at bedtime. Carbon is strongly attracted to Epsom salts (magnesium sulphate). When taken this way, the salts saturate the lining of the digestive tract and, by osmosis, attract and remove the carbonaceous wastes out of the bloodstream and into the digestive tract— eventually reaching the intestines and being eliminated by the body. If the space around the cells is clogged, then nutrients and oxygen cannot reach the cells and they starve and die. This is why the accumulations of waste matter and impurities is so detrimental.

A"mono fast," similar to the grape diet outlined on page 80, is also possible. In this fast, you eat just one food type throughout the period. You may choose to eat nothing but apples, which should be peeled, grated, and left to turn brown (once oxidized the apple loses its acidity and won't harm the stomach) before eating.

Ideally, all fruit and juices should be organic and water should be pure spring water or low in minerals, especially sodium, such as Evian. Alkaline waters, like Vichy, are the most beneficial if they are available. You can increase the effectiveness of your elimination functions during the cleansing period by taking daily doses of vitamin C and extract of globe artichoke. These supplements stimulate the liver and enhance the elimination process.

GUIDELINES FOR FASTING

- Do not fast if you are under a lot of stress.
- Do not fast if you are pregnant.
- Do not fast during a physically demanding or active patch.
- Do not fast if you are ill, unless advised to do so by your doctor and your naturopath.
- Do not fast if you are menstruating or if you are breastfeeding.
- Children should not fast, but a wholesome cleansing diet, rich in organic fruits and vegetables, is always a good replacement to all the junk food they love to eat!
- Do not do a water fast if you eat mostly flesh foods and packaged and refined foods. Try a preliminary two to three day fast, ingesting only fresh, organic fruit juices and raw vegetable juices, together with your choice of mineral water and cups of herbal tea, to which you can add lemon juice and a little honey.
- Fast only when you have the time and freedom to rest whenever you feel like it.

raw food diets

Sprouts and seeds

These comparatively unrecognized superfoods are wonderfully easy to grow and can help immeasurably on the road to optimum health and wellbeing. They can be grown in any climate and take only three to five days to reach maturity. Since they do not require either soil or sunshine, they can be grown indoors by anyone, in any environment. There is no correct growing "season," as sprouts may be grown any time of the year. Because they are a live, raw food that is ingested in its purest state and uncooked, their nutritional value is extraordinary: they compare favorably to meat and have as much vitamin C as tomatoes.

Raw sprouts have a regenerative effect on the body and are one of the essential foods in the diet of the Hunzas, Himalayan tribesmen who are renowned for their longevity and vitality. The sprouting seed is a storehouse of food energy; its rich enzyme concentration stimulates a heightened enzyme activity in the metabolism, leading to regeneration of many of the body's processes, particularly the digestive and circulatory systems.

According to nutrition expert, Dr. Francis Pottenger Jr., sprouted legumes and grains contain a complete protein, and they are easily and completely assimilated

HOW TO SPROUT SEEDS

You can buy sprouting jars and kits or you can make your own using large mason jars or unpainted flowerpots with a lid made of a stainless-steel screen or cheesecloth. Wash the seeds well and soak them overnight in a container of lukewarm, untreated water, preferably distilled or well water.

For the best nutritional value, use organically grown seed. Use two parts water to one of seed. Small seeds, like alfalfa, need to soak for only 3 to 6 hours, while the larger seeds, like chickpea and mung, may be soaked for 15 to 20 hours. Drain off the water and wash the seed in fresh water; then drain off the water again. Place the seed container in a warm, dark place, preferably 60–70°F in temperature.

While the seeds are sprouting, rinse them twice a day in lukewarm water and drain off, placing the container back in its warm, dark place. Remove the seed hulls that come away from the seeds; they will usually float to the surface for easy removal while you are rinsing the seeds.

into the body. A seed's vitamin content increases dramatically when sprouted; they are a very good source of the antioxidant vitamins, A, C, and E, plus the B vitamins. Sprouted wheat, for instance, is less mucus-forming and more easily digested than wheat prepared in any other way, plus the vitamin E content of the wheat increases 300 percent after four days of sprouting. The best seeds for sprouting are: oat, soybean, alfalfa, mung bean, aduki, and wheatgrass.

The principles of a raw food diet

Advocates of raw food diets vary from athletes to those afflicted with cancer to the overweight. All argue that raw food has put them on the right track to gain strength and stamina, and improve recovery rates, or help to cure cancer or lose excess weight. Eating 50 to 100 percent raw food helps with everything from general day-to-day aches and pains to curing long-standing and chronic conditions.Avoid meat, fish, dairy, and any cooked food.

Dr. Ann Wigmore, founder of Hippocrates Health Institute in Boston, was one of the most noted proponents of the raw food diet in the 1950s and '60s. She said, "In conventional nutrition-school curriculum there is little room for a discussion of either the value of enzymes and life forces in foods, or the merits of live (raw) versus cooked foods. Yet the difference, when translated into health terms, is the difference between being vitally healthy and alive, and just breathing." Raw food possesses live, vital energy and it is this that our bodies crave. We are used to eating "dead" foods, foods that are so refined, or cooked until all the natural goodness has been drawn out of them, that we have forgotten what food is supposed to be like and do for us.

Our body's cells must be supplied with food that also possesses energy. Of course we can survive on cooked and refined foods, but our health will continue to deteriorate, and various degenerative processes will occur, with the loss of energy and vitality. It does not need to be this way. "Eating raw foods ensures that you get optimal levels of vitamins, minerals, and fiber, easily assimilated proteins, and top-quality essential fatty acids," writes Leslie Kenton in *The Raw Energy Bible*.

She further advises, "Most of the health-boosting plant ingredients exist in perfect form in raw plants, not in cooked ones. Raw foods also contain a virtually unlimited variety of health-enhancing factors in pristine conditions. These range from the carotenoids (which enhance immune functions) to the powerfully detoxifying isothiocyanates to flavones (which inhibit the spread of cancer and guard against premature aging)."

Many professional athletes claim their strength and endurance are enormously improved by dramatically reducing the presence of cooked foods and greatly increasing the amount of raw food in their diets. Some people are put off the raw food diet because they believe they will have to survive on tasteless green leaves,

FOOD COMBINING

Early this century, Dr. William Hay, a sufferer of Bright's disease, devised food combining as a means of self-cure. In principle, food combining means not eating starches and sugars at the same time as proteins and acid fruits, in order to allow the body's own natural, curative processes to work unhindered. Because food combining also stresses eating less proteins, starches, and fats, and much more whole food, especially vegetables and fruits, it is basically a very healthy regime that helps people lose weight and return to good health.

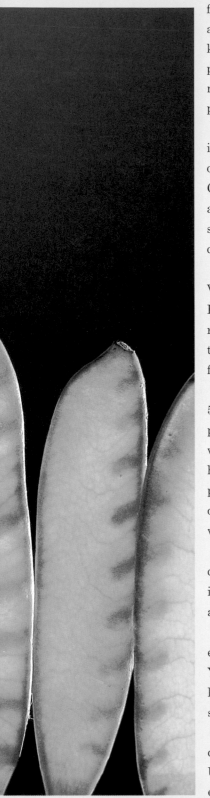

fruit, and a tomato here and there—"rabbit food." This would be unbalanced and detrimental to the body in the long run. Arming yourself with some knowledge of the components of food often helps to awaken you to the potential of raw food dieting. For example, green leafy vegetables contain as much calcium as cheese; fruits provide carbohydrates; fatty plant foods provide calories; nuts and seeds contain essential fats and protein.

Raw food diets used for fasting, for example, can be wonderfully beneficial in clearing out toxins from the body and increasing the efficiency of the body's organs. However, long-term 100 percent raw food diets, according to Catherine Reynolds of the Institute of Food Research in Norwich, England, are "... not healthy, nor balanced. You need to get food from a variety of sources and eating this way stops you doing so." Reynolds believes a raw diet could turn into an unhealthy obsession rather than a normal part of life.

Tom Billings, ex-raw fooder and editor of the website 'Beyond Vegetarianism' says, "I lived for a while on fresh foods of superior quality, but I experienced serious health problems." He goes on to say that 100 percent raw food diets seem to boost energy and make you feel good in the short term, but have a dismal record of failure long-term. He accuses many raw food gurus of making "simplistic and over-idealistic claims" about its powers.

Generally it is accepted that increasing your intake of raw food to about 50 to 70 percent of daily intake is wonderfully beneficial. It is all a matter of personal choice, and learning what suits your body best is imperative. It is widely accepted that those of us living in the colder climates of the Northern hemisphere cannot live on raw food alone. We need hot, cooked foods to provide energy and warmth in the cold winter months. In the hotter months of summer, plenty of cooling foods, such as salads and green vegetables, are a wonderful tonic for the body and for health generally.

For some, eating plenty of citrus fruit is the "be all and end all" of cleansing and an integral part of their daily diet, but for others, citrus means internal discomfort and eliminations. It really is all about what suits you best according to the climate you live in and your body type.

At the end of a long winter, you can feel run down and sluggish from eating lots of meat and heavy meals, and getting less exercise than usual. You may suffer from constipation and other bowel conditions, skin problems like rashes, eczema, or acne, or just have a dull, lifeless complexion that shows you need some nourishment and a breath of fresh air.

There are any number of persistent small symptoms like bad breath, cellulite, and foot odor that suggest we have an overload of toxins in the body. Unfortunately it is all too easy to pollute ourselves, creating a toxic inner environment that we are not even aware of until the damage manifests itself.

detox: a spring clean for the body

Many experts believe that excessive toxicity of the body creates all types of serious illnesses, from osteoarthritis (where toxins settle in the joints), to heart disease, cancer, and diabetes. To prevent such illness, you need to be in tune with your body, aware of its condition and its needs, and be committed to giving yourself a good, thorough, internal "spring clean" at least once a year. Also at that time, implement the good eating and exercise habits that will help prevent subsequent build-ups of a toxic state. A spring clean for the body is an essential part of any preventative system of health care.

Spring is a time of rebirth and renewal—what better time to put into action a detoxifying program that revitalizes and strengthens your body? Give your energy levels the boost that only a clean, toxin-free body can achieve. To restore the balance, you will need to flush out the toxic substances that have built up in the main cleansing organs of the body—the intestines, liver, kidneys, gallbladder, spleen, and skin.

The ideal way to start a detox program is to begin with a 24-hour fast, but only if you feel up to it and are not on any medication. Seek your doctor's or nutritionist's advice if you are unsure. Choose a day when it is not necessary to be very active — preferably a day when you are not physically challenged. You also need to drink lots of fluid during a fast, as dehydration must never be allowed, but drink only water or hot water and fresh lemon juice. To aid inner cleansing, a good health habit is to both begin and end the day with a drink of hot water and fresh lemon juice. This has a cleansing effect on the liver and kidneys, as well as on the rest of the digestive system.

After the first stage in your detox program, your 24-hour fast, the idea is to eat as much raw food as possible for the rest of the week. Raw fruit and vegetables are not only the easiest foods for the body to digest, and the means of getting the most nutrition from food, but they also have a marvelous cleansing effect on the body. Cooked food is more complicated for the digestive system; uncooked food enhances the metabolism and strengthens the immune system. Instead of a slow sluggish constitution, the body finds its best level for peak performance.

Eucalyptus is an aromatic herb and a folk remedy. It can be used as an antiseptic and decongestant, and it has excellent detoxifying properties. Eucalyptus stimulates the circulatory system and is diaphoretic (stimulates sweating), which aids in getting rid of toxins. Teas made from eucalyptus leaves can benefit your health by increasing blood flow to the skin, encouraging sweating and a detoxifying action.

The high fiber content of fruits and vegetables is excellent for flushing toxic residues out of the body. If you try this approach, you will see an improvement in your overall health, with many minor annoying symptoms disappearing altogether. Whether you suffer from skin rashes, headaches, or heart disease, you owe it to yourself to build your body with the right materials.

Try to buy produce that is as fresh as you can get it and buy organic fruit and vegetables where possible, as they obviously have fewer toxins. A good farmers' market will have much fresher fruits and vegetables than large supermarket chains. The fresher the food, the higher the nutritional value. Fresh herbs are also full of healthful properties, so use them liberally. The ideal, of course, is to grow your own herbs and vegetables, but this is not possible for many of us.

Today we are lucky to have a wide range of ingredients from all over the world at our disposal; however, the mainstay of your diet should be fresh food from close to home and in season—at least, this is the purist's view. Do remember, though, that rules are made to be broken. For example, exotic tropical fruits such as papaya and mango contain enzymes that have an excellent effect on the digestive system.

When you prepare your vegetables, keep in mind that many vitamins and minerals are destroyed by the heat in cooking. With boiling, the nutrients are leached out into the water and poured away down the sink. Instead, whenever possible, gently steam or stir-fry vegetables for just a few minutes, until they are crisp-tender, to preserve their nutritious goodness. Also aim to eat a good variety of fruits, salad, and other vegetables every day.

detox action plan

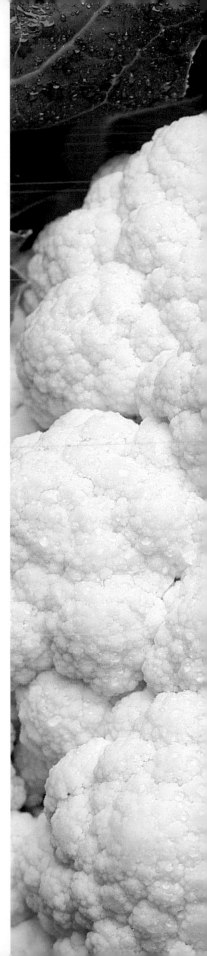

- Begin your detox at the weekend or during a time when you don't have too much going on.
- Walk for at least 15 minutes every day.
- Drink two quarts of water a day—purified, distilled, filtered, or bottled. You can also drink herbal teas.
- Have at least ½ pint of fruit or vegetable juice—either carrot and apple juice (you can buy these two separately and combine with one-third water) with grated ginger, or fresh watermelon juice—every day. The flesh of the watermelon is high in beta-carotene and vitamin C. The seeds are high in vitamin E, as well as in the antioxidant minerals zinc and selenium. You can make a great antioxidant cocktail by blending fresh fruit and seeds in a blender into a great-tasting drink.
- **Eat in abundance:** Fruit—the most beneficial fruits with the highest detox potential include fresh apricots, all berries, cantaloupe, citrus fruits, kiwifruits, papayas, peaches, mangoes, melons, and red grapes.
  Vegetables—especially good are artichokes, bell peppers, beets, Brussels sprouts, broccoli, red cabbage, carrots, cauliflower, cucumber, kale, pumpkin, spinach, sweet potato, tomatoes, watercress, and beansprouts.
- **Eat in moderation:** Grains—choose brown rice, corn, millet, and quinoa, but not more than twice a day.
  Fish—choose from salmon, mackerel, sardines, bluefish, and tuna, but not more than once a day.
  Oils—use extra-virgin olive oil for cooking and instead of butter, and choose cold-pressed canola, sesame, and other seed oils for dressings.
  Nuts and seeds—a handful of raw, unsalted nuts and seeds a day should be included. Choose from almonds, Brazil nuts, hazelnuts, pecans, pumpkin seeds, sunflower seeds, sesame seeds, and flaxseeds.
- **Avoid:** All wheat products, all meat and dairy produce (including eggs), salt and any food containing it, hydrogenated (trans) fats (most margarines), artificial sweeteners, food additives and preservatives, fried foods, spices, and dried fruit. Limit potatoes to one portion every other day and bananas to one every other day.
- Don't be surprised if you feel worse for a couple of days before you start to feel better.
- Take a double dose daily of quality multivitamin/mineral supplements, plus two 1,000 mg vitamin C capsules and antioxidant complex.

supplements

& herbs

Although healthy eating is essential to our wellbeing, there are often times when the food we eat is just not enough and we have to boost our intake of nutrients from other sources. We should be able to get all we need from a balanced diet, rich in whole grains, fruits, and vegetables, but many leading nutritionists believe that, since modern life is so demanding and stressful and our food and environment so polluted, nutritional supplementation is an essential part of healthy living. In many vitamins, herbs, and natural tonics, we have an amazing treasury of totally natural preventative medicines that we can use to fend off everything from colds and flu to heart disease and cancer, as well as help us boost our immune system, deal with stress, and generally improve our frame of mind.

In this section, we take a detailed look at each of the vitamins and minerals, in addition to the more important herbal infusions, Chinese herbs, and the many other natural remedies available, both those that have been around for centuries and some more recent discoveries.

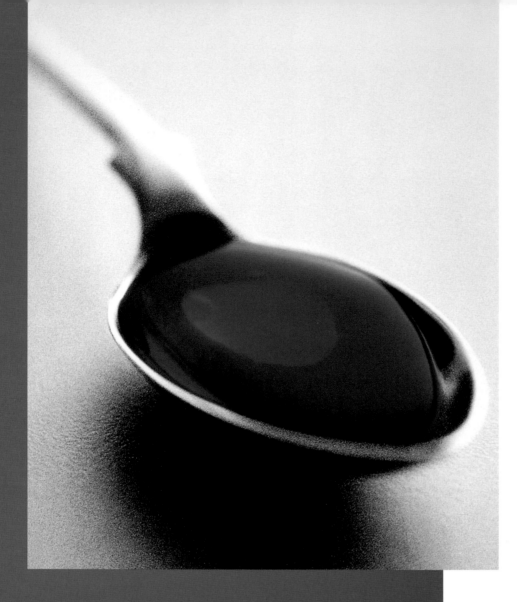

vitamins

supplements

What role do vitamins and minerals play in our lives? How and why are they so important that our total wellbeing is dependent on a sufficient daily intake of these nutrients? How do we achieve a way of eating that makes sure our intake of vitamins and minerals meets the Recommended Dietary Allowance (RDA)?

In order to prevent nutritional deficiency diseases, like scurvy, and set health standards, the Food and Nutrition Board of the National Research Council established RDAs in the 1940s. Since then they have become the authoritative standard on healthy nutrient levels. To include recent research and widen the scope of nutrition's affect on disease, new guidelines, Dietary References Intakes (DRI), have been established. The Food and Drug Administration has developed another set of recommendations called Reference Daily Intakes (RDIs). The World Health Organization (WHO) sets Recommended Dietary Intakes, although these tend to be lower than RDAs. All these guidelines are not designed to create optimum health, but simply to impart information.

It is much more difficult than we realize to eat a diet that meets the RDA levels. Even when we are very conscientious about eating a well-balanced diet, we can fall short of the mark. It is important to remember that the RDAs reflect an average and are not tailored to individuals. Whereas some people may be able to meet the RDA levels with their average daily diet, many others have greater needs and different physiques, genetic makeup, and lifestyle, which place more demands on nutrition.

The RDA guidelines are also intended as advice for healthy people, and not for those who are ill or are athletes, who may need additional supplementation. Because the American diet is so high in saturated fats, sugar, sodium, and alcohol, there is little likelihood of attaining the full RDA standard, unless you

WHEN TO TAKE SUPPLEMENTS

The best time to take most supplements is with the first meal of the day or just after it. If you have difficulty sleeping, don't take B vitamins late at night. However, taking some minerals, particularly calcium and magnesium, in the evening can aid sleep.

SUGGESTED OPTIMAL VITAMIN ALLOWANCES COMPARED TO RDAS

	SUGGESTED OPTIMAL INTAKE	RDAS Male	Female
Vitamin A (retinol)	1500 mcg RE	1000 mcg RE	800 mcg RE
Vitamin C	100–1000 mcg	60 mg	60 mg
Vitamin E	67–500 mg alpha TE	10 mg alpha TE	8 mg alpha TE
Vitamin B1 (thiamine)	5–10 mg	1.5 mg	1.1 mg
Vitamin B2 (riboflavin)	5–10 mg	1.7 mg	1.3 mg
Vitamin B3 (niacin)	10–100 mg	16 mg	14 mg
Vitamin B6 (pyridoxine)	2–50 mg	2 mg	1.6 mg
Vitamin B12	11–100 mcg	2.4 mcg	2.4 mcg
Folic acid	400 mcg	400 mcg	400 mcg
Biotin	30–300 mcg	30 mcg	30 mcg

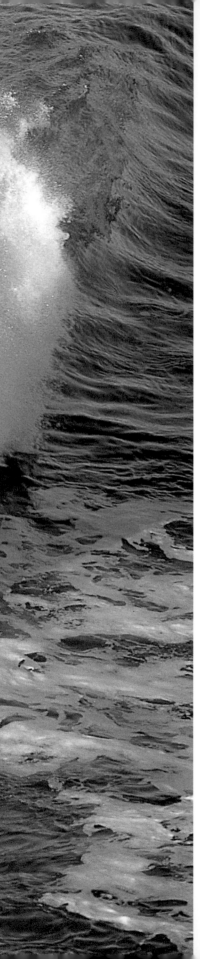

follow a nutritious and careful diet. If you drink alcohol, smoke heavily, live in the center of a polluted city, or are pregnant, premenstrual, on the pill, or menopausal, or just simply in a particularly stressful patch, your nutritional needs can easily double. The way you cook and prepare food, as well as the types of food you choose to eat and the amount, will affect your ability to get the necessary nutrition from your diet alone. Your requirements also vary according to age, with older people having greater needs than younger, especially because lack of appetite, reduced metabolism, and illness can contribute to malnutrition.

A few years ago, Dr. Emanuel Cheraskin from the University of Alabama, USA, was part of an international think tank on the subject of optimum nutrition and supplementation. Over a 15-year period, he and his researchers carried out in-depth studies of the health of 13,500 people living in six different parts of America. They found the intake of nutrients associated with optimum health was many times higher than RDA levels. The people who were the healthiest were eating a nutritionally rich diet and taking vitamin and mineral supplements that far exceeded the RDAs.

Dr. Cheraskin and his colleagues had so much evidence that they established new guidelines, called SONAs (Suggested Optimal Nutrient Allowances), to promote the idea of achieving and maintaining optimal health, rather than intake levels that suggest we will not get a deficiency disease but that not much else will be achieved either.

Recent research confirms the view that vitamins and minerals play an important role in making and keeping us healthy. However, there are two quite contradictory schools of thought concerning intake. What is the best way to make sure we meet our individual vitamin and mineral requirements? One school believes that if we eat a balanced, nutritious diet we don't need to take supplements, and in some cases too much of a good thing is bad, and even dangerous.

Synthetic vitamins and minerals are considered useless—or worse, toxic—by some nutritional therapists, who advise that natural, organic supplements are the only ones to consider. Of course, the purists believe even these are quite worthless and harmful, that fresh raw fruits and vegetables contain most of all our nutritional requirements in their most healthy, accessible state. (Remember that boiling and soaking food considerably reduces the mineral and vitamin content.)

Mother nature, of course, did not intend to nourish our bodies with manmade supplements alone, but largely with fruits and vegetables that are full of natural water, cleansing the insides at the same time. Foods with a high content of water can catalyze this "inner bath." Our bodies are made up of at least 70 percent water and, obviously, we need to replenish our supplies regularly. Water, food, and air are absolutely vital for our survival and optimum health.

In just the last few years, research has started to catalog a whole new level of "micronutrients" present in fruit and vegetables, which have a wide range of powers to combat disease. Among these phytochemicals are the organosulphides present in such high quantities in the onion and garlic family and the glucosinolates found in broccoli and other greens, which stimulate the immune system and help fight cancer and heart disease. The rich content of such chemicals has led to some produce being termed "superfoods." Most of the benefits offered by such micronutrients will not, of course, be obtained by supplementation.

The other school of thought believes that because so many people live at a very fast pace, with a lot of stress and little access to fresh fruit and vegetables, and they also perhaps drink alcohol or smoke, our nutrient needs double. Environmental pollution, sick buildings, whether we are male or female, young or old, all these factors and more influence our individual vitamin and mineral requirements.

There is a consensus of belief in one area only—the only one where all the experts agree—eating more fresh, raw, and organic (pesticide free) fruits and vegetables is a great booster to better health and a real sense of wellbeing.

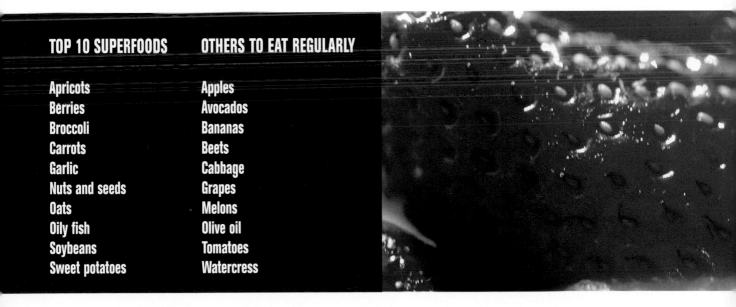

TOP 10 SUPERFOODS	OTHERS TO EAT REGULARLY
Apricots	Apples
Berries	Avocados
Broccoli	Bananas
Carrots	Beets
Garlic	Cabbage
Nuts and seeds	Grapes
Oats	Melons
Oily fish	Olive oil
Soybeans	Tomatoes
Sweet potatoes	Watercress

Vitamin A

Vitamin A is very important for good vision, skin, nails, and hair. It helps maintain healthy tissues throughout the body, including the skin and retina, and is crucial in the formation of strong teeth and bones. Because vitamin A is fat soluble, excesses are stored in the liver, where it can build to toxic levels; for this reason, you should not take too much.

The RDA guidelines use RE, retinol equivalent, units. One RE is equal to 3 ⅓ iu from animal sources, and 1 RE equals 10 iu from plant sources. Safe, daily, regular intakes should be 800 µg RE for women and 1,000 µg RE for men. Pregnant women should consult their doctor before taking supplements, and lactating women should have 1300 µg RE in the first six months of breastfeeding.

GUIDELINES FOR VATA TYPES (see pages 11–15)

Vatas have a need for all antioxidants, especially vitamin C and beta-carotene. They also benefit from nervous system regulators, like vitamins B5 and B6, and the minerals calcium and magnesium, which are all excellent for stress.

Deficiency signs: mouth ulcers, poor night vision, acne, frequent infections, flaky skin, dandruff, thrush, and diarrhea.

Food sources: organ meats, dairy products, fish oils, eggs, melons, mangoes, and vegetables—spinach, broccoli, lettuce, asparagus, squash, pumpkin, tomatoes, carrots, bell peppers, and sweet potatoes.

Beta-carotene

This is an important nutrient with antioxidant properties that inhibit the activity of "free radicals" in the body. It is also thought to help reduce the risk of cancer and heart disease, and is easily converted by the body into vitamin A. Although there is no RDA for beta-carotene, many experts recommend a daiy intake of 10 to 30 mg.

Food sources: fruit—particularly yellow- and orange-fleshed varieties—and dark green vegetables.

Vitamin B1 (Thiamine)

Vitamin B1 is crucial in the digestion and metabolism of fat and carbohydrates in food, and helps to maintain the healthy function of the nervous system. Because it is needed to burn calories, the amount you need depends on the amount of carbohydrates you eat. The RDA is 1.1 mg for women and 1.5 mg for men.

Deficiency signs: this is the vitamin that prevents beriberi. Thiamine deficiency can be highly serious and is linked to depression, sleep disturbances, chronic fatique, irritability, confusion and poor memory, eye pains, stomach pains and constipation, anemia, impaired immune system, water retention, sore muscles,

and even heart failure and lung damage. A principal cause of thiamine deficiency is alcoholism, as Vitamin B1 is destroyed by alcohol. It can also be attacked by environmental conditions.

Food sources: wheatgerm, soybeans, nuts, brown rice, whole grains, wholewheat pasta, bran, pumpernickel bread, lean pork, liver, brewer's yeast, potatoes, milk, eggs, and orange and grapefruit juice.

Vitamin B2 (Riboflavin)

One of riboflavin's most important contributions is to enzyme activity that controls chemical reactions within the body, including digestion, energy release, and the synthesis of fatty and amino acids. Riboflavin forms the essential coenzymes for converting nutrients into energy and helps cell growth. It factors into the maintenance of healthy eyes, mouth, and skin, and can be an effective treatment for migraines. The action of the adrenal glands is influenced by riboflavin levels. The RDA is 1.3 mg for women and 1.7 mg for men. Although it is not easy to overdose on riboflavin, excess will turn urine bright yellow.

Deficiency signs: may manifest in or around the mouth, in a sore tongue or cracked lips, and sometimes lesions of the skin, mouth, and genitals. Burning, itchy eyes, blurred vision, sensitivity to bright light, and even cataracts, have been associated with deficiency, as have dull or oily hair, eczema, dermatitis, and split nails.

Food sources: mostly meat, dairy products, bread and cereals, breakfast cereals, cheese, eggs, liver, kidneys, almonds, green vegetables, and avocados.

Vitamin B3 (Niacin)

Together with thiamine and riboflavin, niacin is a pivotal factor in the release of energy from carbohydrates.

Too much of this vitamin can result in serious liver damage. Niacin has been successfully used to improve blood cholesterol status by raising "good" cholesterol, HDL (see pages 40–41). However, the doses required are "megadoses" and you need to be under the supervision of a doctor or nutritionist to use the supplement this way. The RDA is 14 mg for women and 16 mg for men.

Deficiency signs: long-standing deficiency can lead to pellagra, a very serious and ultimately fatal illness, the symptoms of which are all kinds of mental conditions, from depression, anxiety, confusion, hallucination, and memory loss to dementia, along with serious dermatitis, diarrhea, and vomiting, leading eventually to emaciation. More minor deficiencies show symptoms of depression, exhaustion, a dulled memory, insomnia, headaches, bleeding or tender gums, acne, eczema, and dermatitis. Those who drink too much alcohol are commonly deficient in niacin, in addition to other vital B vitamins.

Food sources: poultry (chicken and turkey), fish (particularly salmon, tuna, and halibut), oysters, lean red meat, liver, eggs, nuts, seeds, and wholewheat bread.

Vitamin B5 (Pantothenic acid)

It is virtually impossible to be deficient in vitamin B5 because it is found in such a wide variety of foods and is essential to so many vital bodily processes. It is converted into the coenzyme A, which plays a major part in the metabolism of nutrients in food and, therefore, in the release of energy. It also affects the functioning of the adrenal glands and helps in the formation of antibodies. Large quantities are required to repair tissue damage. As a supplement, B5 is often called pantothenic acid. The RDA is 5 mg; take a 5 mg daily supplement, perhaps more if you eat lots of protein.

Deficiency signs: symptoms of fatigue, muscle tremors and weakness, apathy, poor concentration, and a propensity to get headaches, dizzy spells, and an upset digestive system. Burning feet or sore heels, nausea or vomiting, and teeth grinding may also be exhibited.

Food sources: brewer's yeast, eggs, poultry and meat (particularly liver), lobster, peanuts, wheat bran, and wheatgerm.

Vitamin B6 (Pyridoxine)

Vitamin B6 is converted into coenzymes that are crucial to a variety of metabolic processes. It aids the action of the many neurotransmitters that directly affect the brain, assists in the absorption of several minerals, helps to break down proteins and fats in food, and affects hormone production. This versatile vitamin also helps to manufacture red blood cells. Research is being done into the vitamin's value in treating asthma, cancer, and heart disease. Many women are successfully treated for premenstrual syndrome (PMS) with this or the entire B complex. Diabetes and food intolerance may respond well to pyridoxine therapy.

Exceedingly high doses of B6, above 500 mg, may result in nerve damage, so seek a doctor's advice when considering B6 therapy. The RDA is 1.6 mg for women and 2 mg for men. The general rule is not to take more than 50 mg per day.

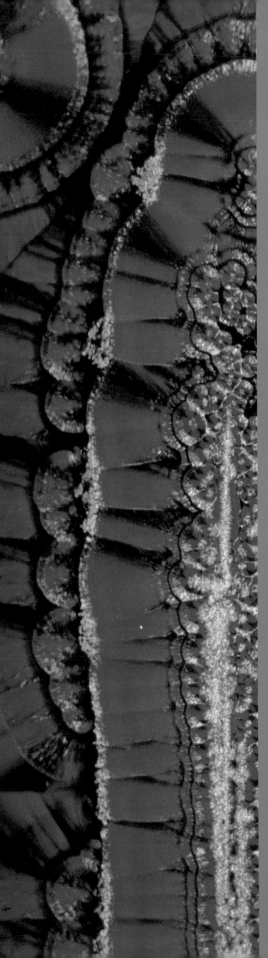

Deficiency signs: water retention, tingling hands, depression or nervousness, irritability, muscle tremors or cramps, lack of energy, and dry, flaky skin.

Food sources: eggs, nuts, cereals, grains, legumes, white meat and fish, beef, bananas, broccoli, peas, beans, cauliflower, and wheatgerm.

Vitamin B12

This vitamin plays a key role in cell production and protection, particularly red blood cells, and in maintaining a healthy nervous system. Most water-soluble vitamins are not stored in the body, but B12—also known as cobalamin because it contains cobalt—is stored in body tissues, so a deficiency may take a long time to show up. When it does, it can result in anemia. It helps to synthesize DNA, in order to metabolize fatty acids and it works with folic acid to control an amino acid, which, in excess, can create the conditions for heart disease. Because the body cannot manufacture B12, we must have it in our diet. The RDA is 2.4 mcg for both men and women.

Deficiency signs: symptoms are pernicious anemia and menstrual problems. A deficiency can be difficult to detect and neurological health may be compromised over time. Signs include poor hair condition, eczema or dermatitis, a mouth oversensitive to heat or cold, irritability, anxiety or tension, lack of energy, constipation, and sore muscles. Vegans and those who drink a lot of alcohol are at risk.

Food sources: lean red meat, especially liver and kidneys, fish and seafood, brewer's yeast, eggs, and cheese.

Folic acid

Essential for blood cell formation and cell division, this B complex vitamin helps to maintain a healthy nervous system. It is an important growth nutrient, and is thought to be particularly crucial in the preconception and early pregnancy stages to help prevent spina bifida and birth defects. It also helps the body manufacture the iron-carrying component in blood and to synthesize nucleic acid. Alcoholics benefit from a folic acid supplement (or B complex with folic acid), since they tend to have depleted levels. A daily amount of 200 μg is recommended for men and women.

Food sources: beans, wheatgerm, yeast, leafy green vegetables, like spinach, citrus fruit, watercress, cereals, wholewheat bread, and poultry.

PABA (Para-aminobenzoic acid)

PABA is a component of folic acid, rather than a vitamin in its own right. It has antioxidant and skin protection properties, and helps to produce red blood cells and to metabolize amino acids. High doses, under professional care, are used to treat some serious skin disorders, such as vitiligo, a condition of skin depigmentation, lupus, and scleroderma, in which the skin thins. Because of its ability to protect the skin, PABA is a common ingredient in sunscreen to protect against ultraviolet rays. It is best to take PABA in a B-complex supplement, rather than on its own. There is no RDA for PABA.

Food sources: wheatgerm, whole grains, bran, molasses, eggs, and liver.

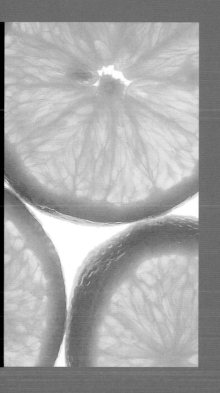

- **Aspirin increases the need for vitamin C, and may lead to deficiencies in iron, folic acid, thiamin, vitamin B12, and potassium.**
- **Antibiotics increase the need for B vitamins and beneficial bacteria.**
- **HRT and birth control pills increase the need for vitamins B6, B12, folic acid, and zinc.**

Biotin

Biotin is the last in the B complex vitamin group, and it is an essential acid for growth and general wellbeing. It aids in several bodily processes, including the metabolism of carbohydrates and formation of fat, and it helps the body use carbon dioxide. Biotin is thought to help prevent the yeast *Candida albicans* from developing into its fungal form, which then becomes much harder to treat. The RDA is 30 mcg for men and women.

Deficiency signs: can lead to anemia, muscle pain, dermatitis and skin conditions, and premature graying or hair loss, especially in babies. Extreme deficiencies are very rare, but may be manifest in depression, hallucination, anorexia, and nausea.

Food sources: egg yolk, kidney, liver, oatmeal, chicken, brewer's yeast, nuts, beans, and wheatgerm.

Vitamin C (Ascorbic acid)

This vitamin is a carbohydrate-like substance that aids various metabolic processes in the body, such as the release of hormones from the adrenal gland, the maintenance of cell structure strength, and the metabolism of several amino acids, including folic acid. Perhaps best known for its role in maintaining an efficient immune system, it is a powerful antioxidant. Many people take vitamin C supplements to protect against, and reduce the severity of, colds and flus and to fight the effects of free radicals, which attack healthy cells and are thought to be a contributing factor in many serious degenerative conditions, including heart disease and cancer. Breast cancer research shows that women with diets rich in vitamin C are least at risk.

Vitamin C helps maintain the skin because it is important in the formation of collagen (the cellular glue), and for tissue repair, growth, and healing wounds. It helps your body absorb iron, aids energy release, and even helps your breathing and heartbeat.

As this is a water-soluble vitamin and the body cannot manufacture or store it, vitamin C needs to be taken daily, preferably in food sources (see below). It is highly unstable and easily destroyed by water, heat, air, and cooking. Smokers need more vitamin C, too; just one cigarette can use up about 25 mg of the vitamin!

In addition to smoking, stress, and alcohol consumption, antibiotics also deplete the body's vitamin C. The levels of the vitamin are also considerably reduced during times of illness. Although the RDA is 60 mg daily, there is good evidence that large doses of vitamin C, such as 1,000 mg, help prevent the common cold.

Deficiency signs: include frequent colds or infections, scurvy, slow wound healing, red pimples, bleeding, inflamed gums, loose teeth, bruising and nose bleeds, general weakness, irritability, chronic fatigue, and muscle and joint ache.

Food sources: fruit, especially citrus fruits, strawberries, nectarines, mangoes, and black currants; and raw vegetables, such as bell peppers, broccoli, and greens.

Vitamin D (Calciferol)

This vitamin is converted in the body into a hormone that controls calcium and phosphorus metabolism, particularly important for the teeth and bones. Vitamin D is formed in the skin when exposed to sunlight, and it is particularly important for children, who need more of the vitamin for proper growth. The RDA is 200 iu for men and women.

Deficiency signs: hair loss, tooth decay, skeletal deformity (rickets in children), painful bones or joints, muscle cramps and weakness, and tenderness in the pelvis, spine, shoulders, and ribs.

Food sources: dairy products, eggs, fish, and fish oils (especially cod liver oil).

Vitamin E (Tocopherol)

The fat-soluble vitamin E is a powerful antioxidant and is believed to slow down the aging process in cells. It helps repair the skin and promotes the growth and formation of new blood cells. Vitamin E also works to prevent nerve and muscle degeneration, promotes healing, and combats atherosclerosis and thrombosis. Other conditions it is said to help prevent include: cancer, cataracts, circulatory problems, fibrocystic breast disease, heart disease, and Parkinson's. The RDA is 12 iu for women and 15 iu for men.

Deficiency signs: lack of sex drive, easy bruising, slow wound healing, varicose veins, loss of muscle tone, and infertility.

Food sources: sunflower seeds, peanuts and peanut butter, almonds, wheatgerm, whole-grain cereals, and leafy green vegetables.

Vitamin K

Vitamin K helps to manufacture the coagulant proteins the body needs for blood clotting. The vitamin is required for bone formation and kidney function. Digestive bacteria synthesize around half the needed amount. The RDA is 65 mcg for women and 80 mcg for men.

Deficiency signs: may manifest in nosebleeds or excessive bleeding.

Food sources: liver, some dark leafy greens, like spinach, and some dairy products.

Bioflavonoids (Vitamin P)

These are a large group of antioxidants that help the body assimilate vitamin C, strengthen capillaries, and speed up the healing of wounds, and muscle injuries. Some flavonoids are credited with strong properties against cancer and heart disease. The best types of supplement are citrus bioflavonoids and rosehip and berry extracts. There is no RDA.

Deficiency signs: bruising, frequent muscle pain or sprains, and varicose veins.

Food sources: berries and citrus fruit.

Inositol

The brain and spinal cord require this "semiessential" nutrient. It is needed for cell growth and for the formation of nerve sheaths, and to help reduce cholesterol and maintain healthy hair. Lecithin and brewer's yeast are the best sources. There is no RDA for inositol.

Food sources: eggs, fish, liver, legumes, nuts, wheatgerm, melon, and citrus fruit.

Choline

This component of lecithin helps break down fat in the liver, aids movement of fat into cells and the synthesis of cell membranes in the nervous system, and also helps protect lungs. The RDA is 425 mg for women and 550 mg for men.

Food sources: eggs, fish, lecithin, liver, nuts, legumes, whole grains, soybeans, peanuts, wheatgerm, and citrus fruit.

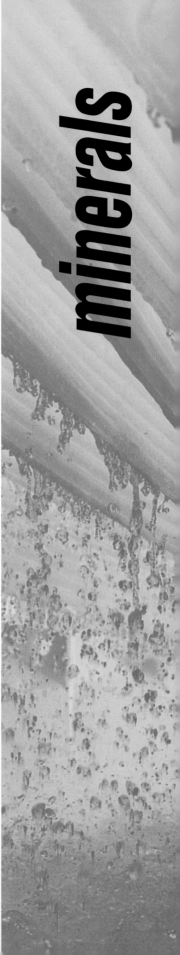

minerals

Minute but mighty, the elusive mineral plays a big part in good health. A natural substance, minerals are inorganic. Many are actually elements, the basic building blocks of all matter. The amount of minerals you need may be small, but their influence on your wellbeing is huge; only about 1 percent of your total nutritional needs is for minerals, but without them you wouldn't last long!

Minerals not only help the body perform some crucial functions, but also contribute to general wellbeing and help prevent the onset of disease. Recent research suggests the role of minerals in your continued health is crucial and often underestimated. Minerals come to us from the earth's crust, and it is the earth's erosion over time that results in minerals seeping into the sea, soil, and groundwater, which is how they are absorbed into the fruits, vegetables, and grains we eat. Your body needs minerals to efficiently absorb and utilize vitamins, enzymes, and amino acids, as well as to build healthy new cells.

Many experts believe that mineral deficiencies that cause cell breakdown, resulting in weak and vulnerable cells, may cause degenerative disease. Every day we lose millions of cells, and to stay healthy, we must replace them. Your body can only do that efficiently if it contains the right mineral balance. Minerals play a major part in every internal function and are found in every part of your body, from blood to bones to brain, and are crucial to your ability to keep well and prevent illness.

There are more than 50 minerals commonly in the body, but only 22 are considered essential. Of these, seven (calcium, chlorine as chloride, magnesium, phosphorus, potassium, sodium, and sulfur) are major minerals which are required in a substantial amount on a daily level to maintain healthy body functioning. The other 15 "trace minerals," or "trace elements," so named because you need only tiny amounts or traces of them, are also extremely important on a daily level. These are crucial for the absorption of the major minerals, as well as the vitamins, amino acids, and enzymes.

In an ideal world it should be possible to get all your mineral requirements by eating a diet rich in vegetables, fruits, grains, and meat and fish. Unfortunately, the soil that produces much of the produce we eat is undernourished and overfarmed—not as mineral-rich today as it probably was in the past. So even if you eat a totally nutritious diet, you may still need a mineral supplement because the food is from a poor or polluted soil area. Also, remember that how you prepare food affects its nutrition; boiling and soaking food considerably reduces the mineral and vitamin content. A multimineral supplement made by a reputable manufacturer should help readdress any mineral deficiencies, but ask your doctor or nutritionist for help if you feel you need some advice—especially if you have special health needs or are taking medication.

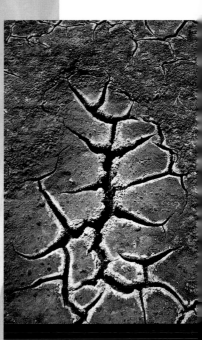

SOME SYMPTOMS OF MINERAL DEFICIENCY

- dull, dry, and lifeless hair and skin
- weak teeth, prone to cavities
- brittle and easily broken fingernails
- very pale (not pink) tongue
- slow-to-heal bruises and cuts
- chronic fatigue
- muscle cramps
- premature aging and menopause
- depressed immune system
- PMS
- painful and exhausting periods

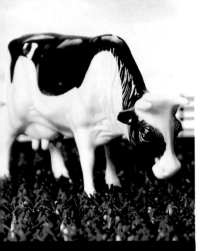

SUPPLEMENTS AGAINST OSTEOPOROSIS

Calcium and magnesium are vital in maintaining bone density. Other bone-building nutrients include vitamin D, vitamin C, vitamin K, boron, phosphorous, silicon, and zinc. Natural progesterone cream has proved four times more effective than synthetic estrogen HRT in restoring bone density.

Calcium

Calcium is both the most abundant mineral in the body and the mineral most likely to be deficient. Calcium is crucial for building strength and density in the bones and teeth—99 percent of the body's calcium is held there. The rest of the calcium supply circulates in the blood and plays a role in some important bodily processes, including blood clotting, nerve impulse transmission, and heartbeat regulation. Malabsorption of calcium resulting from a vitamin D deficiency can lead to rickets—stunted bone growth. Long-term calcium deficiency can also place adults at risk of osteoporosis (loss of bone density, making bones easy to break and fracture) or osteomalacia (the softening of bones). Although calcium-rich foods are abundant, supplements are often recommended. Calcium helps the metabolism of iron and, in combination with magnesium, aids muscle movement.

This essential mineral is also known to protect the body from the effects of pollution and the presence of damaging heavy metals, such as lead and cadmium. When combined with potassium and magnesium, it helps to lower blood pressure and cholesterol levels and protects against intestinal cancer.

Depleted calcium levels are a characteristic of several very serious conditions, such as osteoporosis. Over 28 million Americans—mainly women—suffer from osteoporosis or the low bone mass that leads to the disease. Women can lose up to 20 percent of their bone mass in the 5 to 7 years following menopause. The National Osteoporosis Foundation recommends an intake of 1,000 to 1,200 mg of calcium a day.

Deficiency signs: calcium deficiency may manifest in PMS, severe period cramps, depression, irritability, insomnia, nervousness, muscle ache or cramps, arthritis, stiff joints, high blood pressure, fluid retention, bowel sensitivity and irregularity, and, in extreme deficiency, rickets and malformed bones.

Food sources: dairy products, such as milk, cheese, and yogurt; green leafy vegetables, like broccoli, spinach, and cabbage; root vegetables; seeds, including sesame, sunflower, and pumpkin; salmon and sardines (with bones); and foods fortified with calcium, such as fruit juice, bread, and cereal.

Supplement dose: 500 mg calcium; 250 mg magnesium.

Chlorine as chloride

Chloride works with potassium to normalize water and sodium levels in the cells, and it is a factor in breathing and digestion. It also helps form healthy hair and teeth.

Deficiency signs: difficult digestion, muscle weakness, and poor hair and teeth .

Food sources: salt, kelp, olives, and yogurt. Because it is abundant in most food, there is normally no need to supplement.

Chromium

Chromium plays a crucial role in the prevention of diabetes by enhancing the effect of insulin on the metabolism of glucose and blood sugar levels. It helps growth, reduces blood cholesterol levels, and helps to prevent against high blood pressure and arteriosclerosis. It is difficult to absorb in excess because it is often lost during food processing.

Deficiency signs: excessive or cold sweats, cold hands, dizziness or irritability after six hours without food, excessive thirst, addiction to sweet food, diabetes, chronic fatigue syndrome, mood swings, and hardening of the arteries.

Food sources: liver, kidney, wheatgerm, whole grains, broccoli, brewer's yeast, mushrooms, legumes, nuts, and seafood.

Supplement dose: 100 µg a day.

Cobalt

This helps the body synthesize insulin and other enzymes essential to the process of breaking down carbohydrates and fats. It also helps protect against anemia. Cobalt occurs as part of vitamin B12 (see page 96).

Food sources: milk, liver, oysters, and clams.

Copper

Copper is important in the formation of hemoglobin, the oxygen-carrying component of blood cells, and helps the body absorb iron and vitamin C. It also affects the action of many enzymes and contributes to skin pigmentation. Too much copper can be toxic, while a copper-deficient diet may cause anemia.

Food sources: shrimp, liver, peas, legumes, mushrooms, prunes, and whole grains.

Deficiency signs: anemia and edema (too much fluid in the tissues), hardening of the arteries, cirrhosis of the liver, hepatitis, and osteoporosis.

Supplement dose: take as part of a balanced vitamin and mineral supplement, not on

its own. There is normally no need to supplement the diet with copper.

Symptoms of excess: anemia, eczema, rheumatoid arthritis, hyperactivity, manic depression, high blood pressure, and insomnia. Supplement with zinc and manganese to bring copper levels down.

Fluorine

In its natural state in food, this mineral can help strengthen your teeth, bones, and tissues. The synthetic version can be toxic and should not be taken.

Deficiency signs: tooth decay.

Food sources: seafood, egg whites, cabbage, radishes, beets, lettuce, garlic, whole wheat, and gelatin.

Iodine

This mineral burns off excess fat, aiding a balanced metabolism and efficient energy release, and stimulating growth. An iodine deficiency may impair the thyroid function, resulting in dry skin, fatigue, and weight gain.

Deficiency signs: underactive thyroid, lack of energy, unusual and excessive weight gain, and hair loss.

Food sources: seafood, kelp, iodized salt, vegetables grown in rich soil, and onions.

Supplement dose: kelp, and seek advice.

Iron

As with copper, iron is a key factor in the production of hemoglobin, the oxygen-carrying component of blood. It also helps to produce the enzymes that regulate the metabolism and it aids muscle activity. Iron is essential for the good absorption of B vitamins.

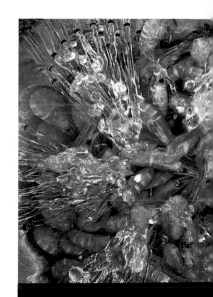

CAN YOU OVERDOSE ON MINERALS?

At exceedingly high doses all minerals are toxic to some extent. Taking only high-quality, balanced formula, multimineral supplements is advised. Excessive copper must be avoided. A strong antagonist of zinc, copper also depletes manganese. Do not take supplements containing copper unless they contain at least 10 to 15 times as much zinc, which will help prevent copper accumulation.

Iron deficiencies are common because iron is often hard to absorb and it is easily lost. Tannic acid in coffee and tea inhibits iron absorption. Iron deficiencies are usually easy to treat.

Deficiency signs: anemia and hemorrhage, pale skin, inflammations, weakness and fatigue, loss of appetite, nausea, and sensitivity to cold.

Food sources: red meat and liver, leafy green vegetables, wholewheat bread, eggs, nuts, seeds, cereals, beans, and molasses.

Supplement dose: females, puberty to menopause, can take 15 mg a day with vitamin C after or with heavy menstrual periods; all others take 8 to 10 mg a day.

Magnesium

A large proportion of magnesium in the body is associated with calcium, and each needs the other to function properly. These interdependent minerals control muscle activity—magnesium forms charged particles that stimulate nerves and muscles. It is known as the "nerve mineral" because it is so important in keeping the nervous system in balance. Magnesium plays a part in countless processes around the body, from DNA function to the release of energy, where it aids in cell nutrient breakdown. A steady balanced intake of magnesium and calcium can help prevent and treat stress, insomnia, depression, PMT and cramps, and sugar cravings. Magnesium is sometimes called the "antistress" nutrient because it has tranquilizing properties, but stress affects the body's ability to use magnesium dramatically. In times of pressure, take a magnesium supplement that also includes calcium.

Deficiency signs:

sleeping problems, anxiety and irritability, nervous energy, hyperactivity, fits and convulsions, depression, insomnia, confusion, poor memory, PMT, high blood pressure, irregular heartbeat, headaches, muscle spasms, tics, constipation, kidney stones and gallstones. Heavy and regular tea, coffee, or alcohol drinking can cause a deficiency, and being deficient is much easier than you may think.

Food sources: cereals and wholewheat bread, green vegetables (particularly dark, leafy ones like spinach), tropical fruit (also apples, figs, grapefruit, and lemons), some nuts, seeds, and legumes, seafood, and dairy products.

Supplement dose: 250 to 400 mg a day, with at least an equal amount of calcium.

Manganese

This mineral promotes normal and efficient cell functioning. Manganese aids the transmission of nerve impulses, calms the nerves, and reduces irritability

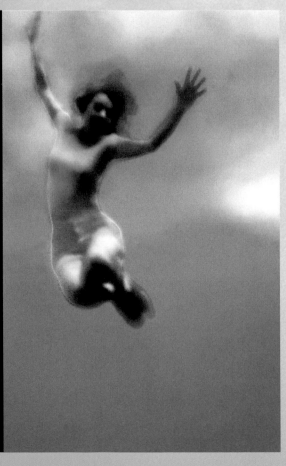

IRON DEFICIENCY IS ON THE INCREASE

A recent American survey found that 90 percent of children between 1 and 2 are getting less than the RDA of iron. They also found 50 per cent of 3–5-year-olds and 95 percent of women aged 20–45 do not get the RDA. Eating a diet rich in whole-grains and vegetables, and limiting cups of coffee and tea, should help avoid iron deficiency.

when necessary. As with many other minerals, manganese is involved in processes around the body, including the synthesis of cholesterol, the metabolism of blood sugar and fats, the release of thyroid hormones, and the formation of bone and tissue. It also helps blood clotting and can be substituted for magnesium for the release of energy. Manganese may help to reduce fatigue and poor digestion.

Food sources: leafy green vegetables, egg yolk, avocados, seeds and nuts, whole-grain cereals, some tropical fruit, and green teas.

Deficiency signs: although rare, the lack of this little-known mineral can lead to that "tired all the time" feeling and to such complaints as excessive irritability, dizziness, chronic fatigue, poor digestion, muscle twitches and convulsions, childhood growing pains, sore joint pain, poor memory, infertility, and diabetes.

Supplement dose: 2 to 4.5 mg a day, taken with B and C vitamins to redress the body's balance and build strength.

Phosphorus

Phosphorus is the second most abundant mineral in the body (after calcium, with which it works closely), and it is essential for growth, maintenance, and repair processes around the body. This crucial mineral helps to synthesize proteins, to produce energy in cells, and to transfer nerve impulses. It plays a major role in the maintenance and repair of cells and tissues. Phosphorus is the "mood mineral." It helps the formation of strong, healthy teeth and bones (where

most of the body's phosphorus is stored), and also aids heart regularity.

Research shows that adequate phosphorus intake plays a part in the prevention of stress disorders, stiffness in the joints (including arthritis), and even cancer. However, it is important to balance phosphorus and calcium intake, because excess phosphorus can reduce the performance of calcium and lead to depleted stores in the body; over time, this imbalance can create the environment for osteoporosis.

Deficiency signs: gum disease, osteoporosis, rickets, a general feeling of weakness and oversensitivity, loss of appetite, arthritis, aching joints, and stress disorders.

Food sources: dairy products (the most balanced ratio of phosphorus to calcium), eggs, tofu, soy, fish, poultry, meat, and nuts, seeds, and grains.

Supplement dose: generally, there is no need to supplement because there is an abundance in most diets. However, for those with any of the signs above, 500 mg each of phosphorus and calcium, and 225 mg magnesium, can be taken daily. Sufferers of arthritis or osteoporosis may need to double the amount, but always seek advice from a doctor or nutritionist.

Potassium

Potassium helps regulate the delicate equilibrium of the cells by maintaining the balance of water and sodium inside and outside the cells. This process is crucial for nerve and muscle efficiency, ensuring the healthy functioning of the nervous system. Potassium is the "brain mineral' because it helps send oxygen to

the brain. It also helps convert blood sugar into a form that can be stored in the liver. Because of its role in balancing the body's water levels, it also plays a vital role in eliminating waste products and reducing blood pressure.

It can be useful in treating allergies and relieving bloating due to water retention. Hypertension or fluid retention sufferers may need to supplement their potassium intake, as may those with high blood pressure or at risk of stroke. Because potassium and sodium are intricately linked in cells, maintaining a balanced intake is important—research shows that high-sodium, low-potassium diets may create the right conditions for cancer and heart disease. Processed, refined, and fast foods contribute to high salt (sodium, see page 105) intake, so extra potassium is needed to counteract this effects. Also, potassium is very easily

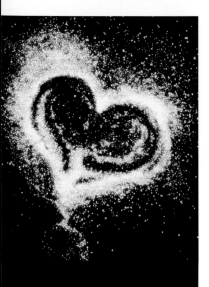

SUPPLEMENTS FOR A HEALTHY HEART

The renowned biochemist Linus Pauling found that vitamin C, together with the amino acid lycine, helped reverse cardiovascular disease. Vitamin C protects against the oxidation of the arteries. Vitamin E is important for healthy heart muscle. In Great Britain, a Cambridge University study showed a minimum of 400 iu a day reduced heart attacks in patients who already had heart disease by 77 percent!

lost in cooking and in the body's excretion processes. Some doctors may prescribe potassium supplements for patients on diuretics, since these medications promote potassium excretion.

Deficiency signs: rapid irregular heartbeat, irritability and oversensitivity, depression, fatigue and confusion, apathy, muscle weakness, "pins and needles," slow reflexes, bloating, cellulite, nausea, diarrhea, hypoglycemia, and a malfunctioning neuromuscular system. If you drink a lot of alcohol, coffee, and tea, you may lack potassium, since these neutralize this important mineral.

Food sources: bananas, potatoes, garlic, onions, leafy green vegetables, citrus fruits, legumes, nuts, dried fruit, fish, tomatoes, barley, whole grains, and dandelion and mint leaves.

Supplement dose: again, there is generally no need to supplement this mineral because it is so abundant in most diets. In fact, it is not normally included in a standard multivitamin/multimineral supplement. Those exhibiting any deficiency signs should eat more fruit and vegetables.

Selenium

This mineral is a key antioxidant that works with vitamin E to protect the cells from free radicals and improve immunity. In addition to antioxidant properties, it contributes to the efficiency of the immune system by aiding white blood cell production. Selenium also protects the skin: it guards against UV radiation to minimize sun damage and prevents premature aging, drying skin, and scalp conditions, such as dandruff.

Selenium also helps maintain good eyesight, has an anti-inflammatory effect that relieves the symptoms of rheumatoid arthritis, and is important to the functioning of the male reproductive organs. It is thought to alleviate some menopausal symptoms. Research has linked selenium deficiency with some forms of cancer.

Deficiency signs: diabetes, cataracts, premature aging, male infertility, a sluggish immune system and energy level, high blood pressure, frequent infections, dandruff, and lowered liver function.

Food sources: Brazil nuts, fish (especially tuna), eggs, garlic, onions, wheatgerm, bran, whole grains, seeds, and liver.

Supplement dose: 60 to 70 µg a day.

THE 10 MOST COMMON SOURCES OF HIDDEN SALT

Potato chips
Cookies
All packaged, processed foods
Precooked convenience meals
Breakfast cereals
Mass-produced sauces and soups
Most canned foods
Smoked fish
Yeast extracts

Sodium

Sodium, in combination with potassium, helps regulate water and pH levels in the body and aids efficient nerve and muscle function. Sodium deficiency is very unlikely because it is found in almost all foods, and only excessive perspiration can seriously deplete sodium levels. The link between sodium and the hypertension epidemic in the Western world is well documented. High sodium intake may also contribute to calcium depletion. The general recommendation is to reduce intake of salt (40 per cent of which is sodium—see box, bottom left).

Food sources: kelp, salt, meat, fish, seafood, and salted, cured, and smoked foods.

Deficiency signs: headache, dizziness, heat exhaustion, low blood pressure, rapid heartbeat/pulse, apathy, loss of appetite, nausea, indigestion and heartburn, and muscle cramps.

Sulfur

Sulfur helps keep skin, hair, and nails healthy and disease-free. It is essential for the maintenance of the "elasticity" of proteins. Sulfur is a "purifying" mineral that helps to detox the liver and fight bacteria to prevent infection. It also helps the brain to function.

Food sources: dried beans, fish, eggs, onions, and garlic.

Deficiency signs: jaundice, liver ailments, headaches, psoriasis, and acne.

Zinc

Zinc is one of the body's most important trace minerals and plays a role in more body functions than any other mineral.

It is an important component of many enzymes in the digestive and reproductive systems, and it is found in the brain, eyes, heart, lungs, spleen, skin, hair, and bones.. It is essential for the maintenance of the body tissues and the immune system, for the functioning of the reproductive system, and for good growth and development. Zinc, like iron, is easiest to absorb when ingested in animal foods, within which it is bound to proteins that aid its absorption. This "healing mineral" speeds up the healing process, and helps to reduce cholesterol levels and to synthesize insulin.

Zinc is often used to treat depression and loss of sex drive, and it is important to the health of the reproductive organs— it may prevent prostate problems.

Food sources: seafood, lean red meat, poultry, egg yolk, milk, yeast, wheatgerm, bran, pecans, seeds, maple syrup, mustard, chili, and cocoa.

Deficiency signs: poor sense of taste and/or smell, loss of appetite, pale skin, skin problems like acne, stretch marks, dandruff, arteriosclerosis, enlarged prostate, slow healing, depression, poor concentration, learning disabilities, anorexia nervosa, lack of sexual function, and infertility.

Supplement dose: 15 mg a day; seek professional advice for larger doses.

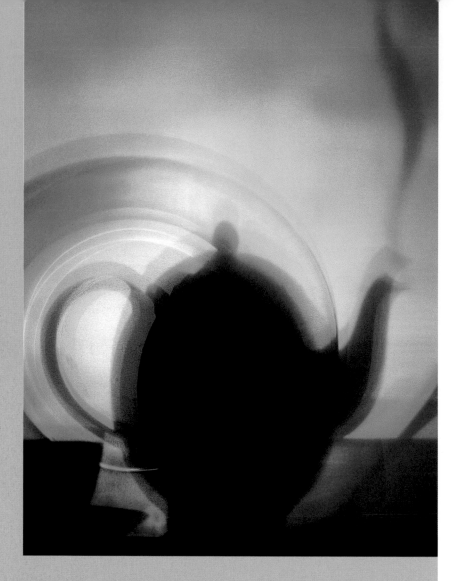

herbs

Ancient physicians and shamans used herbs to cure the sick; the recorded use of this natural form of medicine can be found as early as 2,500 BC. Today we still appreciate refreshing, healthy, and therapeutic herbal teas. Herbs can even provide the stimulating pick-up we all need from time to time, in an easy and safe form. They are also available in tinctures, extracts, powders, capsules, and tablets. You can only enhance your health if you explore the delicious nutritional and medicinal plants that are the original inspiration for most modern, orthodox synthetic drugs.

*"The Lord created medicines out of the earth
and a wise man will not abhor them."*
ECCLESIASTES

In addition to the medicinal value of herbs, administered as extracted medicines mixed by a professional herbalist (see Herbalism, page 269), there are many very different herbal teas you can drink safely on a regular basis. It is important to vary them, as they all also have medicinal properties. Herbal infusions, or tisanes, are delicious, healthy drinks which are easy to prepare. To make them, pour hot, freshly boiled water over 1 to 2 teaspoons of dried or ground herbs per cup and allow to infuse for 5 to 10 minutes. Many herbal drinks are available as tea bags and can be found in your local supermarket or health food store. Herbal infusions are usually made from the leaves, flowers, and sometimes the root of the herb; herbal medicines tend to use the seeds, stems, fruit, resin, and bark.

Herbal infusions can be taken hot or cold. If you follow the instructions, they are harmless and healthy. There are many herbs from which to choose, but the following are the more common ones in everyday use. If you want to treat any major or persistent symptoms, seek the advice of your doctor a professional herbal practitioner, who can prepare a complex combination of herbs into a remedy that is individually suited to your needs, symptoms, and body type. Professional herbalists are trained, and believing you can treat yourself herbally other than using the popular herbs is unwise—some herbs have potent effects and can interact with other medicines. The following herbs are nontoxic and beneficial when used in cooking or taken as a tea.

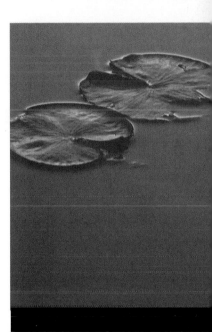

HERBS TO SOOTHE AND RELAX

Camomile
Gotu kola
Kava
Lemon balm
Peppermint
Skullcap
Valerian

Borage

This cooling herb stimulates adrenaline production, helping raise spirits, fend off depression, or cope with grief. A borage infusion made from the dried flowers or leaves is good for treating colds with accompanying fever and bad coughs. Breastfeeding mothers sometimes take borage in combination with fennel to increase their milk flow.

Camomile

A relaxing herb, camomile is also very good for the digestion, helping nausea, morning sickness, and a poor appetite,

and aiding those who are suffering from overeating. A cup of tea at night is good for insomnia and reputed to ward off nightmares. Externally, the tea can be used to lighten hair and to relieve conjunctivitis and skin inflammations.

Dandelion

This is one of nature's strongest diuretics, making it highly useful in detoxing and cleansing your system. The herb gently stimulates the digestive system, liver, and kidneys, and is beneficial for treating many conditions where there is a build-up of toxins, such as in skin impurities.

Elder

An infusion of elderflowers is reputed to be excellent for the prevention and treatment of colds and flus, along with any excessive catarrh and upper-respiratory inflammation, such as that caused by hayfever and sinus infections. The cold tea makes a good eyewash and is reputed to be effective in preventing and treating conjunctivitis. The bark of the elder, used in infusions, helps eliminate uric acid and relieve gout.

Fennel

This pungent, warming, sweet herb is known to aid digestion, to stimulate the circulation, and to act as a diuretic and an expectorant. Its essential oil quickly relieves asthma attacks. The root can be eaten in salad; use the seeds in a tea or infusion to alleviate period pains.

Lemon balm

The reputed soothing effect of this delicious herb has brought it to the forefront of the natural medicine cabinet. It makes a refreshing tea, which helps soothe muscular cramp—a good reason to use it for period pain. It helps encourage sweating, making it useful for fever or flu symptoms. It is also excellent for its calming effect on nervous stomachs and the entire digestive system. Rich in essential oils, it is also used to treat anxiety.

Marjoram

A lightly bitter herb, warming as well as astringent, sweet marjoram has the reputation of being helpful in the treatment and prevention of menstrual cramps, along with soothing indigestion, coughs, and asthma attacks. Externally, the oil can be used to ease varicose veins, rheumatism and stiff joints.

Parsley

One of the most popular herbs in cooking, parsley also has many medicinal properties. Applied directly onto a contusion, it reduces inflammation; it can also reduce an abscess. Its diuretic and detoxifying properties are well documented; parsley can be useful in the treatment of urinary infections and stones, and hypertension. It should not be ingested in large quantities during pregnancy.

Peppermint

This popular, refreshing herb is widely used to help the digestive process, particularly indigestion and gas. It can help treat nausea (especially the kind brought on during traveling) and bad breath, and is used to promote cooling when treating fever. When combined with lavender, peppermint can help to soothe migraine headaches.

Rosemary

Rosemary is used to treat and prevent a wide range of conditions, including indigestion, headaches, fatigue, cold, flu, rheumatic symptoms, and depression. This warming, pungent, and bitter herb is a very good natural antiseptic; a salve made from the essential oil is good for wounds, bruises, and eczema.

Sage

With strongly antibacterial properties, sage was traditionally used as a mouthwash, and fresh sage leaves were used to clean teeth. Sage infusions are excellent for colds and flus, sore throats, digestive problems, menopausal hot flashes, and asthma. A handful of fresh sage leaves thrown into the bathtub has a tonic effect on the body and a calming effect on the nervous system.

Thyme

Its strongly antiseptic properties make an infusion of thyme an excellent gargle for sore throats and coughs and an effective mouthwash for bad breath and gingivitis. Thyme is a popular culinary herb and can improve digestion.

Vervain (Verbena officinalis)

Mainly used for nervous exhaustion, depression, and liver and gallbladder problems, vervain has sedative, nervine, and antispasmodic properties. It should not be used in pregnancy.

Yarrow

Astringent, cool, and bittersweet, this herb is good for treating PMT and menstrual symptoms. Yarrow is also good for the prevention and treatment of catarrh and colds, and is even reputed to help alleviate high blood pressure.

SPICES TO SPEED UP HEALING

It's no secret spices are healthy, giving us more antioxidants and all kinds of nutrients. Experts at Dartmouth Medical School in Rhode Island, USA, recommend including more spices in our diet. These are the top four according to USDA

Ground cloves
Ground cinnamon
Dried oregano
Tumeric

Chinese herbal medicine is part of one of the oldest medicinal systems in the world, traditional Chinese medicine or TCM. One of the early holistic systems, TCM has the aim of restoring and maintaining equilibrium and harmony within the whole person. Chinese doctors believe that, like everything in the universe, humans, too, are governed by the laws of yin and yang—the "Great Principle." There are two complementary forms of *chi* or energy: "*yin*" reflects the feminine, receptive, dark, cool, soft, and moist; and "*yang*" the masculine, creative, bright, warm, hard, and dry. We need a healthy balance of *yin* and *yang* energy to maintain general good health and wellbeing.

Traditional Chinese medicine practitioners believe that clearing and stimulating the channels of energy within the body helps restore balance, thereby restoring health. They consider illness to be the result of the loss of balance between *yin* and *yang*, or that the circulation of *chi* through the body is blocked.

Chinese herbs have been used for their medicinal value and tonic properties for many millennia. Mixtures of herbs are created that can cleanse, cool, or warm the blood, strengthen the immune system, and balance and regulate all the systems of the body to enhance mental—as well as physical—wellbeing. In their herbal formulas, the Chinese include the roots, seeds, stems, twigs, and sap, along with the berries, flowers, and leaves.

Please note that traditional Chinese medicine experts take the ingestion of herbs and tonics very seriously and advise you to seek the advice of a qualified practitioner who can create a formula for your unique needs and requirements. Even ginseng and ginger may be too much of a stimulant for certain types of people and could be dangerous for those with high blood pressure.

Astragalus (Huang Chi)

This traditional Chinese herb is derived from the root of the perennial *Astragalus membranaceus*. In China astragalus is used in traditional medicine to strengthen the *wei chi,* or "defensive energy" of the immune system. The herb is antibacterial, and it is used for "outer energy," in much the same way that ginseng is used for "inner energy."

Combined with ginseng, it is helpful for young adults in order to stimulate energy production and endurance. Its warming energy also helps hypoglycemia and fights off infections and colds.

Among the most popular herbs in the Orient, astragalus is a tonic, used specifically for toning the lungs and spleen. One of the most powerful blood tonics in the Chinese pharmacopoeia consists of an infusion of Dang Gui (see page 110) and Huang Chi; although the quantity may vary, the proportion is always five to six times the amount of Huang Chi for Dang Gui. This simple formula is recommended for those suffering from anemia,or recovering from a long illness or cancer treatment.

Scientists have isolated a number of active ingredients contained in astragalus, including bioflavonoids, choline, and a polysaccharide called astragalan B. Animal studies have shown that astragalan B is effective at controlling bacterial infections, stimulating the immune system, and protecting against a number of toxins. A great immune-enhancer, astragalus boosts production of white and red blood cells, interferon, immunoglobulins, and the adrenal cortex function. The herb is being investigated for use with cancer treatment and AIDS.

Chinese angelica root (Dang Gui or Dong Quai)

Growing profusely throughout Asia and called the "female ginseng," Dang Gui is an all-purpose herb for a wide range of female gynecological complaints. For centuries, Chinese women have used this herb to regulate the menstrual cycle and subdue painful menstrual cramps caused by uterine contractions. Modern herbalists use Dang Gui to eliminate the discomfort of premenstrual syndrome, PMS, and to help women resume normal menstruation after going off the pill. Rich in vitamins and minerals, including A, B complex, and E, it also helps prevent anemia. Dang Gui has been used to treat insomnia and high blood pressure for both sexes. Both men and women use it as a blood tonic.

Researchers have identified in Dang Gui several coumarin derivatives that are known to act as antispasmodics and vasodilators. Use with caution: don't take Dang Gui during pregnancy or menstruation (when you typically experience a heavy blood flow).

Chinese liquorice root (Gan Cao)

This remarkable root can detoxify the ill-effects of drugs, balance blood sugar levels, and relieve digestive pain and spasms. Liquorice also stimulates the action of other herbs.

Codonopsis pilosula (Dang Shen)

As famous as ginseng in China, this herb helps strengthen the lungs, spleen, and stomach. A twining and climbing herbaceous perennial that is native to China, codonopsis is sometimes known as "poor man's ginseng" or "bastard ginseng" because it builds vital force and tones the blood. It is also nutritious, sweet, and warming, containing high levels of immune-enhancing polysaccharides. Dang Shen roots are used for energy deficiency, strengthening the immune system, lowering blood pressure, helping lack of appetite, and invigorating the spleen.

Cordyceps fungus (Dong Chong Xia Cao)

Also known as "caterpillar fungus" or "deer fungus," this is a very effective herb for treating circulatory, respiratory, immune, and sexual dysfunction. The herb is popular as a general health tonic because of its capability to improve energy, stamina, appetite, and endurance, and to stabilize sleeping patterns. In traditional Chinese medicine, cordyceps is used for the kidney and lung meridians.

Female Chinese athletes, who used cordyceps as part of their training program, surprised everyone when they broke the 10,000-meter World Track Record in 1993.

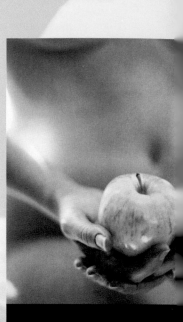

CHINESE HERBS FOR FEMALE REPRODUCTIVE HEALTH

Astragalus, Chinese angelica root, lycium, and codonopsis support female reproduction. (Always remember to consult a qualified practitioner of traditional Chinese medicine.)

Western herbal formula for the menopause: 1 part each black cohosh, goldenseal, life root (*Senecio aureus*), oats, St. John's wort; 2 parts each chasteberry and wild Mexican yam.

Foti root (He Shu Wu)

He Shu Wu is said to possess almost magical rejuvenating properties and is especially popular with the elderly, who believe it can help maintain hair color, preserve youthfulness, and restore fertility.

The root replenishes vital essence and nourishes the blood; it is a powerful liver and kidney tonic, clearing away toxins. It is used to relieve constipation, usually with Dang Gui (see page 110) and hemp seed (see page 121). He Shu Wu is also employed as a remedy for insomnia, diabetes, and skin problems.

He Shu Wu contains a number of glycosides that account for the herb's use as a remedy for stomach disorders. In Chinese *materia medica*, it has been used effectively for neurasthenia, insomnia, excessive sweating, dizziness, elevated serum cholesterol, coronary disease, weakness, pain, backache, and tuberculous adenopathy.

Ginger (Sheng Jiang)

Because of its ability to help prevent blood clotting, ginger offers substantial protection from stroke and heart attack. For centuries, traditional Chinese medicine has valued ginger as a digestive tonic. It is still commonly used for indigestion today, because ginger absorbs and neutralizes toxins in the stomach. As the ginger eases the transport of various substances through the digestive tract, it decreases irritation to the intestinal walls. Ginger also improves the production and secretion of bile from the gallbladder. Bile aids in the digestion of fats, which helps to lower cholesterol levels.

In traditional Chinese medicine, ginger is used to reduce the toxicity of some herbs. Ginger relieves motion sickness, morning sickness, and nausea. Ginger is also used for: colds and coughs, colon and stomach spasms, constipation, indigestion, gas or flatulence, headaches, and sinus congestion.

Ginkgo biloba (Bai Guo, Xin Xing)

The ginkgo is one of the oldest living tree species, dating back over 300 million years, and individual trees can live for over 1,000 years. In China, extracts of the fruit and leaves of the ginkgo tree have been used for over 5,000 years to treat lung ailments, such as asthma and bronchitis, and as a remedy for cardiovascular diseases.

Recently, Western researchers have been studying Ginkgo biloba as a treatment for senility, hardening of the arteries, and oxygen deprivation. Its ability to improve blood flow has been demonstrated in numerous studies with the elderly, leading researchers to study ginkgo as a treatment for atherosclerotic peripheral vascular disease. More than 34 human studies on ginkgo have been published since 1975, showing, among other things, that it can increase the body's production of the molecule adenosine triphosphate, commonly known as ATP. This activity has been shown to boost the brain's energy metabolism of glucose and increase electrical activity.

Ginkgo flavonoids act specifically to dilate the smallest segment of the circulatory system, the microcapillaries, which have a widespread effect on the organs, especially the brain. Researchers have also reported that ginkgo extracts effectively increase blood circulation and increase oxygen levels in brain tissues. Ginkgo is a powerful antioxidant that prevents platelet aggregation inside arterial walls, keeping them flexible and decreasing arteriosclerotic plaque.

Ginseng (Ren Shen)

The ancient Chinese believed that the root of the ginseng plant was the crystallization of the essence of the earth in the shape of a man and that ginseng had rejuvenating, recuperative, revitalizing, and curative action. The first Chinese *materia medica*, written by Shen-nong, stated that ginseng was used for its tonic and tranquilizing effects; ginseng increased alertness, brilliance, and concentration, improved memory, and prolonged use brought longevity.

Ginseng's other claimed benefits include: increased physical stamina, enhanced blood flow, slowing of cell degeneration, reduced stress, calming of nerves, increased metabolism, and strengthening of the immune system.

There are two major ginseng species: Asian ginseng, often called Korean ginseng, (*Panax ginseng*, Ren Shen) and American ginseng (*Panax quinquefolium*, Xi Yang Shen). The name "panax" is derived from the Greek, meaning "cure-all." Ginseng, meaning "wonder of the world," has been known and respected by the Chinese for centuries. The action of ginseng is neither local nor specific; it increases the

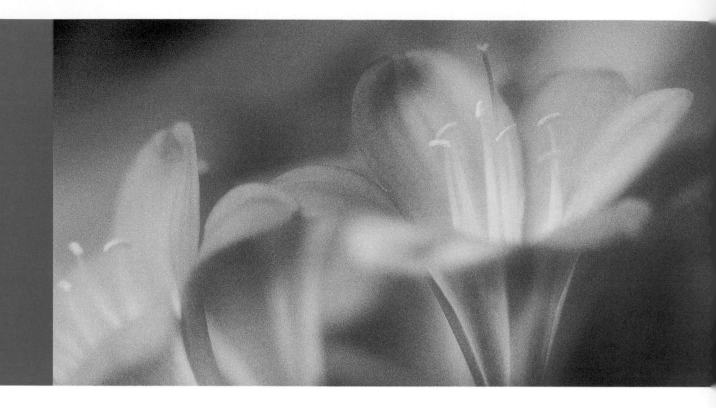

body's strength and capacity for resistance to adverse stress or damage (by chemical, physical, or biological agents). Ginseng stimulates physical and mental activity and protects the human body from severe or prolonged physical or mental stress. It stimulates the function of the endocrine glands and has been used in traditional Asian medicine as a general tonic and cardiotonic agent.

American ginseng has "cooling" properties, while Asian is "warming." Those with "warm" energy should, therefore, take only American ginseng, but those with "cool" energy, only the Asian. American ginseng is often used to reduce stress and fatigue, but the Asian variety has a stimulating effect. The former is effective against high blood pressure and cardiovascular diseases.

Lycium fruit (Gou Qi Zi)

Lycium fruit, derived from *L. chinense* and *L. barbarum*, is also known by common names lycee, lycii, and wolfberry. For thousands of years, Asians have used lycium fruit and liquorice to help maintain good health. Lycium helps improve vision and prevent headaches and dizziness caused by liver and kidney deficiencies. It has been shown effective in mild forms of diabetes. It contains vitamins, minerals, and phytonutrients, beta-carotene, polysaccharides, and amino acids.

Rehmannia root (Shu Di Huang)

Used to treat anemia and fatigue, and to promote the healing of injured bones, rehmannia is also a demulcent and laxative. It stops bleeding, provides energy, and helps strengthen the immune system. Rehmannia also strengthens blood, bones, and tendons.

The rehmannia roots are prepared with wine, amomum fruit (Sha Ren), and tangerine peel (Chen Pi). The roots are steamed and dried in the sun several times until they become black, soft, and sticky; then they are cut into slices.

Rehmannia nourishes blood and replenishes *yin*. The raw or dried root is a cooling herb often used in skin formulas. Rehmannia is a strong blood tonic, often combined with Dang Gui (see page 110) for women's conditions.

Reishi mushroom (Ling Zhi)

Shown in recent studies to be helpful for treating high blood cholesterol levels, normalizing blood pressure, regulating the circulatory system, and helping cure allergies, reishi mushroom contains a high amount of polysaccharides, which are essential for the healthy functioning of the immune system. It is used as a tonic and a sedative, and as an aid for chronic fatigue syndrome, diabetes, liver disorders, hypertension, arthritis, and nervous exhaustion. Reishi has a strong antihistamine action that can help control allergies. Extracts of reishi mushroom have been shown to exert many beneficial effects, which endorses its historical use as an "adaptogen"—a substance that increases resistance to stress and generally improves the tone of the body and mind. In addition to reishi's anticancer and immune-enhancing properties, it has been used to treat insomnia, altitude sickness, high cholesterol, and chronic hepatitis.

In pharmacognosy, reishi mushroom is actually the powder inside the spores of the fungus Ling Zhi, which are formed as Ling Zhi matures. The powder collected from these spores, the essence of reishi, consists of 18.5 percent high-quality protein, with all 18 essential amino acids, plus a combination of vitamins and critical trace elements essential for the functioning of the immune system; the remaining components are polysaccharides.

Schisandra (Wu Wei Zi)

Highly prized by the Chinese as a youth tonic, schisandra is also reputed to increase sexual stamina among men. Until recently, it was coveted only by the wealthy and a favorite among Chinese emperors. Schisandra is considered an adaptogen and, like ginseng, is believed to increase stamina and fight fatigue; it also improves night vision.

Schisandra (*Schisandra chinensis*) is a creeping vine with small red berries, native to northern China. The dried berries are used as an astringent for the treatment of dry cough, asthma, night sweats, nocturnal seminal emissions, chronic diarrhea, and as a tonic for the treatment of chronic fatigue.

During the early 1980s, Chinese doctors began researching schisandra as a treatment for hepatitis, based on its potential for liver-protective effects. Schisandra is now a recognized "adaptogen," capable of increasing the body's resistance to disease, stress, and other debilitating processes. Eastern herbalists commonly recommend schisandra for the lungs, liver, and kidneys, and to help with depression due to adrenergic exhaustion. Schisandra is also used to treat eye fatigue and increase acuity.

Caution: Schisandra should not be used during pregnancy, except under medical supervision to promote uterine contractions during labor. Schisandra should be avoided by those suffering from peptic ulcers, epilepsy, and hypertension.

White peony (Bai Shao Yao)

In traditional Chinese medicine, white peony root is used for heavy bleeding, menstrual pain, and premenstrual syndrome. White peony root is the single herb that will most help with menstrual pain, and is often used with Dang Gui (Chinese angelica, see page 110) and Shu Di Huang (rehmannia root, see page 112). It is also relied on to cure epilepsy. It nourishes the blood, helps with hot flashes and night sweats, is antispasmodic, and alleviates cramps.

Ziziphus spinosa, Jujuba seed (Suan Zao Ren)

The seed of the Chinese red date nourishes the heart and the liver. Its natural tranquilizing properties are used to treat mental fatigue. It helps reduce sweating, especially anxiety sweating, and can be used effectively for insomnia and palpitations.

GUIDELINES FOR KAPHA TYPES
(see pages 11–15)

B complex vitamins are good for kaphas, as are the antioxidants, especially vitamin E. Ginseng and ginger are also excellent herbal supplements because they stimulate more sluggish digestive systems.

tonics & elixirs

Throughout history, all cultures have used various herbs and plants to purify the body and mind, to restore energy to a tired, overstressed physique, and to prevent illness in the future by building up the body's present strength. People require these same remedies today, and the hunt for the ultimate and most effective stress- and age-buster continues globally. Tonics and elixirs are rapidly gaining in popularity—both with the general public and health researchers worldwide.

The demands of modern living make us all feel a little below par at times. Nature has conveniently created an interesting and wide range of natural tonics that act as pick-me-ups to boost energy and rebalance the body.

If you feel tired over a prolonged period, consult your family doctor to determine if there is any apparent physical cause for your "chronic fatigue." Otherwise, you may like to try some of the popular tonics widely available from health-food stores and pharmacies. The following herbal tonics are the most popular and widely available. Also included are suggestions for the form in which to take them. However, remember that, unless you are taking the preparation under the supervision of a doctor or another qualified practitioner, you should *always* follow the manufacturer's instructions and heed any warnings they give.

Acidophilus

This is a probiotic, meaning that it is rich in beneficial bacteria. Acidophilus can help reinstate healthy bacteria in the intestines, lost after an infection or a course of antibiotics.

Alfalfa

Chinese and Indian physicians have long used alfalfa sprouts to treat digestive disorders, and Native Americans used it for its blood-clotting qualities. Alfalfa contains *all* the major vitamins and minerals, and is rich in chlorophyll and enzymes. It assists in the detoxification of the body and, because it is rich in vitamin K, it is an excellent supplement for pregnant women, helping to promote blood clotting during birth.

Aloe vera juice

The rubbery leaves of the aloe vera plant, native to the tropical Americas, are filled with a gel-like substance that is reputed to heal both external and internal wounds. Held to be one of nature's most potent healers, it is especially good for

the digestive system and an effective preventative or treatment for irritable bowel syndrome and related disorders. All kinds of conditions respond to aloe taken internally: acne, arthritis, colds, candida, chronic fatigue, inflammations, ulcers, viral infections, and irritable bowel syndrome, to name just a few. It is available in fresh juice and capsule form, but make sure you buy full-strength rather than the adulterated versions.

Barley grass, see Grasses

Black cohosh

Traditionally used for many problems associated with the menstrual cycle, this root originated in North America, where Native Americans called it "squawroot" or "black snakeroot," because it was also used to treat snake bites. It is a normalizer of the female reproductive system, and helps regulate the cycle and reduce heavy bleeding. Because it contains plant estrogens, it is ideal for balancing female sex hormones and treating premenstrual tension as part of

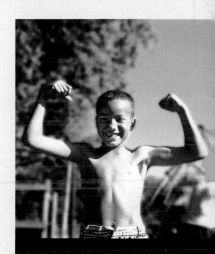

BEST IMMUNE BOOSTERS

Alfalfa
Aloe vera juice
Cat's claw
Coenzyme Q10
Echinacea
Ginseng
Glutamine
Kombucha
Propolis
Reishi mushroom
Royal jelly
Sambucol
Selenium
Zinc

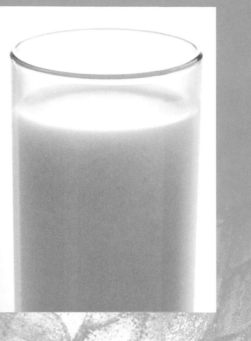

BEST SUPPLEMENTS FOR HEALING

Aloe vera
Cat's claw
Chlorella
Coenzyme Q10
Echinacea
Floradix
Sambucol

Only the potent red inner bark should be used for tea. The dried bark is sold, but increasingly it is available in tea bags and also in capsule form, sometimes mixed with aloe vera to great effect.

Catuaba

The bark of this Amazon shrub or tree is used to brew a tea, with a peculiar bitter taste, that stimulates the central nervous system and the desire for sex. This is one of the ingredients in the tonic "Love Bomb," which also contains Korean and Siberian ginseng, muirapuama, and guarana, and has gained some renown as an aphrodisiac in recent years.

a tonic formula. It is also used in the treatment of arthritis, muscular pain, anxiety, and mental stress.

Cat's claw

This herb from the Peruvian rainforest may turn out to be one of the most important herbal discoveries yet made. Cat's claw is a large creeping vine with the botanical name *Uncaria tomentosa*. It bears strong thorns shaped like a cat's claw, hence its name. The local Indians have used it for thousands of years, but only in the last few decades have Western researchers taken serious notice of this amazing plant. It seems that cat's claw works at so many levels in the body that it can potentially help everything from cancer and candida to allergies, intestinal disorders, depression, and HIV. Studies around the world are now revealing that cat's claw is highly antioxidant, antiviral, antitumor, and anti-inflammatory, and

that it has a pronounced healing effect on the digestive system and seems able to relieve chronic fatigue.

The first Western knowledge came when a German researcher, Dr. Klaus Keplinger, brought specimens back to Germany in the 1970s. He has since obtained patents isolating six alkaloids from the root. The most active one, Isopteredin, is a powerful immune stimulator. Four others markedly enhance the ability of white cells to digest bacteria, viruses, cancer cells, and other toxins.

The shamans of Peru recognize cat's claw as a premier herb for cancer, arthritis, rheumatism, and digestion, with the power to combat infections and inflammation of all kinds. So far the Western catalog of clinical reports adds a beneficial effect on all forms of herpes, Epstein-Barr (mononucleosis), asthma, acne, circulatory and intestinal problems, toxin poisoning, lupus, and diabetes.

Chasteberry (Agnus castus)

Women have long used this herb, also known as Vitex or monk's berry, for combating menopausal symptoms. Containing estrogen-mimicking substances, it has a balancing effect on hormone production and tends to normalize hormone levels. It can, therefore, function like a natural hormone replacement therapy. The active part lies in the berries, which are dried and ground in a tincture. It also had a reputation for reducing the sex drive, earning it its name.

Chlorella

A green algae, chlorella comes from Japan, where today it is one of the most popular supplements. It has a very high protein content and is also rich in beta-carotene, B complex vitamins, zinc, and iron. Chlorella is high in RNA and DNA nucleic acids—responsible for the growth and repair of tissue. Because it contains chlorophyll, it helps to prohibit germs from spreading and assists in the speedy healing of wounds. It is also an excellent booster and tonic for the immune system.

Cider vinegar

Made from fermented apple juice, apple cider vinegar has been used for centuries to aid digestion. It is useful for those who lack stomach acids, such as the elderly. It is rich in potassium and other trace minerals, and may be used in shampoos to make hair glossier.

Clary sage

The essential oil of clary sage contains sclariol, which mimics estrogen and thus provides excellent natural HRT. It is very powerful in its effects and must not be taken during pregnancy or internally, but rather as one or two drops placed on the inner arm at the elbow joint to allow absorption of the oil through the skin.

Cod liver oil

Cod liver oil is a traditional supplement taken for its rich source of vitamins A and D. Vitamin A is good for the skin, eyes, bones, and mucous membranes, while D helps the body to absorb calcium, so helping to strengthen bones. It also reduces arthritic pain and inflammation. Research is being done in Strasbourg, France, into the effectiveness of the oil in reducing fatty tissue around the abdomen.

Coenzyme Q10

Coenzyme Q10, a viral component of every cell and found in the mitochondria, is involved in cellular energy production. Coenzyme Q10 has potent antioxidant properties, which is how it earned its reputation for being an antiaging and immune-boosting supplement. Clinical application includes against chronic fatigue syndrome, diabetes, cardiovascular disease, congestive heart failure, high blood pressure, immune deficiency, and breast cancer.

Damiana

This potent energy and sex tonic was originally used by the Aztec and Mayan Indians as a cure for impotence or as an aphrodisiac. It gets its reputation as a reproductive organ rejuvenator because it increases blood flow to the capillaries. This is a herb that is stimulating to the reproductive organs and may be used to enhance sexual performance. Damiana may be helpful for men in the treatment of impotence and, combined with saw palmetto, would be a useful tonic to ensure prostate health.

Damiana is also known to be useful in treating depression, reducing anxiety, and as a rejuvenator. Damiana is available in capsule form or as a dried loose herb for making into a tea.

Echinacea

Echinacea increases the production of white blood cells, making it a valuable herb in fighting viruses, bacteria, and infection. Echinacea is a popular herbal remedy and is frequently used as a booster for the immune system during the winter months, either as a prevention against colds and flu or in

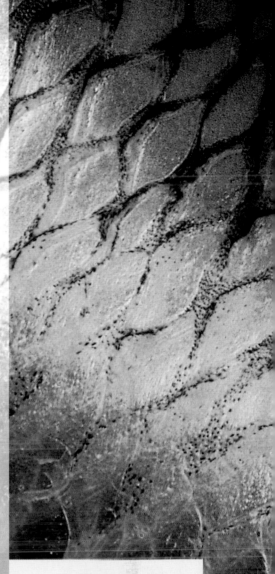

SUPPLEMENTS FOR A HEALTHY SEX LIFE

Vitamins A, C, and E, and B complex vitamins with biotin
Magnesium
Zinc
Damiana
Ginseng
Evening primrose oil
Flaxseed oil
Olive oil
Saw palmetto

their treatment, as well as helping to treat herpes and other infectious diseases. The exception, however, is the HIV virus, which attaches to immune cells—therefore, echinacea may stimulate replication of the virus, too.

As a tea, echinacea improves circulation and may help bronchitis and sore throats. Cancer patients undergoing chemotherapy may find that supervised echinacea supplementation helps restore their immune systems and alleviate the side-effects of the therapy.

Evening primrose oil

We now know that certain types of fats are actually essential for health. The omega-6 essential fatty acids are important for healthy hair, skin, and nails, brain function, immunity, hormone production, and most importantly for the production of anti-inflammatory mediators. Evening primrose oil is an important source of these fatty acids, as well as the hormone-like substances prostaglandins, which combat pain and inflammation, reduce blood pressure, prevent platelet clotting (keep blood thin), reduce cholesterol levels, and prevent water retention. Although an important source of the essential fatty acid GLA (gamma linolenic acid), you have to look further to avoid deficiency of the essential omega-3 fatty acid.

Generations of women have successfully used this supplement to alleviate menopausal symptoms, such as hot flashes, and premenstrual symptoms, such as breast tenderness. Conditions that evening primrose may help to treat include arthritis, acne, eczema, psoriasis, chronic fatigue syndrome, depression, allergies, hyperactivity, alcoholism, and diabetes.

Eyebright

Used internally, this plant extract is a powerful anticatarrhal, and can be used to treat sinusitis, catarrh, and other congestive disorders. As its name suggests, it is best known for its ability to treat eye conditions, particularly acute or chronic inflammations, stinging or weeping eyes, conjunctivitis, and oversensitivity to light.

Feverfew

A plant extract known to help relieve a number of conditions, including dizziness, tinnitus, period pains, sluggish menstrual flow, migraine headaches (in conjunction with hot compresses to the head), and arthritis in the inflammatory stage.

Fennel

Fennel is excellent for toning up a sluggish digestive system and for stimulating the appetite. An infusion of fennel on its own, or mixed with camomile and hops, helps constipation. Mix 10 to 20 drops of extract with one teaspoon of honey in warm water.

Flaxseed

The Cherokee Indians believed that flax was sacred and vital to the life processes of the body, and that its seed captured energies from the sun. They used the flaxseed to nourish pregnant women and to treat malnutrition, arthritis, skin diseases, and fertility and virility.

Flaxseed is one of the best sources of the essential alpha-linolenic acid, an important member of the omega-3 group of fatty acids, so important to health and wellbeing. Omega-3 is recognized as an essential nutrient—it is as vital to the body as a vitamin, but we cannot produce it in our bodies ourselves. In recent times we have lost many sources of fatty acids

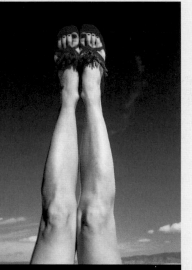

SUPPLEMENTS AS AN ALTERNATIVE TO HRT

Black cohosh
Chasteberry
Wild Mexican yam
Korean ginseng
Dang Gui
Natural progesterone
  cream
Clary sage

from our diet, and some experts believe many of our chronic, modern physical and mental woes may be attributed to a deficiency of these fatty acids. Today it is widely recognized that the omega-3 fatty acids are important in the prevention of arteriosclerosis, cancer, heart disease, depression, mental illness, immune disorders, and allergies. In addition to the vital omega-3 acids, flaxseed oil contains omega-6 (linoleic acid) and omega-9 (oleic acid) in the right balance, which is so important to health.

You should take flaxseeds that are organic and fresh on a regular basis. The pressed oil from the seeds is available from health food stores, usually in the refrigerator cabinet, since it has a short shelf life. You can't cook with it, but it does makes an excellent salad dressing, as well as a simple way of taking the supplement.

Floradix

This internationally renowned vegetarian food supplement, rich in an easy-to-absorb iron compound, combines selected herbs with vitamins, minerals, and fruit concentrates to create a tonic drink that is widely used for people recovering from any long-term debilitating illness. The liquid tonic is also useful in late autumn or early winter to build up the immune system so that you can fight off seasonal colds and flus.

Ginger

This is the herb the Chinese use for treating morning sickness, travel sickness, indigestion, and nausea. Peel and grate the root to make an infusion of ginger tea for treating these digestive complaints, or take one capsule up to three times daily. An infusion of ginger is also helpful in treating most forms of arthritis, as well as cheering those suffering from depression. Tablets may also be used for treating period pains: take one up to three times a day. Ginger is said to stimulate lung function, and your health practitioner may prescribe a tincture for treating bronchitis. An infusion of ginger and scallions is a natural remedy for colds and flu.

Ginseng

Renowned for its stimulating effect, ginseng improves the body's tolerance to stress and is believed to possess aphrodisiac properties. Ginseng provides a natural source of steroids and boosts immunity and mental performance. Despite its stimulating properties, it is also known to have a soothing, calming effect on the digestive system.

There are three main types of ginseng. Siberian ginseng is not a member of the ginseng family, but has very similar properties—it may be used to revitalize you if you feel run-down and it is good for chronic fatigue sufferers.

American ginseng may help calm a nervous or upset stomach as a result of work pressure or other stress.

Korean, or "red," ginseng has been used medicinally in the Far East for over 4,000 years, and it is thought to be the most stimulating of all the ginseng

family. Menopausal women may find it helpful in controlling hot flashes.

The normal dosage is one 600 mg capsule per day; 5 to 10 g powder, mixed with liquid per day; or one cup of ginseng tea per day. If you are taking a vitamin C supplement, allow two hours between taking it and taking ginseng, since vitamin C can interfere with the body's ability to absorb ginseng. Ginseng is not recommended for children, pregnant women, or anyone suffering from a high temperature (through fever or flu, for example) or high blood pressure. It should not be taken continuously or for more than two months at a time.

SUPPLEMENTS TO WARD OFF COLDS AND FLU

Vitamins A, C and E, and beta-carotene
Selenium, zinc
Aloe vera
Cat's claw
Echinacea
Sambucol
Garlic
Ginger
Goldenseal
Mushrooms (maiitake, reishi, and shiitake)
Propolis
St. John's wort

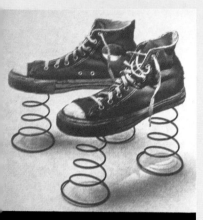

TONICS FOR ENERGY

Vitamin B
   complex
Vitamin C,
   choline
Iron
Copper
Chromium
Calcium
Magnesium
Zinc
Cat's claw tea
   with ginger
Coenzyme Q10
Ginseng
Propolis
Royal jelly

Glutamine

Thanks to ten years of intensive research, glutamine is the new "superstar" amino acid being pursued by expert specialists in everything from cancer and ulcers to depression and rheumatoid arthritis. Illness, surgery, and continued stress can depress stores of glutamine and, in doing so, body functions. In the absence of this amazing amino acid, immune cells do not function correctly or even grow.

"It took researchers a very long time to consider the importance of glutamine," says Judy Shabert, a doctor, dietician, and the author of *The Ultimate Nutrient Glutamine*. "With our current level of understanding, it seems rather naive not to have studied glutamine more closely. It is the most abundant amino acid in the body, especially in the brain, skeletal muscle, and blood. In fact, it is proving to be the most significant amino acid known."

It is only in the last decade or so that glutamine was found to be the primary nutrient for the digestive system, the fuel for the immune system and the brain, important for muscle metabolism, and vital for healing and tissue repair. Because it reduces craving and addiction, in addition to acting as an effective healing aid, it is very effective in treating and preventing alcohol problems. In Japan most people now take it before drinking to prevent hangovers. Glutamine is most commonly available as a powder, for sprinkling on food.

Goldenrod

This plant extract has many uses, including as a gargle to treat laryngitis and pharyngitis and as an anti-inflammatory in cases of urethritis, cystitis, and urinary infections in general. Its carminative qualities make it useful in treating dyspepsia, but its most important use is in the treatment of upper respiratory tract infections, such as acute or chronic catarrh and, with other supplements, flu.

Goldenseal

The extract of the root and rhizome of this plant is useful in the treatment of catarrhal states. A powerful tonic for all the mucous membranes, it may also be used for all digestive problems. Its tonic and astringent qualities also make it good for uterine conditions. It can be used externally for earache, eczema, conjunctivitis, itching, and ringworm.

Grapefruit seed extract

This extract, known by the commercial name of Citricidal®, may turn out to be the most potent, and benign, antimicrobial yet discovered. As well as bacteria, it has been shown to inactivate viruses, yeasts, parasites, and worms.

Grasses

Wheatgrass and barley grass are cereal grasses grown in nutrient-rich soils. Because they metabolize and absorb all the nutrients from the ground, they are a rich source of vitamins, minerals, and fiber. In fact, they are higher in fiber than bran and contain more iron than spinach. They also supply protein, chlorophyll, and beta-carotene. Wheatgrass has been shown to be useful in the treatment of anemia and high blood pressure, and it is also a good liver tonic. These grasses may be eaten as vegetables or in salads, but are most often pressed for their juice.

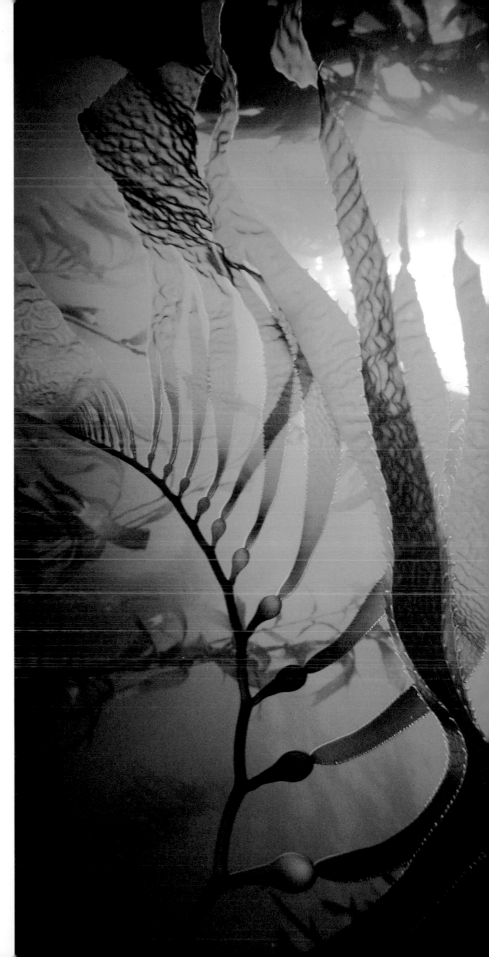

Guarana

A native plant of Brazil, this is a wonderful natural "upper" because of its caffeine content. It helps maintain good concentration, memory, and energy, possibly because its caffeine action lasts twice as long as that of tea or coffee.

Hemp seed

Hemp seed is widely acclaimed as one of the most complete sources of vegetable protein. In addition to providing protein, minerals, and vitamins, hemp seed is also rich in essential fatty acids. All are present in a form that is easily digested. Hemp seed is useful in reducing cholesterol and protecting against heart disease. It also stimulates the hair and nails, and encourages healthy skin.

Kava

Traditionally made into a drink for ceremonial occasions in the South Pacific islands (before the introduction of alcohol), this potent root extract makes you calm, relaxed, and full of optimism. The Tahitians also credit it with the power to aid concentration, promote healthy lungs and digestion, ease the joints, and help maintain normal weight.

Kelp

This seaweed contains a rich concentration of minerals, including calcium, potassium, magnesium, and iron, as well as vitamins A, C, D, E, and B complex. High in iodine, it aids digestion, soothes ulcers, and helps thyroid function and metabolism.

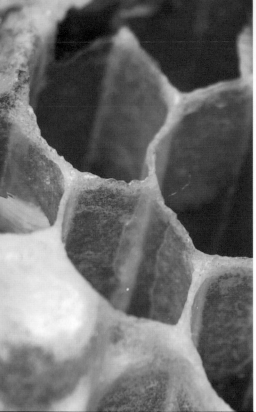

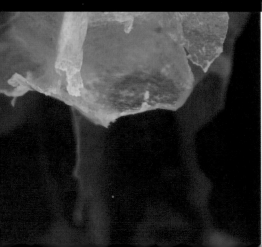

Kombucha

Millions worldwide are convinced this lichen-like fungus has a rejuvenating and strengthening action. For more than 2,000 years the Chinese have brewed and drunk this mixture of bacteria and yeast to stimulate the immune system.

The slimy pancake-like culture floats on the surface of a sweetened tea which, after fermentation, produces a nutrient-rich solution full of good flora and organic acids. This tea is quickly gaining the reputation as an "elixir of life," which can help prevent most serious illness because of its immune-enhancing properties. It is

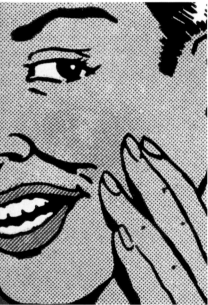

reputed to slow aging, recharge your sex life, reduce the risk of cancer or the size of existing tumors, and cure arthritis!

Lecithin

Extracted from soy, lecithin's most important ingredient is phosphatidyl choline (see also page 196). It has been used to help Alzheimer's, Huntington's chorea, and to lower cholesterol.

Mexican yam

This root, also called wild yam, is valued for its high concentrations of steroidal saponins, including diosgenin, vital for the commercial production of cortisone and progesterone. It was, in fact, the pharmaceutical industry's only source of diosgenin until 1970. As a botanical medicine, it is considered completely safe and nontoxic. You can apply it topically as a cream or oil, or take it internally as a supplement or tincture. It is excellent used in combination with chasteberry for reversing menopausal symptoms.

Milk thistle

The seed shell of this herb yields a group of flavonoid-like compounds that are excellent for restoring and maintaining liver function. The liver is an impressive hormone-filtering system. If it is congested and sluggish, the delicate hormonal balance of the body is disturbed. Milk thistle features in many hormone tonics, but it is also used for treating cirrhosis, hepatitis, psoriasis, and any form of toxicity—even emotional. Its flavonoids help protect the liver against damage from chemicals and speed up production or regeneration of enzymes and proteins. Tea is made from a decoction of the seeds, and tinctures are available.

Motherwort

The Latin name for this plant, *Lenourus cardiaca*, indicates its usefulness against

DAILY SUPPLEMENTS FOR HEALTHY SKIN

Multivitamin and multimineral
   complex (with 300 mg
   magnesium and 15 mg zinc)
Two 1,000 mg vitamin C
Antioxidant complex
GLA (300 mg), evening
   primrose oil
Vitamin E (500 iu)
Fish oil or flaxseed oil

heart problems. It is used for any heart condition that is primarily brought on by stress and anxiety, and it is an excellent remedy for an over-rapid heartbeat. The plant's common name also betrays its uses in treating of female conditions, such as menstrual and uterine flow. In the latter case, it can encourage flow where menstruation has been delayed by stress or anxiety. Menopausal women may also benefit from this herb, as it is a relaxant. It can also be used for false labor pains.

MSM

Sulfur and molasses was a traditional folk remedy, and a growing body of research focused on MSM—a natural form of organic sulfur—suggests that sulfur has powerful nutritional benefits. MSM, which is found in rainwater and has been part of the food chain since life began, is beginning to be recognized for the relief it offers to an exceptional number of health problems.

Can we really have overlooked a nutrient that offers relief to so many challenging ailments? This seems to be the case with sulfur. MSM relieves the pain of inflammatory conditions, such as arthritis, joint pain, swelling, tenderness, osteoarthritis, and bursitis. It also appears to help ease allergies and skin, eye, digestion, diabetic, and lung conditions.

People with chronic to severe allergies report substantial to complete relief of their symptoms with daily doses of MSM, and a majority of subjects with allergic asthma reported that they were able to reduce their medication by 75 percent when taking MSM. It is available in both powder and tablet form, plus as a cream for the treatment of skin allergies.

Nettle

This "spring" herb is thought to be an excellent natural blood cleanser and good all-round tonic. It stimulates the digestion and produces a feeling of wellbeing. It is available in fresh leaf and tablet form.

Phosphatidyl serine

Phosphatidyl serine (PS) is unlike any other product currently available. Clinical studies have shown that it can help support brain functions that tend to decline with age. PS appears to play an important role in the function of brain cell membranes, including the conduction of the nerve impulse. As we grow older, cognitive functions can slow down; recognizing names and faces, learning and remembering information, and maintaining concentration are more difficult. Now extensive scientific research has shown that real improvement is reported after only a short course of phosphatidyl serine.

As a dietary supplement, PS provides nutrients that can positively contribute to enhanced memory, learning, concentration, and behavioral balance (including negative moods and coping with stress). It has also been shown to reduce stress hormone production. PS was once only available from animal sources; now there is an enriched vegetarian form, derived from soy.

Pomegranate

Throughout history this fruit has enjoyed rare, elevated status among foods and its consumption has been associated with strength and longevity. The seeds and juice of this fruit of the ancients are packed with all kinds of nutrients and strong antioxidants. In fact, it has three times more antioxidant strength than green tea, red wine, cranberry or orange juice. Pomegranates are a great source of potassium, vitamin C and polyphenols (which promote heart health). Recent research indicates that the juice from this fruit may help keep fatty deposits from building up on artery walls.

Propolis

A resin obtained from the buds of some flowers and trees, propolis is thought to contain a natural antibiotic, galangin. The bees collect the propolis along with the pollen and take it back to the hives. There, they spread it around to protect the hive from bacteria and viruses. Propolis is thought to be rich in nutrients and minerals. It is used in various complementary remedies to treat low-grade infections, especially among those who want to avoid taking antibiotics.

Pycenogenol

This is a well-known herbal antioxidant made from French maritime pine bark. Scientific literature shows it to have powerful anti-inflammatory effects and for this reason it is an excellent, and a safe, natural pain reliever. Pycenogenol is a patented complex of about 40 antioxidants. Its efficacy as a powerful antioxidant has been supported by many studies, including research by the antioxidant expert and professor emeritus at the University of California, Berkeley, Lester Packer, Ph.D. He found Pycenogenol not only excellent for quenching free radicals, but in addition, that it turns off some of the genes involved in producing inflammation. The supplements can have dramatic effects in people with rheumatic diseases.

Reishi mushroom

Another "wonder tonic" from the East, this mushroom has been the focus of a lot of research and attention in recent years. Like royal jelly and ginseng, it is considered important for increased energy. It stimulates the immune system and is officially listed in Japan as a substance for treating cancer. Reishi mushroom is used to bolster the poor resistance of those with AIDS, for deficiency conditions, and to fortify the body's natural vigor.

Royal jelly

Queen bees are known to grow to a much greater size than other worker bees and it is the consumption of royal jelly that is the reason. Those in the East have known of the beneficial effects of royal jelly for centuries. It is reputed to have countless beneficial effects: it enhances wellbeing, stimulates stamina and the immune system, and increases energy levels. It has a natural diuretic action and also may help diminish the pain—and then the condition—of crippling arthritis; the

Chinese give routine injections of royal jelly to cure arthritis. It is also helpful in relieving allergies and asthma. Fresh royal jelly is good for healing wounds and for cleaning and enhancing the blood.

Some researchers believe that royal jelly can give some protection against cancer by improving the immune system. It can even benefit cancer sufferers by boosting resistance to the harmful side-effects of chemotherapy and radiotherapy.

People who swear by royal jelly take a capsule regularly first thing in the morning or on an empty stomach. It may take two to three months before you perceive dramatic changes in your level of wellbeing, but converts would advise you persist! You can also take royal jelly with honey in a liquid form, which usually contains bee pollen and vitamin C. This, too, is best taken on an empty stomach or as a nutritious breakfast spread. Do not add it to a hot drink because the heat will destroy its beneficial properties.

Fresh royal jelly can be taken as a liquid tonic for a really fast-acting "pick-me-up." This form is usually packaged in a single-dose phial, which is easy to use and gives an energizing effect that you feel almost immediately and which can last all day. This form is not for everyday, regular use, as you may get more energy than you need, but is ideal for a quick boost. Liquid royal jelly tonics are mixed with ginseng and honey, which add to the energizing effect and the ability to fight fatigue and depression, as well as boost both physical and mental energy. Using fresh royal jelly externally can have an excellent effect on skin and hair.

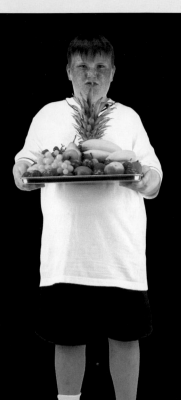

SUPPLEMENTS THAT MIGHT HELP IN WEIGHT REDUCTION

A good high-quality (perhaps true-food form) multivitamin and multimineral, plus extra fat-burning minerals, such as chromium and iodine.
Cod liver oil
Coenzyme Q10

St. John's wort

In Germany tablets of this traditional European herb are now prescribed for depression ten times more frequently than Prozac. Research suggests that, in cases of mild-to-moderate depression, St. John's Wort—or hypericum—is an effective, natural antidepressant. It has been found useful against Seasonal Affective Disorder.

Sambucol

Sambucol™ is a natural product made from a black elderberry extract and has been shown to be effective in inactivating viruses. It is derived from the black elder tree, *Sambucus nigra*, grown mostly in central Europe.

This natural substance has rare antiviral strengths—proven antiviral preparations are rare. Even the pharmaceutical companies haven't been able to come up with an effective antiviral, with the exception of Aciclovir for herpes and the expensive and limited Interferon. Sambucol™ was developed by Dr. Madeleine Mumcuoglu, a prominent French/Israeli virologist, who patented the product, which combines the natural benefits of the plant with other components, like raspberry extract.

Clinically tested, Sambucol™ has been used by thousands with spectacular results. It is safe, nontoxic, and natural. Research shows that active ingredients in the elderberries bind with viruses before they have a chance to penetrate the wall of a normal cell. The liquid extract has been tested on numerous well-known flu viruses and was effective on every one.

Saw palmetto

This small North-American tree has dark red berries that are ground into a powder. It is apparently excellent as an energy and sex tonic, particularly for men with impotence or prostate problems. The Native Americans have a long tradition of using the berries for chronic congestion. They are also used for urinary problems.

Serotone

Serotone is a mood regulator, with a calming effect. It is a natural source of 5-HTP, the precursor of serotonin (the neurotransmitter involved in mood and sleep). Modern antidepressants, such as Prozac, increase the level of brain serotonin by preventing its removal from the system, hence the classification name SSRI—serotonin reuptake inhibitor. One problem of the SSRIs is that serotonin is supposed to be secreted by the body, and by preventing this, many SSRIs cause side-effects. There is no such problem with serotone because it helps you produce more serotonin naturally.

Spirulina

This highly nutritious blue-green algae, traditionally eaten by the Aztecs, is a rich source of protein more easily assimilated by the body than protein from eggs, fish, dairy products, or meat. It is also rich in a wide variety of trace minerals, vitamins, enzymes, chlorophyll, and beta-carotene. Available in powder and capsule forms, this is an extremely useful supplement for people who are on a diet, because it can suppress the appetite, but at the same time supply important nutrients.

GUIDELINES FOR PITTA TYPES (see pages 11–15)

The minerals calcium, magnesium, and zinc are of benefit to Pitta types, as are sea minerals and algae, such as chlorella and spirulina, and wheatgrass. Mint tea is also excellent.

Valerian

The rhizome and root of this plant are used to make one of the most common relaxant nervines. It is quite safe to use to reduce symptoms of stress, anxiety, over-excitability, and hysteria, and is particularly useful to treat insomnia or poor-quality sleep. An antispasmodic, it also aids relief from cramps, intestinal colic, and period pain. It can even be used in the treatment of migraines and rheumatic pain.

Wheatgrass, see Grasses

Yellow dock root

Useful in treating chronic skin complaints, such as psoriasis and eczema, yellow dock root is also used for constipation, as it has a cathartic effect on the bowel. It promotes the flow of bile and acts as a blood cleanser, and can help in treating jaundice.

natural

exercise

In addition to what we take into our bodies, the other crucial aspect of ensuring our overall health is regular exercise. As with most aspects of the holistic approach, this must be tailored to suit your own body's needs and your lifestyle. You don't necessarily need to join a gym or hire a personal trainer; perhaps all you need to help restore your balance is a few hours of gentle walking or getting back into the daily two or three lengths of the pool you did until a few years ago, or even joining a dance class. Consider what suits you best, or you think you might enjoy, and look at all the possibilities on the following pages. Here you will also learn how to assess your physical state, decide on the right exercise for you, and find the motivation to do it.

There is also plenty of advice on improving your posture and on how to warm up and cool down before and after exercise. This section includes two complete exercise programs for you to follow if you choose; one for basic stretching, strength, and stamina training, and another utilizing the gentle principles of yoga and associated Eastern disciplines.

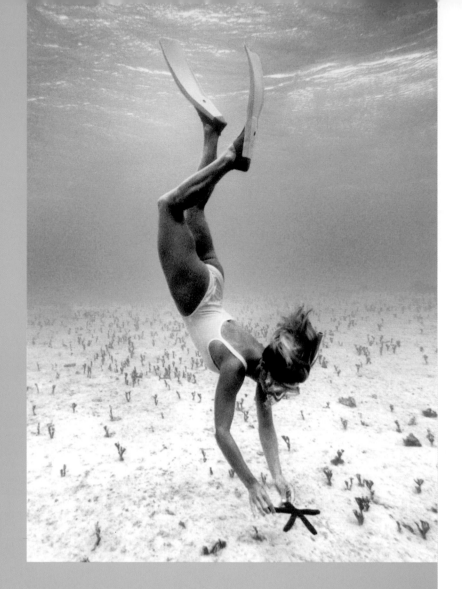

natural exercise

The natural way to a happier and healthier you is to combine a balanced whole diet with regular exercise and adequate sleep. You will then feel good and look good, making you generally more positive and able to tackle the tasks of daily living. The single best thing you can do to protect, maintain, and promote your wellbeing, and prevent serious illness is to exercise responsibly: to stretch and move your body regularly, and within your individual needs and means.

Someone who eats junk food, sits in front of a computer all day, travels home through rush-hour traffic to snack on more junk food, and then veges out in front of the television will look and feel tired, lethargic, and jaded. This lifestyle actually puts a great deal of strain on the body, but the more you use your body, the better it will perform and cope with the tasks you face. The human body was designed for movement. These days, unfortunately, movement can often consist only of the short walk to the mode of transport which takes you from home to work. Even this small amount of movement can be rushed and fraught, and not allow you to reap the benefits of fresh air. The society in which we live today dictates that we actually have to allocate time for exercise.

Fifty years ago, people walked more and could expect to lead more physically demanding and active lives than they do nowadays. Now the average person will probably rarely move at all, except to perform basic functions, such as shopping for food or cleaning. With such dramatic changes to our basic lifestyle, is it any wonder that the huge rise in death from heart disease and other degenerative illnesses continues, in spite of the amazing advances made in modern medicine and our understanding of disease?

Unfortunately, too many of us still lead sedentary lifestyles that can lead to many of the illnesses common in the modern world, including depression, stress-related conditions, and even muscular wastage in those as young as their mid-20s. Not to mention the increasing problem of obesity in children, who take too little exercise and watch too much TV. However, the message does seems to be getting through. From the 1980s aerobic workout on, more and more people are awakening to how vital exercise is to good health and longevity, and how it should feature in daily life. With so much choice of, and greater awareness in, the various forms exercise can take, people are turning their attention to creating a healthier lifestyle that incorporates regular exercise, healthy eating, and enough sleep.

There is no question that people who take exercise feel better and have more energy and vitality than people who don't. It is well known that you experience a rise in alertness for a few hours after a workout, yoga, or dance class, or a good brisk walk. Exercise can help you overcome and treat depression; it raises the levels of endorphins, the body's natural opiates or "pleasure hormones," which reduce the sensation of pain in the body.

The adrenal glands produce hormones like adrenalin and cortisol, the levels of which are elevated in stressed and depressed people, causing sleep problems, belly fat and irritable bowel syndrome. Regular exercise keeps hormones in check, helping to stabilize the overall mood and ability to cope. There is also mounting evidence that people who suffer from too much stress or depression are much more likely to develop serious degenerative health conditions, leading to disease. Anything that so dramatically reduces this threat, as exercise and good diet do, must be a priority.

WHY EXERCISE IS IMPORTANT

- Apart from a healthy diet, it is the best thing you can do for preventative health care.
- Reduces the risk of heart disease.
- Improves circulation.
- Helps prevent the development of cancer.
- Improves breathing and your entire respiratory system.
- Helps alleviate symptoms of osteoarthritis.
- Strengthens your back and reduces lower back pain.
- Increases bone density.
- Reduces your risk of osteoporosis.
- Strengthens muscles, tendons, ligaments, and cartilage, and stabilizes joints.
- Increases flexibility.
- Improves posture.
- Slows down the aging process.
- Increases energy.
- Helps reduce body fat levels.
- Helps maintain your ideal body weight.
- Helps shift and prevent cellulite.
- Improves digestion.
- Helps correct bowel problems, particularly constipation.
- Boosts the immune system, which, in turn, makes you less susceptible to colds, flu, and general debilitating ailments brought on by inertia.
- Improves your self-esteem and body image.
- Reduces depression, anxiety, and stress.
- Improves brain function. You really could become more intelligent or realize just how intelligent you actually are!
- Helps you look better, feel better.
- Stimulates more energy and a positive attitude to life.
- Makes you HAPPIER!

According to the Dunn Clinical Nutrition Centre in Cambridge, England, it could be much easier to adopt a more physical life than we think. For example, walking rather than using the car and carrying groceries home burns off nearly ten times more calories. Losing the television remote and walking across the room to change channels would mean that you walk three miles a year! Housework and gardening are wonderful ways to burn calories. Of course, it is advisable to become as physically active in all areas of your life as you can, remaining aware of how you use your body.

When performing any kind of exercise, consider your unique physical being and its state at that moment, and have the courage to push yourself just enough to know—and move within—your boundaries and limitations.

Creating your personal exercise program

The way we approach exercise and the types of movement that appeal to us is completely individual and influenced by many different factors, whether they are hereditary or social conditioning, or informed by the way our family approaches play and sports. Mix that with your own unique talents, tastes, and experiences and you can see why people express such different interests. It doesn't matter what kind of exercise you decide to implement into your daily regime—as long as your choices reflect your natural inclinations.

If you are getting exercise or playing sports, you are probably in pretty good shape and in a healthy state of wellbeing, unless you simply don't know your limits and overdo it in one area without balancing it in another. For example, you might be incredibly strong through intensive strength-training with weights, but be inflexible and unable to run for a bus. It is important to balance your program to incorporate all three aspects for overall fitness: stretching, strength training, and stamina.

Even very fit, supple young people can push themselves too far, inflicting serious physical damage, or worse, while performing some physical activity or athletic competition. Learn to recognize your limits and the dangers of pushing yourself past the point of pain in the pursuit of excellence—it will only be a hollow victory for vanity. which will not serve you well in the long run. To prevent injury during exercise, do not overdo it—do not strain or push too far. Gently and slowly is always the safest approach, especially if you are just starting to exercise again.

Walking or brisk walking and swimming are very safe, low-injury-risk exercise systems. Regular walking is one of the best exercises you can give your body. After all, we are upright—designed physically to walk—and should do so on a regular basis to prevent any number of health complaints. For good heart- and brain-health, walk briskly, swinging your arms freely, for 10 to 20 minutes a day.

Remember that it is not necessary to go to an aerobics class for two hours every other day to reach your optimum physical health. For many people who can't get to a health club, tennis game, or a dance or yoga class, you can still keep physically active with shorter and more frequent bursts of exercise. A lot of recent research suggests that 10 to 20 minutes of brisk walking, swimming, or bicycling, per day, is as beneficial as a long workout at the gym a few times a week.

Although some experts believe a little every day is the best approach, that may not be true for you. If your regular two to four hours a week has helped you achieve an optimum level of wellbeing, then stay with what works for you—but perhaps weave in new ways of moving your body now and then. On the other hand, if you are athletic and have built up a program over time, your body can handle a longer workout. In these cases, vary the types of exercise and introduce new challenges; not only will this alleviate boredom, but it will also provide a more balanced regime.

Finding motivation

When motivation fails, draw from within. If you are participating in a regime like yoga or t'ai chi (see pages 168 and 182), you will be gently learning about discipline. If not, focus on your inner self and on using the positive will power within, and find the courage to continue to participate, knowing you can only benefit in the long run. If you do find it difficult to make it to a class or session, and have to skip a day, don't beat yourself up for it. Instead, try to make sure that you do manage something, however small—perhaps some gentle stretching to make sure your muscles and ligaments do not tighten and shrink through inactivity. Ease out the stresses of the day with gentle neck, head, and shoulder rolls, and then stretch the limbs, torso, and spine. About 10 minutes of stretching and mild-to-moderate activity is better than nothing at all, and will keep you on track until you can make it to the gym.

For many people, fitness can be something that other people do; the plethora of activities available can be daunting. Some may feel insecure about joining gyms or exercise classes, perhaps believing that they need to be fit before joining! The thought of muscle-bound, toned bodies, perfect physiques, and competition may stop you from doing something that is beneficial. Most of these fears are unfounded, as classes are attended by people in all stages of fitness, and special classes for beginners are the starting point for all of us. Drop-out rates are very high for first-timers at gyms; once the initial enthusiasm has worn off, it can be difficult to maintain a program. You might benefit from the added incentive of starting an exercise program with a friend or a "training partner." Often the impetus to exercise will be enhanced if you are not your own sole motivator!

Keep an exercise journal, however simplistic; it is a useful tool to provide motivation. Instead of writing in what you have done when you've done it, fill out your proposed program for a few weeks ahead. Seeing it in black and white in your diary will be a better prompt for you than a hazy memory of a class or session you were supposed to attend!

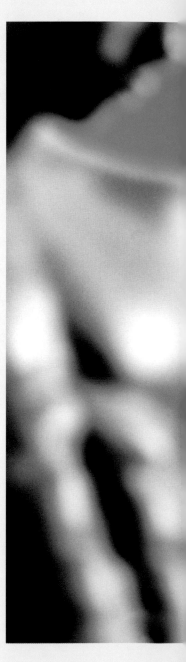

Recovery days

When exercising regularly, it is important to allow recovery days because the muscles continue to tone in recovery. In fact, this rest time is when the repair work is done. It is also vital not to become exercise-obsessive—a common syndrome today. Allowing yourself to rest for a day can be hard, as the desire to make it to the gym can overshadow the need to allow the body time to recuperate. This is all part of the discipline and will only add to your overall fitness. Of course, even on recovery days, gentle stretching after warming up is still recommended, as is walking, yoga, or any activity that you find comfortable and which does not stress your muscles, heart, or lungs.

Jogging five miles a day and training for a marathon or triathalon may feel like the right thing for you, but starting with gentle walking, rehabilitation, and strengthening exercises is much more sensible and beneficial. If you notice any pain or weakness in any part of your body once you start exercising, then you should stop or modify the exercises and get medical attention.

With cardiovascular exercise, get a good health check in order to find out whether or not you are overdoing it and potentially leading to, or causing, injury. A simple test that you can do for yourself is the "talk test." If you have difficulty talking during or immediately after exercise, then you may need to slow down and decrease the intensity.

Be realistic regarding the amount of time and energy you can put into an exercise program. Don't set impossible goals: do something you enjoy and can stick to relatively easily, until it becomes as much a part of your daily routine as showering and eating. If your goal is to lose weight, don't go crazy in the first week, exercising several hours every day and starving yourself. You will almost certainly find yourself unable to stick to such a regime and you could seriously injure yourself by pushing your body too hard and too fast.

Devise a plan that fits in with your lifestyle. Managing your time may seem impossible, but even just 20 minutes of exercise can usually be found in at some point during the day. Increase the goals as your fitness levels increase and gradually build up to an acceptable, manageable level, with the guidance of a qualified instructor where necessary. Plan to exercise for one hour, three or four times a week, and eat sensibly. Don't skip lunch for exercise.

THE GOLDEN RULES OF EXERCISE

No matter what exercise or movement program you subscribe to, there are a few important rules you need to remember. For a healthy, balanced life and wellbeing through exercise:

- Be safe rather than sorry. When in doubt, do nothing.
- Warm up before exercise; cool down after.
- To avoid injury, stretch after warming up and after cooling down.
- Allow yourself to go slowly and gently, whatever exercise you take.
- Make gradual improvements rather than quantum leaps in your physical achievements.
- Breathe properly—evenly and deeply—when exercising, using the exhale for that extra effort or stretch.
- Never overstrain: listen to and watch yourself. Forget about the culture of competition: this is only about you and your body and no one can know better how you feel than you! Work at your own level and pace.
- Be aware of your posture: shoulders down and relaxed, stomach gently pulled in.
- Do your exercises with care, control, and concentration.

ASSESSING YOUR PRESENT PHYSICAL STATE

Before commencing any fitness program, it is important to identify any medical conditions or muscular-skeletal injuries or imbalances that may be aggravated by certain forms of exercise. If you have any doubts regarding your health, or are a man over 40 or a woman over 45, or any of the following apply to you, then seeking medical advice before embarking on a fitness program is advisable.

- A history of heart problems, chest pain, or stroke.

- A history of heart problems in the immediate family.

- High blood pressure.

- Any chronic illness or condition.

- Recent surgery (within the last 12 months).

- Pregnancy (now or within the last three months).

- A history of breathing or lung problems.

- Diabetes or thyroid condition.

- You are a smoker.

- Obesity (more than 20 percent above ideal body weight).

- High blood cholesterol.

- Hernia or any condition aggravated by lifting heavy weights.

- Muscle, joint, or back problems, or any previous injury still affecting you.

After assessing your present physical state, the next important step is to define your goals.

core training

Over the past few years the buzzword of the fitness and physical therapy industries has been 'core training'. Many fitness gurus believe this is the safer way to build a stronger body and at the same time reduce the risk of injury. The 'core' refers to the body's trunk and pelvis and the core muscle group consists of the abdominals, glutes, obliques and lower back muscles. The purpose of core training is to stabilize and strengthen these trunk and pelvis muscles.

The body has three layers of abdominal musculature in front of the spine and an intricate network of deep and superficial muscles in the back. In most people, these muscle groups are under developed and the weakness of these muscles is the cause of many back problems. By strengthening the core of the body, we can enable everything else to function better and longer. Pilates, yoga and many other kinds of exercise are forms of core training. Correct core training will help you use your body in new and safer ways by creating a stronger and more functional frame.

As with any form of exercise, it is important to create a realistic exercise schedule that fits in with your lifestyle – one that you can stick to and that will become an intrinsic element of your everyday life. Build up this exercise schedule slowly, safely and gradually. Exercise should be entertaining, not an ordeal, but make it non-negotiable – think of it as something you do without question, like going to work. Make it a habit!

GENERAL TIPS FOR EVERYDAY EXERCISE AND POSTURE

- Walk to work when possible.
- Get up from your desk every 15 minutes or so to stretch your back and legs.
- Check your desk positioning. Are you slouching because of a chair that is too high or too low?
- Make sure your back is supported.
- If you are on your feet all day, try to give your legs a break to prevent swelling in the ankles and knees. Always wear well-fitting shoes. Sit with feet up and ankles above the knees to assist in blood flow, which acts against gravity in the legs. Rotate ankles, knees, and hips.
- People on their feet and walking a lot may develop lower back problems, especially if walking on hard surfaces, like concrete and wood. Rotate hips and then lengthen spine by standing on tiptoes and stretching arms into the air.
- Driving long distances creates an imbalanced use of the legs and spine, which are often incorrectly supported. When possible, stop the car, get out and walk, even if only for ten minutes every hour or so. Legs also need stretching to avoid tight ligaments or tendons.

good posture before exercise

THE GOLDEN RULES OF GOOD POSTURE

- Feet: stand barefoot, hip-width apart, both pointing forward.
- Spine: lengthen and relax, imagine a line traveling from your head down to the feet.
- Do not flatten natural curves at waist and neck.
- Lengthen the back of the neck.
- Lift up your chin and keep your shoulders down and back.
- Gently ease the shoulders down. Do NOT hold them rigidly.
- Shake out both arms and allow them to hang by your sides; don't hold them rigidly.
- Tilt your pelvis back and forth, until comfortable.
- Keep knees soft.

Good posture can help the body to function better, minimize stress on the spine, and make you look slimmer and healthier. When maintained throughout exercise, it also reduces the risk of muscular imbalances that can lead to injury. Good posture will give you a sense of freedom, grace, and ease of movement.

Posture awareness and correction are integral parts of any exercise program. Gaining and maintaining a good posture requires a certain amount of vigilance and awareness of your daily habits and lifestyle. Improving your posture will increase your energy levels,

Because all nerves travel down through the spinal column and send messages to the brain via the medulla oblongata, a poorly aligned spine will distort the messages they carry. The body's muscular-skeletal systems will overcompensate for poor spinal alignment by tensing—potentially causing the spine to adopt a permanent, though not irreversible, curvature, which will then need a concentrated effort with physiotherapy to correct.

Look at the way children move. Children naturally have perfect posture. To check your posture, begin by standing with bare feet hip-width apart and both pointing forward. Good posture starts with the feet. Be aware of the positioning. Is one foot slightly forward? One turned in and the other turned out? Correct the imbalance. This may feel uncomfortable at first, but persevere until this standing position becomes natural to you.

Next work up the legs. Be aware of any other imbalances. Is one hip sticking out more than the other? Look in a full-length mirror when checking your posture, since ingrained imbalances can often feel quite normal.

The next—and very important—stage of posture checking is with the spine and pelvis. Many imbalances in the rest of the body are caused by misalignments in the spine. If you notice anything serious, then seek the advice of a specialist. A good way to check your alignment is to place a book on your head. A basic rule of posture is that the head, shoulders, and hips should all be in the same vertical plane, in line with each other.

Tension in muscles causes "knots" to develop and creates countertension in surrounding and related areas. Therefore, a misaligned spine can affect the lungs, neck, and brain—even thought processes will be negatively affected if there is excess tension in certain muscles.

All muscles and the entire skeleton, as well as all the body's internal organs, will improve from postural realignment and correction. The increased sense of wellbeing and energy gained from working on the posture will encourage you to be aware of your body at all times, leading to new and improved habits that soon become second nature.

Once you have found the correct posture, it is important to strengthen the muscles that hold you in position, especially those in the stomach and lower back.

The most central structural part of the human body is the spinal column; it is made up of 26 articulated bones, part of a system of 33 small bones called vertebrae that are held together and supported by muscles and ligaments. Most of the vertebrae are separated by discs made of tough, fibrous tissue, which act as protective shock absorbers.

The spinal column serves as the main support to the body and as a protective cover for the spinal cord, the lower part of the central nervous system, running from the base of the skull down to the lumbar region.

The spine is actually the first part of the body to be formed after conception. Indeed, possessing a spinal column with vertebrae capable of a turning movement is what distinguishes

GENERAL TIPS ON POSTURE

- **WALKING:** Keep the head and body balanced, looking ahead. Move from the thighs, as though propelled from behind. Swing arms rhythmically.
- **SITTING:** Make use of the support provided by your chair. Sit back. Lengthen the spine and allow it to be fully supported. Balance the hips evenly with both feet on the ground. Keep feet flat on the floor and don't cross your legs. When leaning forward, do so from the hips, not curving the shoulders and slouching.
- **LYING DOWN:** Keep the spine long. Do not twist. Keep the body symmetrical and lie on your back when possible. If lying on your side, do not bend the legs too high to the chest and keep the back straight. Do not use too many pillows, because this unnaturally curves the neck and spine, and can lead to tension and headaches.

- Stand straight with the shoulders relaxed and firmly supporting the neck and head, stomach held in (but not too tense or tight). Holding a firm, centered, straight, but not rigid, spine, neck, and head is an important exercise in its own right.
- Both overarching your back and collapsing into a curved slump are bad for back health, causing strain by throwing you off balance. Your weight should be balanced between both feet.
- Sleep on a firm mattress.
- When lifting anything heavy, don't bend over from the waist or stoop down and hunch your back. Always bend the knees and get down as close to the object you are lifting as possible. Keep your back straight and use your leg muscles when lifting. Hold the object close to you when carrying it any distance.
- When carrying anything heavy, always distribute the weight as evenly as possible. Don't carry heavy loads that will strain your neck, shoulders, or back. Use a cart with wheels instead.
- Make sure that your office chair provides you with the right support. Remember: you spend a lot of time in that chair!
- Those who slave before a computer for long periods should move around or stretch every 15 to 20 minutes.
- Get your work heights right. Stooping over a work surface too low for your height can be bad for your back.
- Do stretching exercises regularly to reach and maintain your optimum degree of suppleness.
- Always warm up before you exercise.
- Avoid being overweight: this is never easy on the back.
- Avoid wearing high heels, wedges, or platforms. These shoes force an imbalance in the alignment of the spine and throws good posture out.
- Aromatherapy and massage treatments are the best gifts you can give a stressed back.
- Osteopathy and cranial osteopathy are excellent for redressing the balance of a back and neck that are out of alignment.

"When a man is born, he is soft and flexible;
When he dies, he grows hard and rigid.
So it is with all things under Heaven,
Plants and animals are soft and pliant in life;
But brittle and dry in death.
Truly, to be hard and rigid is the way of death;
To be soft and flexible is the way of life."

TAO TEH CHING

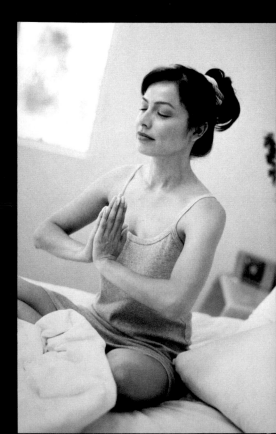

"higher animals" from the rest—hence the term "vertebrates." Humans are the only vertebrates that stand absolutely erect. It is the distinctive characteristics of the spine that enable us to carry ourselves upright and make us capable of an enormous range of movement.

Backache affects at least 80 percent of the population. If you are in the habit of getting regular exercise, you are probably in the 20 percent of the population not suffering from some kind of back pain. Most health professionals are aware of the great value of exercise in preventing spinal problems, but getting patients to participate in a regular exercise program is not an easy feat!

Back pain is often due to weakness in the ligaments and muscles, and the spasms that result when unused bits are jolted into action! Your movement becomes restricted when unused ligaments shorten. Ligaments are sheets or bands of fibrous tissue that connect two or more bones. As you get older, the backbone stiffens because the ligaments become tighter and shorter. However, this does not have to happen. The best way to keep your spine flexible is by keeping to a regular exercise and stretching program that suits your needs.

Part of the reason for yoga's surging popularity in the West is that the secret is out! Yogic posture (see page 168) focuses considerably on spinal mobility and ligament flexibility, and many of the poses were designed specifically with the spine in mind. A key belief in yoga is that a pliable spine is the key to long life.

Back injuries are the number-one health hazard at work. Billions of dollars in work days are lost every year due to back injuries. Many large companies are addressing this problem with screening and preventative programs—and saving lots of money as a result. Some of them organize yoga and exercise classes at the workplace, while others give employees time off from work to attend some kind of exercise class. Still other companies arrange for massage experts to visit their premises to help staff relax and loosen the spine through massage therapy. These employers know that any kind of physical activity, like walking, or even massage, is far more beneficial to back pain sufferers than drugs or rest.

The couch-potato lifestyle is responsible for all these weak, sloppy spines. At the root of the problem is too little exercise and too much stress—not to mention fashion fascism (the vogue for stiletto and platform shoes is guaranteed to give you back problems if you wear them for more than five minutes after the age of 19!). Weak muscles lead to back pain. To prevent back injury, alleviate pain, and restore your body's balance, you must exercise to strengthen your back.

Regular exercise reaps real rewards and allows you to reach your optimal spinal flexibility. Choose an activity you really enjoy. Walking, dancing, stretching, rebounding, or swimming are all excellent ways to keep in shape. And, of course, yoga and pilates classes can really help. The choice is yours, and so is the opportunity to avoid losing flexibility and mobility throughout life.

warm up and cool down for safe exercise

Although often neglected, warming up and stretching the body to prepare gradually for more intensive exercise, and then cooling down afterward, are essential ingredients of any fitness regime and highly valuable for injury prevention.

Try not to do any intensive stretches right after waking up. The muscles, joints, and ligaments are especially tight in the morning. Wait for at least an hour after getting up before undertaking any deep stretches or conditioning exercises.

A warm-up should be at least five minutes long and, depending on the type of activity performed, should include stretches for those body parts most under stress during the given activity.

Alternatively, go for a brisk walk for at least five minutes. This will get the blood circulating around the body, raise the body temperature, and give the synovial fluid around the joints a chance to start circulating, producing a cushioning effect around the joints and softening the ligaments in preparation for more vigorous exercise. If you are doing a running workout, then a good warm-up is to walk briskly or march on the spot for about five minutes, and then do stretches for the calves, hamstrings, and quadriceps.

When the workout is over, cool down gradually to bring the heart rate down to normal slowly, preventing pooling of blood in the legs.

The best way to cool down is to reduce the intensity of the exercise. For example, run, bicycle, or swim at a slower pace, or walk for five minutes, until breathing is back to normal. Then you can stretch the muscles again that were first stretched in the warm-up, holding the stretches for a few seconds longer than earlier. This helps avoid the build-up of lactic acid and lengthens the muscles, helping to prevent muscle soreness and fatigue.

After walking on the spot in either the warm-up or cool-down stages, try shaking out your whole body, hands, arms, and legs. Then stand stationary, with feet hip-width apart and both pointing forward, keeping the knees soft and slightly bent. Keep the feet firmly planted on the floor and, without letting the area below the hips move, swing your arms from side to side, twisting the torso and loosening the spine. Continue this stretch for about 30 seconds to a minute.

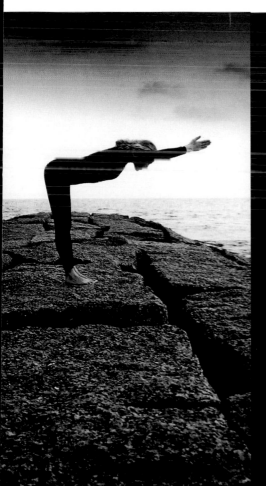

WARM-UP EXERCISES FOR THE SPINE

Head rolls

Sit comfortably with a supported back that is straight, but not rigid and tense—a gentle straightness. Shoulders should be relaxed and hands gently resting on the thighs. Gently drop your chin to the chest and slowly move the head all the way around, first clockwise and then, gently, counterclockwise. Don't let the head roll back, especially if you have neck or shoulder injuries. Repeat twice. The exercise softly massages the upper part of the spine; if you feel and hear a lot of inner crackling, that's the natural by-product of a good neck-and-shoulder massage.

Knee hug and roll

Sitting on the floor, cross your feet and draw the knees to the chest, holding onto your feet or ankles in a relaxed, but firm, knee-hug, and with the chin dropped right down and tucked into the chest. If you are comfortable and supple enough to go onto the next phase, gently roll back as far as you can go without strain, and then slowly roll forward to a sitting position.

stretching, strength & stamina

Good physical fitness is a condition that results from the development of an optimal level of muscular strength, cardiovascular stamina, and flexibility and stretching. These are the three "S"s to remember: strength, stamina, and stretching.

As we age, our bodies inevitably deteriorate, and we realize that tasks we used to find easy become more difficult. Even something as simple as bending down to tie shoelaces is a task that requires flexibility. To stop this gradual deterioration and to enhance your present lifestyle, it is necessary to train your body in each of these three important disciplines.

Stretching for wellbeing

Flexibility is defined as the range of motion of a given joint; inflexibility increases the risk of joint and muscle injury. In order to perform everyday tasks and activities well, such as reaching up for a high object or bending down to pick something up, you must be able to move through the motions specific to the activity with ease and fluidity. You could be very flexible in one area, even "double jointed," but inflexible in another. Attaining overall flexibility is the end goal. With continued practice, your joints will become more supple.

Yoga, stretching, and Pilates are all excellent for increasing flexibility. With training, flexibility can and should be developed at all ages. Flexibility does not necessarily develop at the same rate in everyone. In general, the older you are, the longer it will take to develop the desired level of flexibility. Older people may have to work harder if they have led very sedentary lifestyles, especially if joint stiffening has already become a problem, but perseverance always pays off. Hopefully, though, the wisdom that comes with advancing years will lend a more patient and self-loving attitude to continued exercise.

Stamina or cardiovascular fitness

This describes the health and function of the heart, lungs, and circulatory systems, particularly the ability of the lungs to provide oxygen to the blood and the ability of the circulatory system to carry blood and nutrients to tissues in the body for long periods. It is this process that allows us to sustain any activity for an extended period without excessive fatigue.

There are many benefits to improving one's cardiovascular fitness or stamina. It helps lower blood pressure, strengthens the heart and lungs, increases the ability to burn body fat, helps lower blood cholesterol, and gives you more energy for everyday tasks, like walking up steps.

The principles of basic stamina training are pretty straightforward: at least three times a week you should move continuously and use the large muscles, such as the legs and arms, to keep the heart rate raised for at least 20 minutes. When exercising, you should feel a little bit breathless, but still be able to hold a conversation.

Types of stamina training

Walking, running, jogging, bicycling, swimming, rowing, and aerobic classes are all very good forms of stamina training, as are any athletic sports that involve running or where the heart rate is increased, such as basketball, soccer, and hockey. The key is finding the activity you enjoy and one which is suitable for your body type. If you like, you can cross-train by doing several different activities. In any given week, for example, one day could be devoted to an aerobics class, a second day to swimming, and a third day spent walking.

It doesn't really matter how you combine activities, as long as you adhere to the basic rules of keeping your heart rate elevated for 20 minutes or more, at least three days a week. Avoid overtraining, however, because the body needs at least one day a week for rest and recovery. Also try to alternate your sessions; do not do the same exercises for two or three days consecutively, as you will be overtraining the same muscle groups and could cause imbalance in other muscles, or strain on the muscles repeatedly exercised.

PRINCIPLES OF BASIC STAMINA TRAINING

At least three times a week move continuously, using the large muscles, such as the legs and arms, to keep the heart rate raised for a minimum of 20 minutes. While exercising, you should feel a little breathless, but not so much that you could not talk, if necessary.

basic exercise
program

stretches

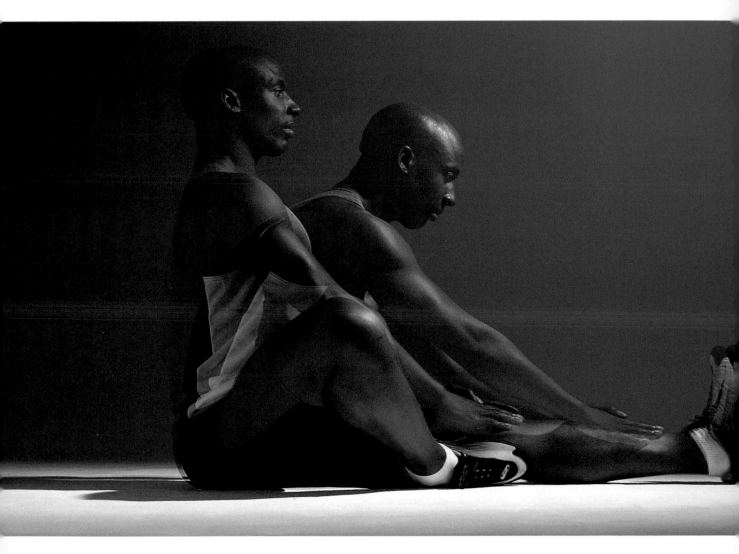

Hamstring Stretch

Stretch your left leg straight out in front, bend the right leg and lean forward from the hips, as if you are about to sit down, sticking out the buttocks. Rest your hands on the right knee for support, making sure both feet stay flat on the floor. Hold for 15 to 20 seconds, and then swap sides.

Calf Stretch

From standing, bend the right knee out in front and stretch the left leg behind you—your feet should be far enough apart that you can comfortably keep your back leg straight. Both feet should be flat on the floor, with the heels firmly planted. Lean forward, keeping the stomach and back straight, and rest your hands on your right knee. Hold for 15 to 20 seconds. Come back up to standing and swap legs. This exercise can also be done with the hands pressed against a wall, or holding onto the back of a chair for support.

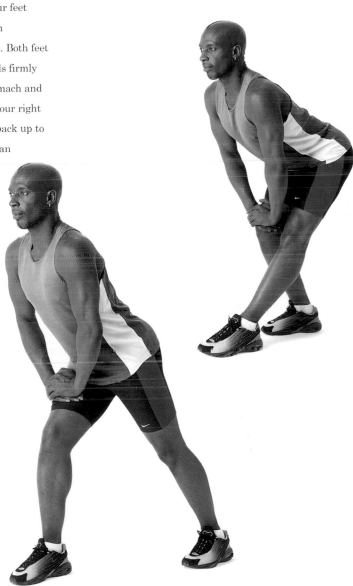

Lower Back Stretch

Sit on the floor with your left leg stretched out in front of you and the right knee bent, so that the right sole rests against the inner left knee (see left). Let the bent knee drop toward the floor to expose the inner thigh. Bend gently forward from the hips over the left leg, keeping the back as straight as possible and bending the left knee if necessary. Hold for 15 to 30 seconds, and then swap sides.

Posture Check and Shoulder Roll

These exercises will help you to correct poor posture and relieve pressure on the spine and neck. Sit on the floor in any comfortable position—either with knees bent outward and feet together and drawn in toward you, or with legs crossed—with the spine erect (see right), as if you were sitting with your back against a wall. (Try sitting against a wall first, to test how this feels.) Keeping your stomach pulled in and the back straight, slowly raise shoulders up toward the ears in a rolling motion, first forward, then back, 4 to 8 times in each direction. Return the shoulders to their natural position, then roll the head, first to the left, then forward, then to the right. DO NOT LET THE HEAD ROLL BACK or force it into any uncomfortable pose because this may strain the neck; allow the head's natural weight to stretch the neck and release tension in the shoulders and upper back. Repeat 8 times.

correct posture

incorrect posture

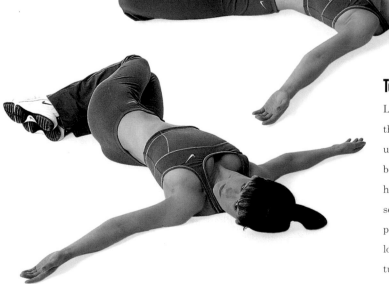

Torso Stretch

Lie on your back with knees bent up and the arms stretched out to the sides, palms up and level with the shoulders. Lower both knees slowly to the left, and turn the head to the right. Hold for 15 to 20 seconds, then return to the starting position. Repeat for the other side, lowering the knees to the right and turning the head to the left.

Inner Thigh Stretch

Sit up straight with the legs stretched
out to the sides (see above), as wide
as comfortable and with feet relaxed.
If this position is uncomfortable, try
this alternative (see right): bend the
knees and place the soles of
the feet together, drawing
them slightly in to the body
and letting the knees drop
open and down to the floor. In
either position, bend slowly forward
from the hips, keeping the back as
straight as possible. Hold for 15 to
20 seconds, then release.

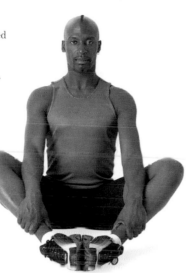

Modified Cobra

If you have a history of lower back pain, do this
exercise very gently and carefully. Lie on your
stomach with the elbows and forearms resting on
the floor and tucked closely into the body. Palms
should be face down and pointing forward, and
elbows roughly in line with shoulders. As you
inhale, push the floor away with the arms, slowly
raising the upper torso as far as the hips—the lower
abdomen and thighs should remain in contact with
the floor. Hold the pose for 5 to 10 seconds, but
release earlier if it becomes uncomfortable.
(The full Cobra is pictured on page 175.)

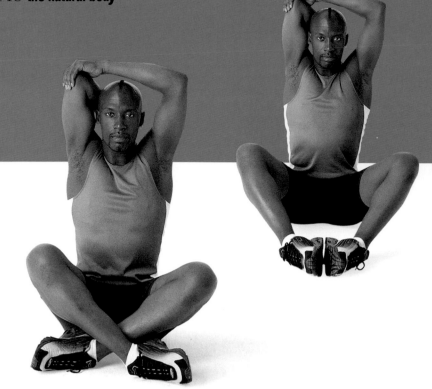

Tricep Stretch

This exercise can be done standing up, sitting on a chair, or on the floor, either with legs crossed (see far left) or with feet together and knees bent outward (see left). Choose whichever position is most comfortable for you. Stretch your right arm above your head, then bend the elbow, bringing the palm down to rest on the left shoulder blade. Grip the right elbow with your free hand and pull the arm to the left until you feel a gentle stretch in the upper arm. Hold for 15 to 20 seconds, and repeat for the other arm.

Hip Stretch

Lie on your back with knees bent and feet flat on the floor, a short distance from the buttocks (see top left). Keep your left foot firmly planted and raise your right leg to rest the right foot on the left knee, letting the right knee drop open. If comfortable, grip the left thigh and pull it gently in toward the body, letting the left foot come off the ground (see left). Hold for 15 to 20 seconds, and then repeat for the other leg.

Pelvic Tilt

This exercise is to prepare for the
abdominal strengthening exercises in the
next section, and ideally should be done with the basic crunch (see page
150). Stay lying on your back with bent knees, as in the hip stretch
(see below left). Exhale and contract the stomach muscles, pressing the
lower back gently into the floor and squeezing the buttocks—you should feel
the stomach hollow out slightly (see top right). When you have squeezed in
as tightly as you can without straining, release the contraction and return
to the starting position, relaxing the buttocks and visualizing the stomach
flattening along the spine. Repeat 20 to 30 times.

Quadricep Stretch

This stretch requires some balance, so to begin with use a wall
or other solid object—maybe a chair back—for support, or even
do the exercise lying down (see below). Stand with feet close
together and pointing forward. Bend the left leg up behind you
and hold the foot with your left hand to stretch the front thigh.
If you aren't holding on for support, stretch the right arm to the
side at shoulder level for balance (see right). Hold for 15 to 20
seconds, and then release and swap legs.

strengthening exercises

Basic Crunch

Lie on your back, knees bent and feet hip-width apart, contracting the abdominal muscles to press the lower back gently against the floor. Clasp the hands lightly behind the back of the head—don't grip too hard or you may strain the neck.

Inhale; then exhale as you slowly raise your head and shoulders, keeping the abdomen pulled in tight at all times. Don't try to lift too high—if you can't control the popping-out action of the stomach muscles, you'll know you've gone too far—and resist the urge to drop back into the starting position. Don't let your feet and knees move around during the exercise, but keep them firmly in place. Repeat 10 to 30 times.

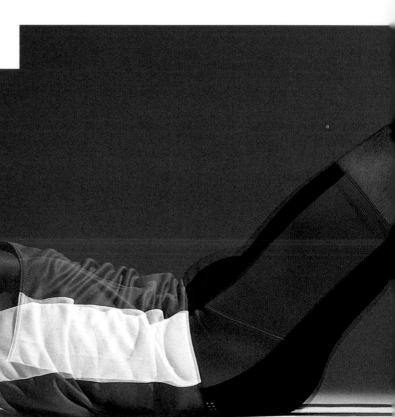

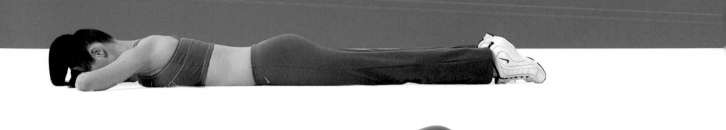

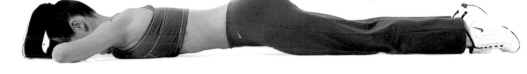

Pulling In

Lie face down on the floor with the forehead resting on the hands (palms down) and the feet shoulder-width apart (see top). Inhale; as you exhale, contract the abdomen, pulling it away from the ground in a movement similar to the pelvic tilt, while keeping the rest of the body still (see above). The movement is very slight—only your stomach should leave the floor—but very effective. Hold each contraction for 10 to 20 seconds and repeat 5 to 10 times.

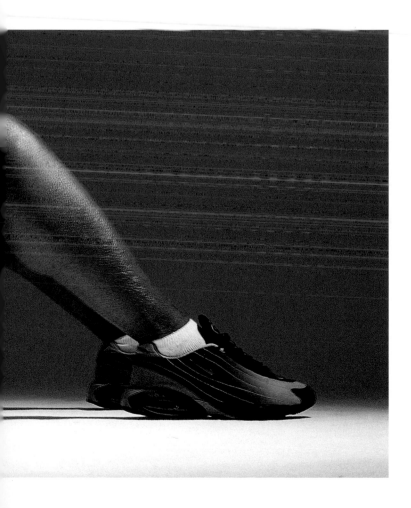

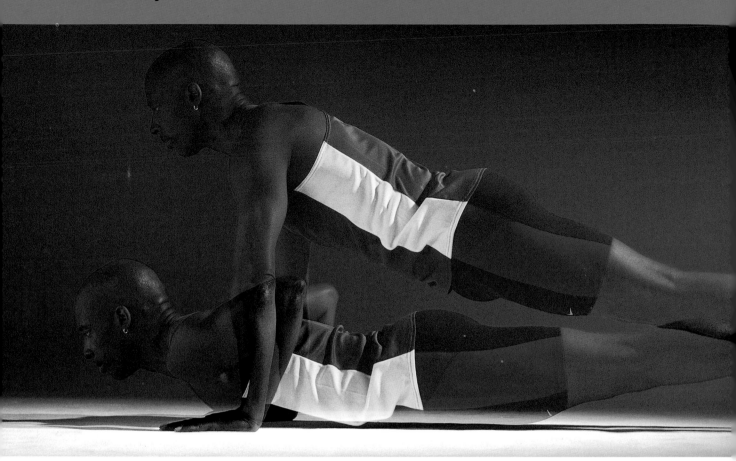

Lower Back Strengthener

Lie face down with your arms and legs extended and palms down. Slowly raise the left arm and leg away from the floor, keeping them straight and keeping the torso in contact with the floor. Hold for 5 seconds, and then slowly return to the starting position. Repeat about 5 times, alternating sides.

Push-Up

Only do this version of the exercise when you can do the push-up comfortably (as shown below). In this exercise, only the hands and toes touch the ground, and the back should be kept straight with the neck and spine aligned. Lower the chest to the ground, then return to the starting position; repeat the exercise 10 to 20 times.

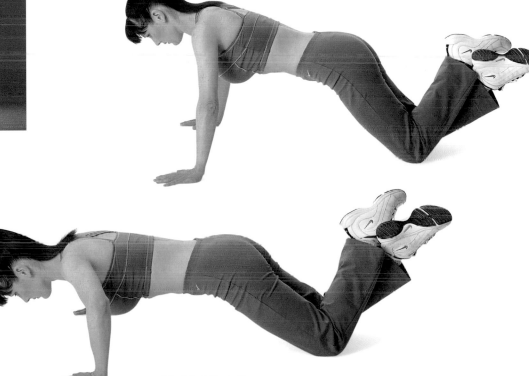

Modified Push-Up

Kneel down and rest forward on the hands, which should be slightly wider than shoulder-width apart. Keep the neck and spine in line, with the back straight and the stomach tucked in. Lower the chest to the floor by bending the elbows, then return to the starting position. Repeat 10 to 20 times, resting in between if necessary.

Inner Thigh Workout

Lie on your right side with the right leg extended in line with the body and the left knee bent, with the foot in front of the right knee and the sole flat on the floor. Keep the stomach pulled in tightly as you stretch the right leg away from the hip, flexing the foot—imagine a thread running from your hip being pulled through the heel. Raise and lower the right leg, pausing at the top of the movement. Keep the leg straight and don't let the foot touch the floor during repetitions. Repeat 20 to 30 times, and then swap sides.

Hamstring Curl

Lie on your right side, as in the inner thigh workout (see right), and bend the knees in front of you, so that the thighs sit at a right angle to the torso (see below). Raise the left leg two or three inches to separate the knees and, keeping the thighs in line and stationary, straighten the left leg and flex the foot, without locking the knee. Keeping the left thigh stationary, bring the lower left leg back, heel toward the buttocks, and straighten up to the starting position. Repeat 15 to 30 times, and then swap sides.

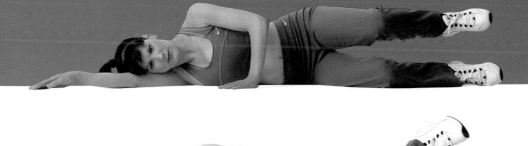

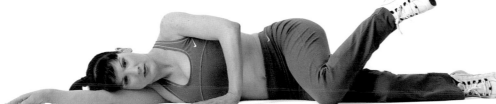

Butt Blast

Lie on your right side, knees bent in front of the body and slightly apart (see top). Lower the left knee to touch the ground in front of the right knee, then return to the starting position. Keep the movements flowing and don't let the knees touch. Repeat 15 to 30 times, and then swap sides.

Outer Thigh Toner

Lie on your right side with the knees bent, as in the butt blast (see left). Extend the left leg in front of you, thighs parallel and knees slightly apart (see below). Steadily raise and lower the left leg, keeping the torso stationary. Repeat 15 to 30 times, and then change sides.

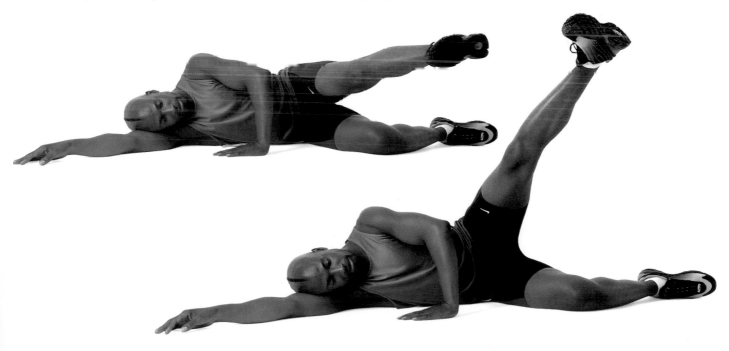

walking for a healthy heart

WALKING IS MORE THAN JUST GOOD EXERCISE!

In a study of sedentary women in California who followed a 15-week regime of walking 45 minutes a day for five days a week, their levels of antibodies increased 20 percent—and if they did come down with colds and flu, these lasted half as long.

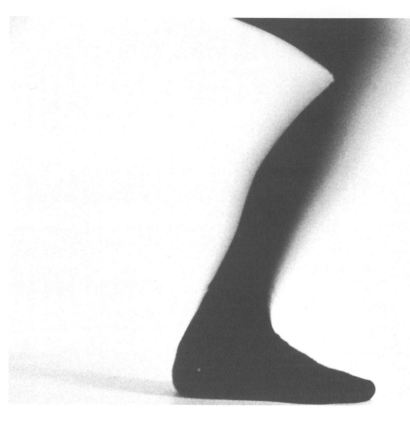

Walking is one of the best, safest, and most natural forms of exercise. You can, in fact, walk your way to a healthier, stronger cardiovascular system. Walking is effective exercise for people of all ages and all states and levels of health. What's more, walking increases your sense of wellbeing. Think about it—we were actually designed for lengthy, regular walking.

Walking is the most underrated exercise and yet the most effective; it is the best starting point if you haven't exercised recently. One of the easiest and safest ways to get and keep fit is a brisk walk of 20 minutes, three times a week. Studies show that regular brisk walking can lower cholesterol levels, stimulate circulation, strengthen the heart, help control weight, reduce high blood pressure, stress, and depression, improve mental alertness and memory, prevent osteoporosis, and develop strength, stamina, and endurance. New research also suggests walking is the best exercise for the brain. The brain is nourished by blood sugar, and walking, unlike high-aerobic exercise, does not rely on blood sugar for energy.

If you haven't taken any exercise for a while, then start off gradually by strolling with a little more determination and a little longer than normal, slowly building up your endurance level. A good idea is to start walking at a fairly relaxed pace until you have warmed up, before graduating to a really brisk gait.

- Strolling walk: walking in a relaxed way, but with good posture, the shoulders down and arms swinging naturally as you walk.
- Brisk walk: fitness, pace, or aerobic walking all mean pretty much the same thing, stepping up the pace and pumping the arms as you walk.
- Power walk: for a very fit, younger, experienced walker, usually working with a personal trainer. Walking with weights, carrying them in the hands and/or strapping them on the waist and ankles.
- Water walk: walking (wading) through water, either in a pool or in the sea. Walking hip- to waist-high in water is a good, low-stress, high-intensity exercise. For greater resistance, run in the water, but you will need a flotation vest or belt to keep you in an upright position.
- Treadmill walk: most gyms have treadmills, but many people are buying home versions that chart distance and speed, and time the walk.

You need to be prepared for walking

If you are doing a lot of serious, committed walking, then you might want to buy a pair of shoes that are actually designed for the purpose. When you walk you land with 1¼ times your body weight on the outside of your heels, then you roll your weight forward on the ball of your foot. A good walking shoe will ease the rolling action of the foot. Older people may be more stable in a shoe with a thinner, hard sole. You should also wear comfortable clothes, which won't restrict your movements. In winter, wear layers that you can peel off as you warm up.

Walking is the most natural, practical, and straightforward preventative exercise program. The ultimate safe, natural fitness routine, walking builds body strength, stamina, and tone. It also works to de-stress you—which is good for the heart and the nervous system. In the later years, it helps slow down the aging process, keeping you fit, agile, and mobile. Walking also allows you to develop better coordination, breath control, self-esteem, and endurance.

Walking should be the primary part of your fitness routine, no matter what other exercise systems, movements, or sports you are involved in. Walk first, then run or dance, take an exercise class, or ride a bike. It's up to you—you can bicycle until you're blue in the face and you still won't get all the benefits you get from a brisk, long walk. If your walking muscles atrophy, the rest of your body will soon follow. Brisk walking is the greatest form of exercise: it is a natural, basic, lifelong conditioning program, protecting the heart and enhancing wellbeing.

TIPS FOR HEALTHY WALKING

- Drink water before and after walking. If very thirsty, stop to drink during the walk.
- Don't walk right after a meal. Leave at least 45 to 60 minutes after eating before going for a brisk walk.
- Avoid the hottest hours of the day (noon to 3:00 p.m.). The ideal time is morning or late afternoon.
- After a long or brisk walk, it is wise to eat some form of carbohydrate within a couple of hours to restore your glycogen levels.
- In summer, if you are taking longer walks, protect your skin with sunscreen. Use sunglasses or a visor to protect your eyes in extremely sunny weather.
- If brisk walking is uncomfortable, alternate it with slower walking.

in the swim

After walking, the next best activity you can do for your body is to swim on a regular basis. Swimming is an enjoyable and safe way of exercising, providing all the aerobic benefits of, for example, running and bicycling without the same wear and tear on the muscles, joints, and bones. Swimming several lengths gives an excellent aerobic workout by exercising most of your major muscle groups.

The natural resistance of water strengthens and tones the muscles, joints, and bones without the risk of injury that is present when you exercise on land. Water is about 1,000 times more dense than air, which is why it offers considerable resistance, resulting in a "double positive" effect on your body. It exercises opposing sets of muscles at the same time—for example, the front and back of your arms in the same movement. Swimming is the ideal exercise for body-conditioning without the sweat. From a body-sculpting point of view, swimming doesn't encourage bulking of muscles; in fact, with the added resistance of the water, muscles often become lean, rather like those of runners. Just walking in water is a fantastic exercise for building up endurance. Walk as briskly as you can in waist- or chest-high water.

Swimming and other water exercises are considered so much safer than working out on the ground or in the gym because water is the perfect cushion of support, allowing you to feel almost weightless. As your body is 90 percent lighter in the water, you are more buoyant and therefore there is much less pressure on your joints than there would be in the gym.

The impact of cold water and the pressure of the water also promotes blood circulation in the muscles. The pulse is slowed down, and there is quicker recovery from exertion than when exercising on land. Despite the exhaustion that can be experienced through exertion, the pleasant tiredness created leaves you feeling very good and, invariably, very relaxed and refreshed.

In fact, swimming is excellent for relaxation, not least because of the enforced deep breathing necessary. Some people even compare it to moving meditation; the sensation of being supported by water, the quiet and freedom experienced by the body while gliding through the water, all add to the sense of inner calm often experienced by those who meditate. Staying focused on the swim encourages the quieting of the mind and forces out all external influences. The natural support of water usually has a very comforting and relaxing effect on your state of mind. As your mind calms down, so does your whole body, improving and massaging the muscles as you effortlessly move through the water.

Water exercise is also excellent for the injured, the disabled, the elderly, and mothers-to-be, because no additional stress is placed on the joints when moving

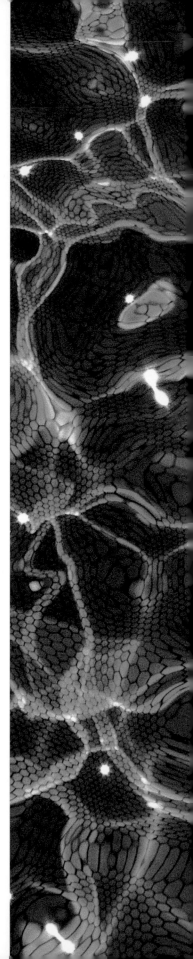

through the water—it is a low-impact exercise. This is the most painless way to exercise, which is why it is recommended for so many health conditions. Water therapy and exercises are beneficial for those suffering from lower back problems, osteoarthritis, and hip injuries; they are also employed for the rehabilitation of serious injuries and to help disabling diseases. After walking, it is the best form of exercise for preventing degenerative health conditions, and a wonderful way of moving, enabling you to maintain the wellbeing of both body and mind throughout life.

Swimming can be enjoyed by people of all ages and levels of ability. Children usually love water from a very early age, and encouraging children to find their feet in water when very young will allay any potential fears of water which they may develop later on. Once children have taught their bodies how to float, there's no stopping them. So much fun can be had just by splashing around and floating, or jumping in, until children are ready to take on the structure of learning different strokes.

The elderly, or those otherwise less mobile, can also benefit greatly from sessions in the pool. The relaxing state of simply *being* in water will induce a feeling of calm. Even if you cannot swim, working out in the shallow end can be highly advantageous to health. Of course, people of any age can enjoy the benefits of learning to swim, even if they have not had the pleasure from childhood. Many pools offer classes for children and adults, from complete beginners to experienced veterans.

It is important to remember that swimming is an exercise like any other, and warm-ups and stretches are just as relevant here as if you were running five miles on a treadmill. Warming up could consist of one lap, followed by stretches of the shoulders, arms, and upper back.

All warm-ups and stretches can be done in the water, and once in the water, it is advisable not to get out until ready to shower, dry, and get dressed again. The muscles cool down rapidly when you get out of the water, which could cause potential problems. Remember to make sure you cool down at the end of your swimming session by

THE BENEFITS OF SWIMMING

- Strengthens the cardiovascular and respiratory systems.
- Maintains and develops bones and muscles.
- Builds stamina and endurance.
- Gentle whole-body exercise with high aerobic value.
- Increases your general level of fitness and wellbeing.
- Maintains flexibility and muscle tone.
- Stimulates the circulation.
- The horizontal position places less stress on your heart in respect of blood circulation.
- Gentle pressure of water on the skin enhances blood circulation.
- The cardiovascular benefits are essentially the same as for running or walking, with all the major muscle groups being worked.
- Lowers blood pressure.
- Water resistance helps to build up muscle strength.
- Weightlessness in water allows effective stretching, using the water as support.
- Excellent for maintaining flexibility and suppleness.
- Creates lean muscles and not heavy, bulky muscles.
- Rehabilitates injured or weakened muscles.
- Speeds up the healing process.
- Relaxes and refreshes the mind.
- Good for overweight people because the body weight is well supported.
- Safe for pregnant women throughout all stages of pregnancy.
- Good for those with joint or back problems.

slowing down during the last few laps and, again, finishing with some stretches.

Once you have gained confidence through a qualified instructor's guidance on the best techniques for each stroke, try to vary your strokes during your swimming session. This way you avoid overworking one particular muscle group and you ensure that all the muscle groups are worked in turn, creating an overall fitness program for the entire body.

Aqua-aerobics

Aqua- or water-aerobics is another wonderful and safe way to give your whole body a really good workout, putting considerably less strain on it than with land-based exercise! Community pools and health clubs usually offer different types of water-exercise classes, which provide a great way to get fit, keep fit, and have fun.

The exercise offered will normally incorporate training the leg muscles as well as the upper body, and may involve the use of special apparatus and music. This form of exercise is suitable for everyone at any age and is particularly enjoyed by older people, as the exercises are gentle and the class often becomes an opportunity to meet friends socially. However, more and more younger people, too, are beginning to realize the significant health benefits of aqua-aerobics. Water exercise is especially recommended for anyone who enjoys working out, but does not like getting sweaty and hot, or for those cautious about using gym equipment, running, or strength-training with weights for fear of coordination problems and joint injuries.

EXERCISE GUIDELINES FOR PITTA TYPES
(see pages 11–15)

Swimming is the ideal activity for pittas, as is walking in nature, which really calms them down.

BASIC AQUA-AEROBIC EXERCISES:

- Stretches using a handrail.
- Running on the spot in chest-deep water.
- Walking in chest-deep water.
- Running in chest-deep water.
- Using aqua weights in water to intensify training. These handheld weights are used when jogging on the spot, walking, and running, to increase fat burning and the heart rate.
- Lifting weights against water pressure increases muscular strength and toning in the arms and the sides of the body, the back, neck, and chest.

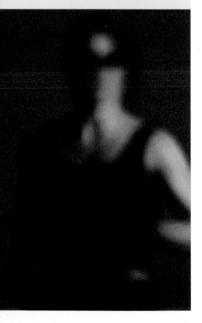

EXERCISE GUIDELINES FOR KAPHA TYPES (see pages 11–15)

Kaphas need to sweat and to be in the open air. Good, brisk walking, skipping, or running are the best forms of exercise for them, but they should avoid aerobics and step classes. They should also steer clear of water exercises (many Kaphas can't swim). They must be careful to control their tendency to oversleep, since this contributes to their inherent sluggishness.

running and jogging

If the thought of getting up at the crack of dawn, sliding into warm and comfortable workout gear and shoes, and braving the elements for a two-mile run is a major turn-off, then think again. You can adapt running to suit your lifestyle and time-scale—and it can transform your body. The benefits of running—including boosting the immune system, respiratory improvements, and benefits to your self-esteem—cannot be overestimated. You also get the advantage of being in the open air, which is something so many of us lack in our daily lives, as we are huddled into crowded commuter trains and stuffy offices most of the working day.

Getting started

Beginning with a realistic program will help. Keep a check on your progress and, if possible, have a fitness assessment before you start. If you have any injuries to the bones, back, knees, ankles, or feet, opt for strength-training exercises and stretches that will correct these problems. Running on hard ground may exacerbate any long-standing or recent injuries, putting you off running altogether.

Start with a program of walking and running intermittently. If you haven't run since you were at school, then begin with just brisk walking, trying to up the pace as you go. Set a goal. Even starting with just five minutes' walking, building to ten, and then on until you reach your goal of, for example, 30 minutes, will be more beneficial to you in the long run than trying to run a mile, finding it impossible, and giving up.

When you are ready to start running, remember to take precautions, as you would with any other exercise. Obviously, it is essential that time and consideration are given to buying suitable running shoes. Most athletic suppliers can advise you.

Always warm up the muscles, especially those in the legs, with brisk walking before you run. Then stretch the leg muscles and the upper body for 10 to 15 minutes. You may prefer to alternate between running and walking until you feel confident enough to run continuously. Wear a watch that is easy to read and run for five minutes, then walk for five minutes, building up to your goal level.

Pace yourself. Don't race ahead at the beginning of your session if you are unfit or planning to walk or run a long distance. If, at any time, you feel out of breath and uncomfortable, do not stop suddenly but slow down and keep moving, gradually settling into a walking pace. Stopping suddenly will be as shocking to your body as running like the wind without having trained, or warmed up and stretched.

Running technique

Hold your arms loosely by your sides, bent at the elbow, and not tight across the shoulders. The arms should move naturally in opposition to the legs, just like they swing when you walk. If this feels strange at first, pay attention to it. Soon it will feel as natural as walking. When brisk walking, and in early training, bring the arm position into the walking motion. You will probably find that walking becomes more fluid and the legs are able to stride from the hip more easily.

Be aware of your breathing. This will come naturally to you after a period of time, but if you are unused to this kind of physical activity, you might experience a tightness in the chest. Try to deepen your breathing until you are breathing rhythmically with the striding of your legs. If you begin with walking, focus on your breathing then. You will naturally breathe more deeply during exertion—training your breathing is as important as training your body, and good practice during the early stages will enable you to utilize breathing more effectively when running. Shortness of breath can often be attributed to poor breathing techniques, such as very shallow breathing that does not allow the lungs to fill properly.

When you have finished your run, cool down gradually, slowly decreasing your pace until you are walking briskly and your breathing has returned to normal. Shake out your arms to release any tension stuck there. When you've reached your goal, do your stretches, gently holding each stretch for at least 30 seconds.

If running is your chosen cardiovascular activity, try to do it at least three times a week. Cross-train with other forms of exercise, including strength-training and stretching. Strength-training is vital to produce the strong leg muscles and abdominals essential for effective running.

Running in the gym is as effective and almost as beneficial as running outside. In addition to the pleasures of being in the open air, however, wind resistance and rough terrain outside can greatly increase fitness. Avoid any risk of injury by being sensible and seeking advice from a personal trainer, coach, or another runner.

A TYPICAL 6-WEEK PROGRAM FOR THE COMPLETE NOVICE

WEEK 1
Warm-up; stretch. Walk 4 minutes; run 1 minute. Repeat 3 times. Stretch.

WEEK 2
Warm-up; stretch. Walk 4 minutes; run 2 minutes. Repeat 4 times. Stretch.

WEEK 3
Warm-up; stretch. Walk 3 minutes; run 3 minutes. Repeat 4 times. Stretch.

WEEK 4
Warm-up; stretch. Walk 2 minutes; run 3 minutes. Repeat 5 times. Stretch.

WEEK 5
Warm-up; stretch. Walk 1 minute; run 4 minutes. Repeat 5 times. Stretch.

WEEK 6
Warm-up; stretch. Run 20 minutes. Stretch.

dance is a natural exercise

The spirit of the dance is within all of us. On hearing music, children will often move their bodies and connect to a rhythm naturally. Dancing is a primal and ancient form of movement that has been part of our lives from the beginning of time. There is also no doubt that dancing is a wonderful exercise, releasing and freeing not just our bones, muscles, and joints, but raising our spirits.

Massively popular across the world, dancing at clubs is a way of releasing the stresses of the week, whether from college or work. High-energy dancing also gives your body a great workout, but be sure to drink plenty of water and do not overdo it—even just going out dancing can cause physical injuries when pounding the floor repeatedly, particularly in the ankles, knees, and hip joints.

There are so many dance forms from which to choose—jazz, swing, ballroom, salsa, modern, tap, and ballet, or how about belly and shamanic dancing or temple dancing? Choose the form that moves and satisfies you, and to which you feel instinctively drawn; however, be realistic about your state of fitness, your age, and your ability. Start at the very beginning, learning steps and form gradually as you build up more stamina and confidence.

TIPS FOR SAFE DANCING

- Always warm up first.
- Wear appropriate clothes and shoes.
- If you are unfit, or unused to exercise, take it gradually and very gently at first.
- Communicate any chronic or present health problems to the instructor.
- If dancing for pleasure at a party or club, pace yourself appropriately.
- Drink plenty of liquids.
- If you expect to be dancing energetically for a period of time, eat slow-release energy foods (see page 43) about two hours before dancing.

Shamanic dance

Free-flowing and impulse-based, shamanic dance is primal, awakening and moving sexual energy to constant rhythmic drum beats. Shamanic dance enables you to enhance the natural renewal and regenerative processes within yourself, and so allow yourself to be reborn and experience elation.

Ecstatic trance dance

This dance-form, which works with techno, ambient, global, and world music, aims to release you through euphoria and move you into higher states of consciousness. It is all about being—or discovering—who you really are, when you are not in competition with others or

trying to be the best. You dance in each of the four elements—earth, water, fire, and air—for about 15 minutes. Your breathing and the music changes with the feeling the elements provoke. The session fills you with energy.

Five rhythms

This is a dance form formulated by New York dance guru, Gabrielle Roth, who says it is "…harnessing the raw power of rhythm into a part of self-realization that gives us a practice, a perspective, and a philosophy that allows us to celebrate the wild, ecstatic dancer within."

Five rhythms dance behaves like a build-up and breaking of a wave—from flowing, through staccato to chaos, where people really let go of stresses and their selves, turning to a lyrical stillness that takes them back to the beginning of the circular rhythmic dance form. It is an excellent way of stretching muscles, while enhancing physical alertness and mental prowess. In addition, it allows free-flowing creativity and helps to shift any ingrained stress.

African dance

This is ritualistic, earthed, vibrant, and ecstatic dance all rolled into one form. Constant drumming puts the primal self back into the forefront and encourages you to move with the beats. Classes in many cities teach some movements and actual ritual dance for the celebration of stages of life and seasons.

Salsa

This is a highly popular form of dance, due to its vibrancy and being just plain, good fun. Dancing with a partner is coming back into fashion, making salsa the preferred form for many. The Latin-American dance is exciting and the music uplifting. The fun and laughter enjoyed in salsa are incredibly beneficial to many who may dislike traditional exercising. Salsa uses a great deal of energy, is profoundly good for the soul and inherently sexy, releasing sexual energy.

Ceroc/Rejive

This dance form is based on traditional dance steps, like the two-step, cha-cha, and waltz, along with modern jive, rock 'n roll, and Latin, performed to modern music and beefed up. Dancing with a

partner makes it romantic and fun. Ceroc classes are often described as Rejive.

Jazz dance

Traditionally learned by professional dancers, many health clubs and dance groups cater for a wide range of abilities. It is a rhythmic, percussive dance that ranges from more traditional jazz, which incorporates ballet and modern dance techniques, to jazz funk.

Ballet

Many dance companies offer ballet classes for adult beginners! It is something that one is never too old to learn and provides an excellent discipline that maintains very high levels of fitness and suppleness. You can't expect to become a prima ballerina, but you can enjoy some of the benefits ballet dancers experience, like grace, poise, balance, well-toned muscles, and a strong body.

Belly dance

This Middle Eastern dance form is traditionally performed by both men and women. Belly dancing is recommended by doctors for the prevention or treatment of many ailments. It is useful for weight problems, toning the body, easier childbirth or premenstrual syndrome, reviving flexibility, and enhancing self-esteem and your love life.

Temple dance

Versions of temple dancing are seen in most Eastern cultures, such as those in Thailand, India, and China, as well as many Middle Eastern countries. Training

in these ritualistic and religious dance forms can take many years, but the basics can be enjoyed by all. Watered-down versions of various forms of temple dance are available and often help to bring a spiritual element into your life.

Dancercize classes

These are taught in community gyms and health clubs by dancers and aerobics instructors. More choreographed than traditional aerobics classes, they incorporate dance routines, which vary according to the age group catered for. Dancercize classes are also available for children and older people. They are fun and good exercise at the same time.

THE BENEFITS OF DANCING

- Builds endurance.
- Increases flexibility.
- Increases agility.
- Builds strength.
- Helps balance.
- Develops coordination.
- Builds confidence.
- Enhances body awareness.
- Develops overall fitness.
- Ideal for all age groups and levels of fitness.

Pilates

Joseph Pilates developed the Pilates system of breath and movement work about 75 years ago. He studied many forms of Eastern and Western bodywork and, as he suffered from a range of disabilities, initially developed the exercises to help his own conditions. He continued studying and refining the techniques, and then began teaching what is now a popular exercise technique. Historically the techniques were a secret known mainly to the dance world, but they are now becoming more widely recognized and practiced by a greater variety of people. When performed regularly, the Pilates exercise techniques constitute a complete fitness method that positively changes bodies. According to Joseph Pilates, "In ten sessions you'll feel the difference, in twenty you'll see the difference, and in thirty you'll have a new body."

Pilates bridges the gap between strength and flexibility training, enabling it to be incorporated into existing physical activities, whether cardiovascular, swimming, bicycling, or any other form of bodywork. Regular practice of Pilates can significantly improve performance in all other athletic activities, as well as enhance your general wellbeing. Pilates combines awareness of the spine, proper breathing, and strength and flexibility training. Where most forms of exercise develop muscles, Pilates is virtually unique in that it slims the muscles, making them more compact by developing slenderness, rather than bulk. Regular Pilates devotees can expect to achieve a balanced body, which is strong and supple, with a flat stomach, balanced legs, and a strong back. Its effects, however, are more than physical—anyone who stays with the routine will feel revitalized, relaxed, confident, invigorated, and more flexible, with a great and new sense of wellbeing.

Pilates works by assisting you in changing the way you use your body. By redressing imbalances and altering movement patterns, your body is brought back into balance. Your posture and coordination will be corrected, and you will learn to move the way nature intended and the way that you used to move as a child, before you developed poor postural habits.

With this newly learned ease of movement, not only the muscular-skeletal system will function efficiently, but also the circulatory and lymphatic systems. In fact, every system of the body is improved through regular Pilates practice, including the nervous system, and in doing, so stress levels are reduced, making a stress-free existence possible. This is an exercise system that affects every part of you, down to cell level. Your body will become properly nourished, with oxygen being replenished and toxic waste removed. Emphasis is placed on mind-body integrity, making it a truly holistic fitness regime.

BENEFITS OF PILATES

- Complements other bodywork and natural therapies.
- Helps prevent injury.
- Provides postural realignment and enhancement.
- Develops grace.
- Increases relaxation.
- Boosts the immune system.
- Has a beneficial effect on osteoarthritis and osteoporosis.
- Benefits knee and shoulder injuries.
- Relieves stress.
- Relieves headache and other pain.
- Purifies the blood stream.
- Permanently changes body shape.
- Provides a totally holistic system of fitness.

Pilates is renowned for its usefulness in both injury prevention and rehabilitation. The technique is often employed to rebuild and strengthen muscles after injury or strain. Because it is a gentle program, it is useful for many cases of rehabilitation—lower back injury, neck and shoulder tension, and even general aches and pains, to name just a few. Exercises can be performed without involving the injury area, as the supporting muscles are worked and strengthened, thereby giving the injured area time to heal.

Pilates classes are held in many gyms and health clubs throughout the country. Qualified practitioners will take you through a series of moves and breathwork, correcting any errors you may make as you work into position. Every class is balanced in its own right, and through repeated attendance at the class, you will learn as many as seventy different exercises. Pilates instructors are highly qualified, and very diligent in correcting errors and encouraging correct breathing during class.

When you feel confident that you have mastered the moves and breathwork, Pilates can be practiced at home on a daily basis to enhance its healing and physical benefits. Pilates can also be practiced before workouts in the gym or other athletic activities, taking the place of a warm-up.

THE EIGHT PRINCIPLES OF THE PILATES METHOD ARE:

- Relaxation
- Concentration
- Alignment
- Breathing
- Centering
- Coordination
- Flowing movements
- Stamina

Pilates breathing

Breathing correctly ensures that the body receives its full quota of oxygen. Pilates breathing is called thoracic, or lateral, breathing. You are taught to breathe in to prepare for a movement; then breathe out, with a strong center to the spine, and move; and finally to breathe in again to recover from the movement. Breathe into the ribcage, expanding the lower ribs and increasing the lungs' capacity to take in more oxygen. "Zip up and hollow" is a much-used breathing and abdominal tightening exercise used in Pilates. To do it, you draw the muscles of the pelvic floor up and in, and hollow the lower abdomen back toward the spine.

"A man is as young as his spinal column."
JOSEPH PILATES

"Above all, learn how to breathe correctly."
JOSEPH PILATES

yoga for keeping well

Yoga is an ancient system of mind-and-body exercises that originated in India over 5,000 years ago. Today, people all over the world are learning the simple techniques of yoga and experiencing the benefits of this holistic approach to exercise. In yoga, the goal is to balance the mind and body through a series of physical, breathing, and relaxation exercises—the word "yoga" literally means "union." Yoga's popularity in the West is increasing all the time; no surprise when you consider the high value placed on a well-honed, well-toned body and mind in our culture.

Hatha yoga is the branch of yoga that concentrates on body postures (asanas) and movement, together with Pranayama, where the focus moves to the breath. Hatha yoga practice encourages awareness of the breath as a channel through which the *prana*—the life force that makes all things possible and manifest, including the restorative practice of yoga—can flow. The very quality of the postures and breathing flow encourages the centering of mental concentration within. Along with the sound of your inhalation and exhalation, you will learn to listen and hear

EXERCISE GUIDELINES FOR VATA TYPES
(see pages 11–15)

Vatas are advised to get involved in yoga, t'ai chi, walking, and anything rhythmic. They have a tendency to overexercise and should take active steps to make sure they have "recovery" days (see page 133).
Activities for Vatas to avoid include high-impact aerobics and step classes.

other internal sounds: muscles, joints, and bones all telling you what they need. We can learn to be more aware of our inner being – so often forgotten in the midst of external demands – and to find a deeper state of peace Yoga can help integrate our inner and outer worlds, helping us process the impact and the interface between our inner and outer realities.

Yoga is not a competitive endeavor, although some who practice the new "power yoga," Ashtanga, would disagree. To begin with, it's a good idea to find a qualified instructor to assist you in attaining the asanas. Instruction in correct breathing can only be given by a qualified instructor and, when enough familiarity with the asanas and breathing is attained, regular practice at home is essential. In the words of Swami Sivananda Vedanta, "Ten minutes practice is worth more than hours of theory."

De-stressing with yoga

Yoga is thought to be an excellent way to de-stress because it not only works on the muscles, bones, and joints, but also on the nervous system. By practicing yoga, you stretch and tone the body, increasing muscle strength and stamina, and correcting posture. At the same time, you learn how to relax the mind, dramatically improving your concentration, sense of wellbeing, and spirituality. Asanas are designed to exercise the body while simultaneously calming the mind. They have both a Sanskrit name and an English translation, and both are given on the following pages. Yoga is always done slowly and thoughtfully, concentrating and breathing into each posture. Stop each pose at a point well before pain and overexertion. Listen to your body and your breathing, taking the postures slowly and gently.

This is where Pranayama is so important—correct breathing supports and strengthens the asanas. Generally, you inhale as you begin the first phase of the posture and exhale while you expand and move into its final phase. To avoid injury, do not force your body beyond its limits. Never push through pain to achieve a more "correct" asana; instead, allow the gentle unfolding of a posture to the best of your ability. In the early stages of your practice, it is always a good idea to take instruction from a professionally accredited yoga teacher. This will help you grasp the basic principles of each pose and avoid developing bad habits.

Inverted postures

Inverted postures, where your heart is above your head, are very powerful and need to be approached with great care. Do not do these postures (asanas) if you suffer from high blood pressure or have a fever or headache. If you have back or digestive problems, consult your doctor before undertaking any but the most simple, basic forms of exercise, like walking. Do try to have some proper yoga classes before attempting these postures, unless you are highly experienced in exercise systems, and are very fit and supple. Inverted postures are so potent because the effects of gravity are reversed. The organs that are in the upper part of the body, usually receiving a smaller flow of blood, are now below. The blood pours into these organs without the least exertion of the heart, which has to overcome the force of gravity in order to pump blood to the neck, head, and brain. The burden on the heart is greatly reduced, giving it a chance to truly rest and relax.

Eastern exercise program

Trikonasana (Triangle Pose)

Stand with the feet wide apart and parallel. Stretch the arms out to the sides in line with the shoulders as you inhale. Turn the right foot out at a right angle, the left foot in slightly, and keep the torso facing forward, as you exhale and lean over the right leg. Bend from the hips, not the waist, and keep the left side flat and in line with the hips. Inhale and stretch the left arm up, resting the other arm on the right leg. If comfortable, turn the gaze up to the left hand; if not, look ahead. Hold for a few breaths, and then swap sides.

Tadasana (Mountain Pose)

This is an excellent warm-up posture and is good for expanding the chest and opening the lungs. Stand up straight with the feet together and arms down by the sides. Stretch the spine by lifting up through the head and chest, but without raising the shoulders—keep them relaxed and down. Pull up the thigh muscles to lift the knees, with legs straight. Keep the gaze soft. Hold for a few complete breaths and relax.

Vrikonasana (Tree Pose)

Stand up straight with feet together and arms by your sides. Inhale deeply; as you exhale, bend the right knee, drawing the foot up toward the groin and resting it as far up the inner left thigh as comfortable. Gaze at a fixed point in front of you to help you balance. Raise the arms above the head and press the palms together in a praying motion. Hold for a few complete breaths before changing legs and repeating on the other side.

Horse Position

The Calming Inhalation

Stand with your feet parallel and firmly placed about shoulder-width apart, with toes slightly turned in and knees bent a little. As you inhale deeply through the nose, raise the arms slowly from the waist, up the torso, palms turned up, and imagine drawing the breath from the base of the spine to the top of the head (see far left).

The Calming Exhalation

Begin to exhale through the nose, turning your hands over and lowering them slowly in time with your exhalation—imagine drawing your breath down through the spine and the center of the body. Repeat the entire cycle two to three times.

Stretch Over One Leg

Sit on the floor with a straight, firm back and your legs stretched out straight to the sides. Inhale and stretch the arms up over the head, lengthening the torso. Then exhale and lean from the hips over the right leg, keeping the back and left side as straight as possible. Rest the right hand on your leg and hold for two to three complete breaths, then return to the upright position and repeat for the other leg.

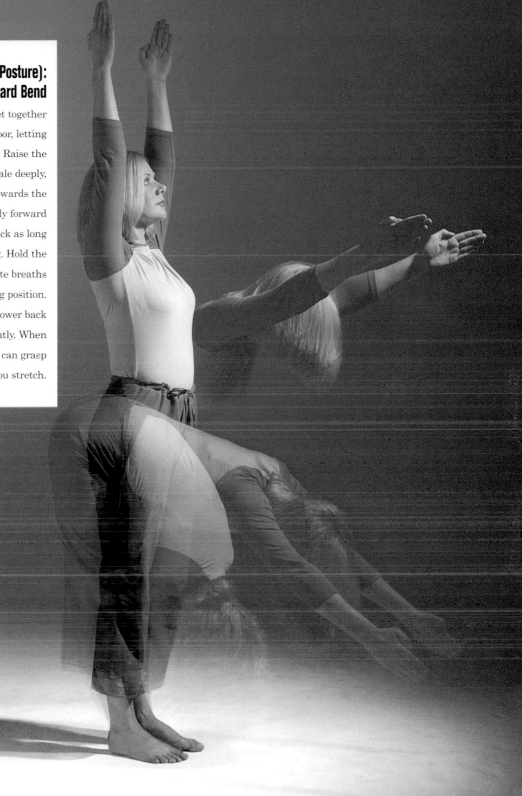

Padahastasana (Stork Posture): Standing Forward Bend

Stand up straight with your feet together and firmly in contact with the floor, letting the arms hang by your sides. Raise the arms above the head as you inhale deeply, stretching the fingers up towards the ceiling. Exhale and bend slowly forward from the hips, keeping the back as long as possible without straining. Hold the position for three to six complete breaths and return to the standing position. If you experience pain, or have lower back problems, bend the knees slightly. When you become more flexible, you can grasp the legs or ankles to help you stretch.

Spread Legs Stretch

Stay in the same upright sitting position as in the Stretch Over One Leg pose (see opposite). Inhale and place the hands on the knees. Slowly exhale as you lower your head toward the floor, bending forward from the hips and keeping your back long and straight. Hold for a few breaths. Never strain the back or legs in this posture, and stop if you feel any pain.

Forward Bend Sitting

Lie on your back with the arms resting by your sides. Inhale deeply and slowly raise the arms until they are flat on the floor above the head. With the exhalation, sit up slowly, bending forward from the hips until you can touch your toes (if you are very flexible) or grasp your ankles or calves. Hold for a few breaths. Avoid any unnecessary strain by keeping your back as long and flat as possible, and by bending the knees slightly if you feel any pain.

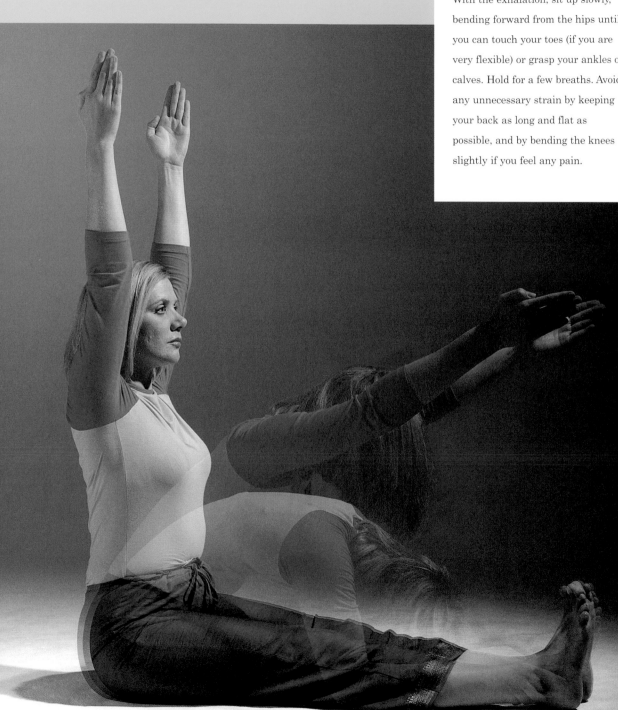

Child's Pose

Kneel with the toes touching and knees
slightly apart, and then bend forward over
the thighs. Rest the forehead on the floor
to take the weight of the head. Rest the
arms by the sides of the body, palms facing
up. This is a good counterpose to the
Cobra and other postures in which your
spine is arched. It also helps to relieve
back strain after doing inverted postures,
such as the Shoulderstand.

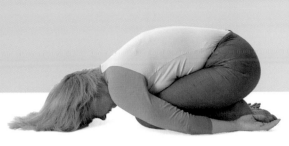

Bhujangasana (Cobra)

Lie face down with the forehead resting on the floor,
legs and feet together, and elbows bent, with the
palms down and roughly parallel with the shoulders
(see above). Inhale and push the floor away with the
hands, so that the back arches and the torso (as far
as the thighs) lifts off the ground. Gaze up, but keep
the face and neck muscles soft. Hold for several
breaths, then lower back to the starting
position. Recover from the Cobra by resting
in the Child's Pose (see top).

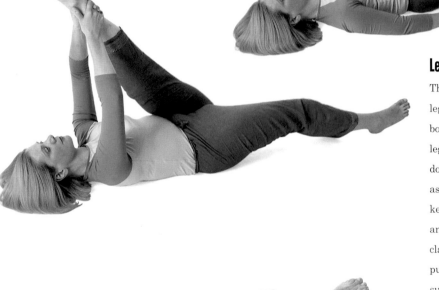

Leg Raises

This pose can be done either by raising one leg at a time, as illustrated here, or with both legs together. Lie on your back with legs straight and arms by the sides, palms down. Inhale, then slowly raise the left leg as high as possible without straining, keeping the other leg firmly on the ground and using your hands for support. Exhaling, clasp the raised calf with both hands and pull the leg down toward your body, making sure that the leg stays straight. Hold for several breaths and release.

Wind Relieving

Again, this exercise can be done one leg at a time or with both legs together (see right). Inhale as you raise the legs toward the chest, clasping the shins. Hold briefly, then draw the legs in even more as you exhale, raising the chin slightly to meet the knees. Hold the pose for a few breaths, then release the legs slowly back to the floor.

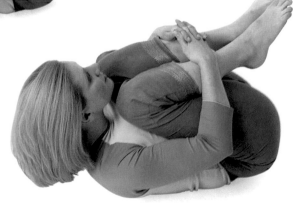

Sarvangasana (Shoulderstand)

Lie on your back on a flat surface—
a rug or mat will help to cushion the
neck—with the arms by the sides,
the palms down, and legs together.
Pushing down with your hands, raise
both legs to an upright position (see
above). Use the arms to help lift the
back off the floor, tilting the legs back
over the head and supporting the spine
by holding under the hips (see right).
Finally, stretch up to bring the legs
vertical and in line with the spine—
imagine that you are being pulled up
by a thread running through your
back, hips and legs (see bottom). Hold
for a few complete breaths, and then
release by placing your hands back
on the floor for support and gently
lowering the torso to the floor. If you
feel any pain in the neck or lower back,
come out of the pose immediately.

Surya Namaskar (Sun Salutation)

1 Stand upright, with feet together and weight equally balanced. Bring the hands together in the prayer position and exhale. **2** Inhale and stretch the arms above the head, arching the back slightly and keeping the legs straight. **3** Exhale as you bend forward, placing the hands at either side of the feet, in line with the toes, and pressing the palms into the floor. Keep the head tucked in and, if necessary, bend the knees. **4** Inhale and squat down. Stretch the right leg back behind you to rest on the toes, and drop the right knee to the floor. Exhale. **5** Inhale and move the left leg back to join the right leg. Keep the head in line with the body, the feet together, and the back straight. **6** Exhale; then lower the knees to the floor and bend the elbows. Lower the chest, and then the chin, to the floor, keeping the hips raised and toes curled under.

start

7 Inhale and lower the hips. Push the floor away with the arms, arching the back and stretching the torso. Roll the toes under (see Cobra, page 175). **8** Exhale; roll back onto the soles of the feet, and push up through the buttocks to form an inverted "V." The hands and feet should be firmly on the floor and the head and spine aligned. Push down into the heels. **9** Inhale and step the right leg forward (mirror of position 4). **10** Exhale; come into a squat by bringing the left leg forward to join the right. Straighten the legs into a forward bend (see position 3). **11** Inhale and come up to standing, stretching the arms up over the head and bending gently backwards (see position 2).

12 Exhaling, return to the prayer pose (see position 1). Repeat the sequence one to twelve times, alternating the legs in positions 4 and 9, and try to maintain a continuous flow between postures.

Padmasana (Lotus)

Sit with the legs crossed, the spine erect, and the palms resting on the legs. This is a meditative pose, so keep the gaze soft and turned down, and concentrate on breathing deeply through the nose. Use the hands to lift the left foot up to rest on the right thigh. Then place the right foot across it to rest on the left thigh. Rest the hands, palms-up, on the knees (see far right). If you find this position too hard, try the Half-Lotus (see right):. stretch one leg at a time into position, hold the pose for a few breaths, and then swap legs.

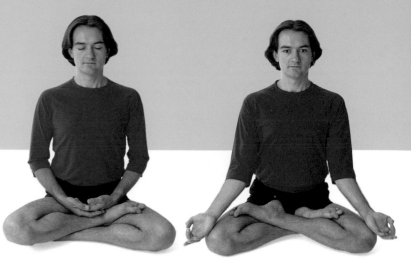

Vakrasana (Sitting Twist)

Sit on the floor with the legs stretched out in front of you, the back erect, and hands palm-down by the sides. Bend your right knee, drawing the leg up until the foot is parallel with the left thigh, and then crossing it over. Inhale. As you exhale, twist your torso to the right, holding the right knee with the left arm and stretching the right arm out behind you. Gently turn your head to look over the right shoulder. Use your breathing to stretch up through the spine and to gently increase the twist. Keep the spine straight to avoid strain. Hold for a few complete breaths, and then swap sides.

Savasana (Corpse)

Lie on your back on a firm surface, such as a rug or yoga mat on a hard floor. Stretch the legs out straight and shoulder-width apart. Rest the hands by your sides, with palms up, and either close your eyes or gaze straight ahead. Rest the back of the head softly on the floor. Let every muscle relax completely. Rest in this pose for a few minutes, or as long as you need to relax, breathing deeply through the nose throughout. When you are ready, roll gently over to your right side, hold for a few moments, and then sit up.

breathing for yoga

In terms of yoga, the art and science of breathing is called Pranayama. Breathing through the nose is a basic rule of health in the exercise disciplines of the East. Breathing through the mouth is a bad health habit, and one which is much more prevalent in the West. If you habitually shallow breath through the mouth, it is vitally important to your health to reeducate yourself. Full deep breathing through the nose will relax you on a much more profound level and, in addition, give you the best protection from infectious diseases.

In Pranayama, the basis of all breathing exercise is complete deep breathing. Each breath combines abdominal, middle, and upper-chest (clavicular) breathing. To breathe correctly, inhale through the nose into your belly, so that your abdomen expands as air is drawn into the bottom of the lungs. The next phase of the inhalation moves up into your middle; and your chest and upper-chest area expands last. As you slowly exhale, your abdomen, middle, and then your chest contract. This powerful exercise should be done three to six times initially. Accomplished regularly over time, Pranayama will enhance vitality and reduce stress levels.

Complete yoga breathing

Sit comfortably, either cross-legged on a mat, in a chair, or on your heels with the spine firm and centered, not tense. Close your eyes, focusing on your navel. After a complete exhale, breathe in through the nose, expanding first the abdomen, then the ribs, chest, and collarbone, raising them as you count to eight. Then exhale through the nose, contracting the abdomen, ribs, and chest, and finally lowering the collarbone and shoulders to the count of eight. Repeat three to six times. The exercise induces relaxation by calming the nervous system, and it also oxygenates the blood and increases lung capacity.

Kumbhaka breathing

This exercise can be done sitting, standing, or lying down. The focus of your attention is on the heart area. This is the same as complete yoga breathing (see above), but you extend the cycle by holding your breath to the count of four after completing inhalation and before exhalation. Always breathe in and out to the count of eight; you can extend this with practice, but you should never strain. Do not do this exercise if you have a heart condition. It is calming for the nervous system, and can regulate the pulse and heartbeat by slowing the heart.

t'ai chi chuan

T'ai chi—literally "grand ultimate boxing"— is an ancient Chinese exercise system that coordinates simple movements into a continuous rhythmic sequence with steady and controlled breathing. The roots of t'ai chi go back thousands of years to early Eastern philosophies, including Buddhism and Taoism. Many of the sequences are based on the movements of animals.

T'ai chi is similar to yoga in that it relaxes both body and mind, prevents tension, and helps build strength and a sense of wellbeing. However, t'ai chi is characterized by continuity of movement, combined with regulated breathing and deep reflection, rather than a series of distinct poses. Practitioners believe this system helps to clear the blocked energy (or *chi*) that causes disease and encourages a free flow of energy through the body to improve health. Research at Johns Hopkins University has proved that regular practice of t'ai chi lowers blood pressure. T'ai chi is especially popular with the elderly because it improves strength and general health through low-impact exercises. With t'ai chi, you can quickly learn where you hold tension and how to release it.

As with most exercise, it is advisable to locate a teacher who is qualified in the form of t'ai chi you want to study. A typical weekly lesson of around two to three hours will often start with a standing meditation to release accumulated stress and will teach you enough to practice at home.

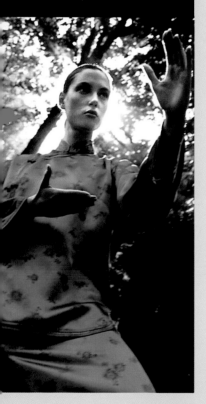

T'AI CHI IS FOR ALL

T'ai chi suits young people with good fitness levels, but it is also especially popular among the elderly because it improves strength and general health through low-impact exercises.

falun gong

This form of meditation and gentle exercises is based on ancient Chinese traditions of health and self-improvement. Practitioners of this discipline aspire to achieve a state of selflessness and inner balance by cultivating compassion, tolerance and truthfulness. Mark Palmer, former US Ambassador to Hungary and 26-year veteran of the US State Department has said that falun gong is 'the greatest single spiritual movement in Asia today. There is nothing to compare with it in courage and importance.' It is practised freely in more than 60 countries, but the Communist leadership in China have attempted to eradicate it and many thousands of people have been detained, tortured and persecuted for their practice of falun gong.

qigong

Qigong is a form of t'ai chi that focuses on healing through "energy cultivation." Two forms of energy are activated—internal *chi* (or *qi*) and external *chi* (or *qi*)—through breathing exercises, movement, and meditation. External *chi* can be emitted to heal others.

There are about 500 forms of qigong practiced around the world. Although each approach generally seeks to improve balance and awareness, there are fundamental differences between them, depending on the philosophy upon which it is based. For example, the Buddhist form aims to release the Self through awareness; the Taoist form focuses on connecting you with nature; and the Confucian form is concerned with establishing your place in society as a whole.

Banned in China for many years, qigong is enjoying a huge resurgence in popularity. Practitioners around the world report on the many medical benefits of qigong, including relief from allergies, asthma, hypertension, liver disorders, and even potentially life-threatening illnesses, such as cancer.

Taijiwuxigong

A particularly interesting form is taijiwuxigong, which focuses on the daily cleansing of negative energy and posture correction. Its creator, Dr. Shen Hongxun, believes bad posture is one of the main causes of disease, creating irritation of the nerves of the spinal column and damaging circulation and metabolism. This system differs from other versions of qigong because it involves a repetition of only a few key postures, consisting of outward movements away from the body. Because of the simplicity of the exercises, taijiwuxigong is accessible to people of all ages.

Results can be dramatic, even after one session, and the student is advised to remain calm and quiet for some time afterward to avoid faintness or shock. Taijiwuxigong can sometimes induce very powerful responses, both physical and emotional, signaling a release of tension and negative energy. The result is a feeling of release from tension and an overall sense of wellbeing. Whatever form of qigong you decide to practice, it is important to find a qualified instructor. During sessions, wear loose clothing in which you can move freely, and take a warm outer layer with you to help retain body heat when the class ends.

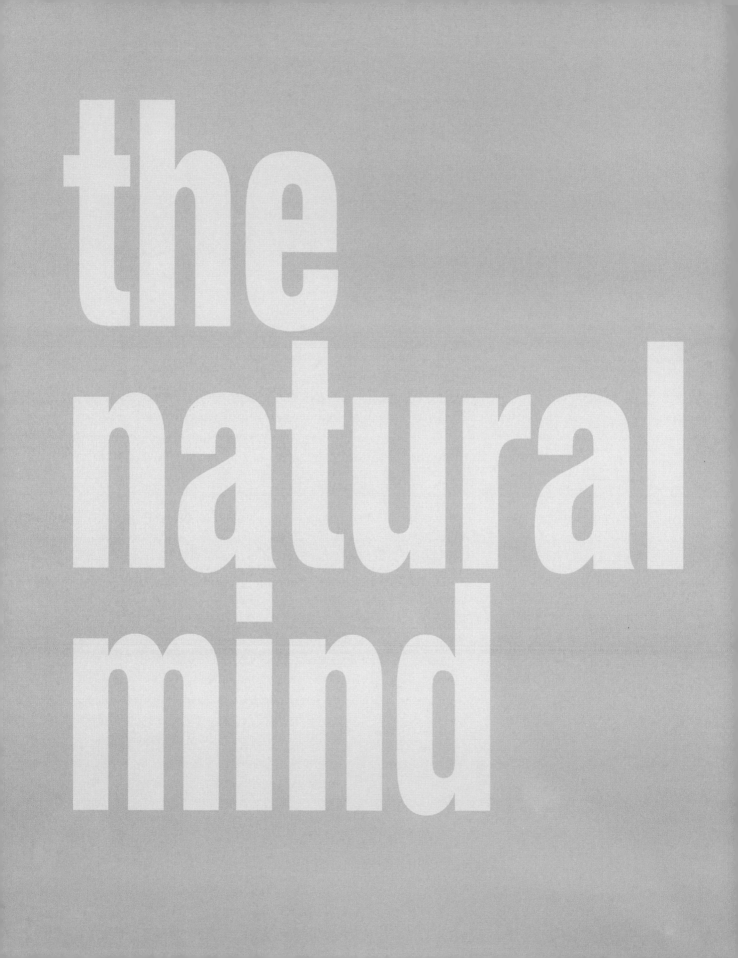

the natural mind

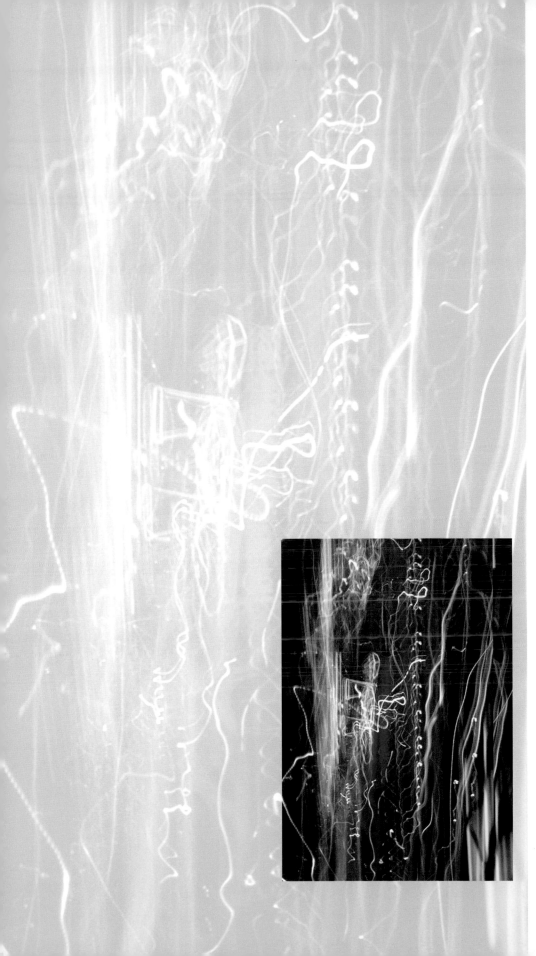

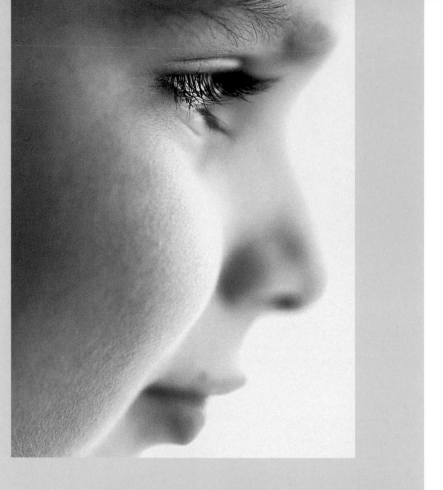

understanding your brain

The latest scientific thinking on the brain suggests great minds are made, not born. Nurture rather than nature determines how agile your mind is. Continual curiosity and learning keeps the mind active, and like any muscle, you have to use it or lose it. Unlike other parts of the body, the more you use the brain, the better it gets, and the more honed and skilled it becomes. The brain is the amazing, mysterious facilitator of all we experience and perceive, the center of our emotions and thoughts.

anatomy of the brain & nervous system

Knowing that new scientific discoveries show you really can change your brain —that nerve endings can grow throughout life and new brain cells can emerge— is exciting and empowering. A young brain may be more malleable than one that is middle-aged, but, even in the middle and later years, good and regular brain training, a sustained brain workout, can make nerve cells flourish.

World expert on the brain, Professor Susan Greenfield, of the Department of Pharmacology at Oxford University, England, says, "Your brain is changing all the time. No single area of the brain is activated exclusively and solely during a specific mental task. Whole constellations of cells become active at different times and in subtly different ways, depending on what you are doing. Indeed, far more brain regions turn out to be involved than had previously been thought possible."

The brain is our most mysterious and mighty organ, weighing no more than around three pounds. Residing within the skull at the top of the body, the brain is capable of running the whole show without using more than a small percentage of its capacity. After decades of intense scientific research, there is still so much we do not understand about this most complex and fascinating part of the body. The command and communications center, it controls the nervous system, an intricate network receiving messages from the senses, processing them, and then coordinating and directing all our actions and reactions.

The brain and nervous system work together with the glands of the endocrine system, which governs the body's hormones, to form a regulation and control system of exquisite refinement and awesome power. The home of our thoughts, feelings, sensations, perceptions, creative imagination, and talents, as well as the instruction headquarters for all the body's functions, the brain's power comes from electrical energy carried in the chemical substances known as neurotransmitters.

The brain is divided into three parts. The largest is the cerebrum, where voluntary action and thought are controlled. This is the reception center for the messages to and from the rest of the body. Speech, muscle control, vision, and touch are dealt with by the cerebrum: the front lobe of the cerebrum deals with planning and complex functions; the back with vision. The second part of the brain, the cerebellum, is located behind and under the cerebrum. This is where the controls for balance and muscle coordination are based. The third part, the medulla, controls involuntary reflex actions, such as breathing, respiratory rate, heart rate, and digestion process. The brain never sleeps—even when we do; it is still processing information from our five senses and beyond.

The nervous system includes the central nervous system, consisting of the brain and spinal cord which are protected by the skull and spine, and the peripheral nervous system, which extends from the central nervous system to the rest of the body via its cranial and spinal nerve network. The central nervous system serves the rest of the body like a central computer system, receiving and analyzing sensory information and then sending out the appropriate response.

Nerves conduct messages to and from the brain and around the body. The messages consist of electrical impulses that travel from one end of a nerve to the other, and are then chemically transmitted to other nerves or to muscles. Motor nerves carry orders from the brain to the muscles; sensory nerves carry messages about feelings, such as itching, pain, coldness, and so on, to the brain.

Impulses travel through the nerves, long tube-like extensions of nerve cells or neurons. Each neuron has a cell body, an axon, and branches called dendrites. The small gap that separates each neuron is called a synapse. The chemical released by each neuron as it contacts the next in the nerve chain is called a neurotransmitter. Released from the end of the axon, the neurotransmitter crosses the synapse and carries the message to the next neuron.

The central nervous system is made up of over 100 billion tiny neurons. Each is connected to around 10,000 other neurons, and they are constantly sending messages to each other. All this activity takes a lot of energy and uses a high level of the body's prime fuel, glucose. The peripheral nervous system consists of the autonomic nervous system, which controls our involuntary body functions, like blinking, shivering or sweating, and the somatic nervous system, which controls the muscles responsible for willed, conscious movement.

The autonomic nervous system mainly controls the organs and glands, and is divided into the sympathetic and the parasympathetic nervous systems. Most of the time these two systems maintain a kind of balance, but the sympathetic system dominates during times of fear, delight, or excitement by stimulating the increased breathing or heart rate required by the body's natural "fight-or-flight" response (see page 205). Everyday functions like digestion and sleep are the concern of the parasympathetic system.

anxiety

Many people experience anxiety in one form or another: from mild to severe, from panic attacks to chest pains, dizziness to breathing difficulty, palpitations to sweating, from loss of appetite to insomnia. All of these effects and more are the symptoms of anxiety, which can, if untreated or ignored, lead to more serious problems when they start affecting normal, everyday life.

Anxiety and panic attacks are often a result of emotional upset. Feelings should be examined and dealt with. Vitamin B deficiency can also cause anxiety problems.

Supportive measures include:

Aromatherapy (see page 261)
Geranium essential oil is emotionally balancing; lavender soothes; and frankincense uplifts and helps you to slow down the pace.

Nutrition (see pages 36–87)
Avoid sugar and sugary foods and drinks; steer clear of coffee or any caffeine-based drinks or foods; but do eat foods rich in B vitamins.

Homeopathy (see page 270)
- Take arsenicum album if anxiety worsens when you are alone or in the dark.
- If experiencing palpitations or "loss of reason", take calcarea carbonica.
- If suffering extreme anxiety, which worsens before a thunderstorm, take phosphorus.
- Take argenteum nitrium (arg-nit) or gelsemium if anxious before a key event.
- For ailments after a panic attack, take arconitum.

Supportive treatments include:

Acupuncture (see page 260)
Alexander technique (see page 260)
Chiropractic (see page 265)
Cranial osteopathy (see page 266)
Massage (see pages 220–29)
Osteopathy (see page 274)
Bach flower remedies (see pages 263–64)
- Mimulus for fear with known cause.
- Rock rose for panic.
- Aspen for fear of the unknown.
- Cherry plum for fear of mental collapse.

MEMORY AND STRESS

The panic stations that go on alert when the body is directly stressed affect the amount of memory you are able to access through the retrieval system. The amygdala, which controls fear, blocks the ability of the body to retrieve stored information. Next time you need to remember something (like information for an exam), make sure you are allowing yourself the necessary tools to de-stress first before trying to access these memory banks.

Now that we have explored the brain in some depth, we are aware of the incredibly complex nature of this organ of consciousness. We can understand how there are two ways of knowing—two ways in which we process the same information—through the brain's two hemispheres.

exercising the brain

The left hemisphere of the brain analyzes, verbalizes, counts, plans, and is rational and logical. The right hemisphere intuits, imagines, relates, integrates, and freely associates. Getting to know and stimulate both sides of your brain is an important step in optimizing your creative potential.

The whole brain theories

The left hemisphere controls the right side of the body; the right hemisphere controls the left side of your body. Your nervous system is connected to the brain in a crossed-over way so the right hand is connected to the left hemisphere and the left hand to the right hemisphere. In terms of function, human cerebral hemispheres develop asymmetrically. This is reflected in our propensity to be either right- or left-handed—it is the rare individual who is ambidextrous and can use both hands with the same ease and control.

In recent years, many experts and theorists have embraced the new "whole brain" theories. These conclude that, even though many human beings seem to be dominated by either the left (and are analytical by nature) or the right (intuitive, creative) hemisphere of the brain, if the whole brain is "switched on," all learning, healing, creating, and gaining of new skills becomes easier. Open, childlike enthusiasm and curiosity are rekindled when we stimulate our whole brain. Whether you are an analytical left-brain type or an intuitive right-brain person, the important thing is more integration of the hemispheres in your daily life.

According to psychologist Janet Goodrich, in her book, *Natural Vision Improvement*, more balanced use of both hemispheres "makes for a self-realized person, who is happy, healthy, and creative in a total sense. When [the brain hemispheres are] integrated, we are able to see an image and describe it as well. We want to maximize the flow of energy from one side of the brain to the other and create dual dominance—full activity and interchange of both hemispheres."

Kinesiologists and natural vision therapists agree on the importance of the crawling stage in human growth for the brain's development, as well as for motor development. Crawling begins our first autonomous exploration of the space around us. It prepares us for eventually learning how to read and write "where our eyes, hands, and mind will flow from left to right across the midline of the paper." It is during this crucial crawling stage that we first move freely from one hemisphere of the brain to the other, as we move left hand in synchronization with right leg (and vice versa).

To exercise the whole brain and stimulate hemisphere integration, you can simply get down on the floor and crawl like a baby. You have to have "crossover"; that is, use alternate hand and leg movements—when the left hand moves forward, so does your right leg. You can also simply march slowly in place (to music if you like), alternating hands and legs (see also Brainpower Boosts, page 194).

LEFT-BRAIN FUNCTIONS

Reason, logic, hearing, right-handedness, number skills, writing, time perception, details, objectivity, extroversion, and tension.

RIGHT-BRAIN FUNCTIONS

Emotion, intuition, ESP, left-handedness, musical skills, sight, seeing whole picture, space perception, subjectivity, introversion, and relaxation.

regenerating the brain

One of the most remarkable recent discoveries about the brain is that it can regenerate. If you suffer any sort of brain damage, you will almost certainly be told by doctors that your neurons can't regrow. While skin, blood, and bones are all constantly replacing themselves, brain cells—so the experts have led us to believe for nearly a century—just grow older.

However, according to recent research, this does not seem as certain anymore. Last year, researchers at Princeton University proved the official version wrong. Using a drug originally developed to detect new cancer cells, Dr. Elizabeth Gould discovered that new cells were growing deep in the cavities at the centers of monkeys' brains, and then migrating up to the top layer of the brain's cortex, which controls memory, thinking, and decision-making.

This discovery is making neuroscientists rethink their theories of how the brain works, and it holds out the possibility of repairing the brain. Within the next ten years, doctors may be able to replace cells damaged by a stroke, restore the covering to nerve fibers stripped off by multiple sclerosis, and even reverse the effects of Alzheimer's.

Neurogenesis, as it is called, is throwing new light on how memories are stored. The old idea was that memories were created by strengthening connections between neurons, but now it looks as if memories may be held in new cells. This explains, for example, how memories are date-stamped —recent memories are actually stored in newer cells.

The scientists are aiming to exploit neurogenesis with all the sophisticated techniques of modern cell biology. Although it's far from perfect—otherwise no one would be permanently affected by strokes— damage to the brain does speed up new cell growth. An epileptic seizure, for example, triggers a spurt of new growth. And, even more exciting, new cells tend to migrate toward the site of the trouble. Currently researchers are attempting to develop drugs that improve these natural processes.

Another approach in research is to exploit the chemical signals that make these cells grow. As far as we know, nerve cells in the spine don't regrow. However, take spinal cells and put them in a part of the cortex that controls memory, known as the hippocampus, and they can renew themselves. Researchers plan to grow new cells outside the body, using the chemicals that stimulate them, and then replant them when needed.

However, we don't have to wait for all these hi-tech approaches to deliver; the good news is that we can influence neurogenesis now. Stress, for example, slows down cell growth. Specially treated rats that can no longer produce stress hormones churn out new brain cells at a much higher rate than usual. This suggests that stress delivers a double

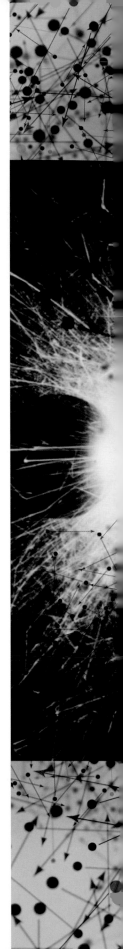

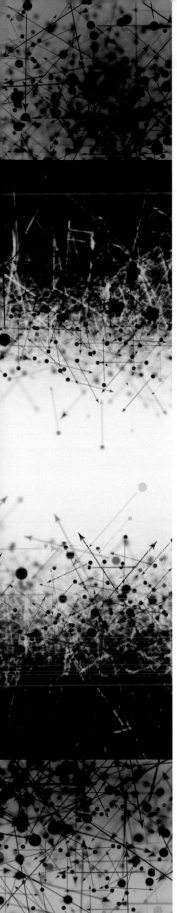

whammy: not only do the hormones involved actually kill off brain cells, but they also knock out the repair system.

The repetitive process of learning new information or behavior patterns stimulates the brain to produce a chemical called 'Calphin'. It builds new tendrils on our neural axons that actually end up constructing new neurons in our brains. When we employ self-help, any new thinking, psychotherapy or new regimes, we produce calphin, which can cause the brain to build new pathways. However, it is not sufficient to simply read new material or do a new behaviour once or twice. There must be repetition in order for the calphin to have an effect on the neural pathways and on the neurons themselves.

You don't even need drugs to keep those new brain cells coming. Experiments by Professor Fred Gage of the Salk Institute, California, showed that rats allowed to exercise whenever they wished, rather than being forced to, and living in a spacious cage with lots of toys, grew more new brain cells. Other researchers have found that having to do important learning tasks, like remembering where seeds are stored, also encouraged neurogenesis.

It is much too early to say how effective the hi-tech approach is going to be, although you can predict that unpleasant side effects are inevitable. In the meantime, neurogenesis provides a fascinating new mechanism to explain why such old remedies as relaxation, exercise, and keeping mentally active are so good for the brain.

Neurobics: the gym where your brain works out

Just as current research shows that cell regeneration occurs, proving that the brain is fortunately more adaptable than we've given it credit for in the past, there are ways to reverse the trend of shrinking cells. Growth in brain cells and in the dendrites (the connection between cells) is promoted/encouraged by learning more and interacting with new people. As your own life experiences become richer, they have a direct effect on the healthful quality of pathways in your brain.

Keep learning: if you shy away from studying a topic you know nothing about, fight the urge to play it safe and dive in at the deep end. Learn a new language or skill, or take a graduate course. And when you next feel inclined to hide away at home, try and make it a point to get out and meet new people every day. Acknowledging new faces and new patterns in routine behavior, as well as

BRAIN FACTS:

Why so wrinkly? While the brain itself could be considered less than attractive, its streamlined design makes the most compact use of available surface/work space.

IN UTERO LEARNING

Scientific evidence shows clearly that *in utero* experiences do affect the development of the brain. Hearing as an active faculty develops in the sixth month, and babies do react to stories they first heard in the womb.

broadening your knowledge, directly influence the expansion of your brain.

Professor Lawrence C. Katz, of the Department of Neurobiology at Duke University Medical Center, North Carolina, has created an exercise program for the brain he calls "Neurobics." It encourages using the five senses to activate different neural pathways, and claims, "Neurobic exercises enhance the brain's natural drive to form associations—putting a name to a face or a smell with a food—which are the building blocks of memory and the basis of how we learn." Katz also says that it is important to focus your attention regularly and to make major breaks in your routine, changing the order or way in which you do things—even going to work by a different route or trying to use your senses in a new way, whatever you are doing.

Brainpower boosts

Attune to the senses and stretch your sensual brain musculature: try getting dressed in the morning with your eyes closed, using your sense of touch to navigate the way around the brain areas which are linked with touch.

Cross-training is not just for the gym anymore: it activates both sides of the brain simultaneously, expanding the nondominant side of the brain at the same time as working the more dominant side. For a neurobic activity, stand tall and march the legs up and down, making sure you lift the knees up high. Now add elbow work: touch the right elbow to the lifted left knee and then the left elbow to the lifted right knee as you walk in place or around a room. Other cross-training activities can be as simple as crossing one foot over the other when walking around a room. Cross-training for a few minutes before doing activities where you need your left and right brain to work together, and see how this simple exercise adds dimension to your work.

How to have a high-powered memory

Take a look at these numbers: 3...6...5...5...2...1...2...4. Now, without looking at them again, see if you can remember them. No cheating!

How well did you do? Did you manage two? Three? Because of the way our brain works, this task is hard to do, and yet our lives are full of numbers we need to remember—ATM numbers, phone numbers, credit card numbers—as well as names, shopping lists, and appointments. Wouldn't it be great to be able to do away with all those notes and memos and be able to reel off your credit card number or hold phone numbers in your head? In fact, there is absolutely no reason why you can't. Look again at that number we started with, 36552124. Now look at it arranged like this 365 52 12 4. There are 365 days in the year, made up of 52 weeks or 12 months of (about) 4 weeks. Bet you could remember it now, because you've taken two vital

We all forget things occasionally, but are you really much better or worse at remembering than other people? This test will give you an idea. Answer each one with "never," "rarely," or "often."

1   Do you intend to watch a TV show and then forget?
2   Do you find yourself wondering if you've turned off the stove or a light?
3   Do people's names slip your memory?
4   Do you find yourself forgetting points you are trying to make in a conversation?
5   When someone has just told you something, are you unable to recall all the details?
6   Do you say, "I don't remember that" in conversations?
7   Do you fail to pass on messages?
8   Do you go into a store, and then wonder what it was you went in for?
9   Do you forget appointments?
10 Do you throw away the thing you want, a matchbook for example, and then keep what you meant to throw away, i.e. the used match?
11 Do you leave things behind and have to go back for them?
12 Do you do something routine, like brushing your teeth, and then find yourself doing it again?

Score 0 for each "never," 2 for each "rarely," and 4 for each "often," and then add up the scores.

If your total is:

0–16: You have an above-average memory and your life is probably well-organized.

17–32: Your memory is average and, although there are occasional lapses, they are not serious. You could probably improve your concentration.

33–48: You have a poor memory, but don't worry too much, since it may be that you are just very busy at the moment. The more you need to remember, the more there is to forget. Try using notebooks to help you while you build up your skills.

steps that make a number memorable—divided it into chunks and then connected them to something else you already know.

Normally memory works best with things it can see, and the odder and more unusual the better. So to fix those phone numbers in place permanently, you need a system with links, digits, and pictures with a rhyme. You could have: One "bun," two "shoe," three "tree," four "door," etc. This will be your special set of connections, so spend a bit of time making each one specific and clear. Then link each number picture with an item on a list; or link the pictures so they tell a story as a way of remembering a number. So 241 might be using a shoe to bang on a door and wherever you hit, a bun appears. The same principle works for remembering names. Make a connection that's vivid and strange.

feeding the brain

CAN NUTRIENTS MAKE US SMARTER?

One of the most exciting areas opening up in nutrition is the discovery that some nutrients can not only make us more intelligent, but also that the right ones can improve our short- and long-term memory. Some also boost mood and energy.

How well we can concentrate affects practically everything we do, not just studying or taking exams. For example, a better memory might improve your performance at work; it could also help you remember people's names, or actually get the shopping you set out for. Most people would like to be better at solving problems and planning—how to get the best rate of return for your money, for example. Then there's mood. How many of us could say that we never get depressed, that we aren't interested in knowing how to influence how we feel?

But are these real possibilities, or just wishful thinking? Pharmaceutical companies are spending a fortune on the development of drugs to aid mental acuity, but drugs are drugs… they are foreign to the body and it is impossible to tell what their long-term effects might be. The good news, however, is that there are natural substances, found in the body and in food, that really can make us smarter. In fact, in many cases, drug companies start with a nutrient and distort it, not because changing it makes it better or stronger, but because that's how they make their profit, since they cannot patent a natural substance.

Lecithin

Lecithin is a superfood (see page 122), which is normally extracted from soy. Lecithin's most important ingredient is phosphatidyl choline, known as PC, which is probably the body's best source of choline. Choline is needed to make acetylcholine, the neurotransmitter that is important for thought transmission, and has been shown to improve performance in intelligence and memory tests.

PC itself is the major ingredient from which all cell membranes are made. The membranes of cells are where most electrochemical activities take place, including those connected with thinking. PC is also the major ingredient of mitochondria, the energy factories inside every cell of the body, where our food is burned for energy. So PC can help us build energy and combat fatigue, as well as enhance brain power.

DMAE

Our grandmothers were right when they said that eating fish would make us brainier. Fish, as it turns out, contains a nutrient called DMAE (dimethylamino-ethanol), which enhances memory, concentration, energy, and mood. DMAE, which occurs naturally in the brain in small amounts, achieves its effects by increasing the production of acetylcholine, important for memory and learning.

People given DMAE report that they feel more wide awake during the day and sleep more soundly at night, often needing less sleep. After two to three weeks, they commonly experience a mild state of stimulation, which (unlike that produced by coffee and other stimulants) has no side-effects and no let-down when discontinued.

DMAE has also been shown to improve memory and learning, increase intelligence, and raise physical energy. Powers of concentration may be considerably increased. In children it has been used to improve learning problems, shortened attention span, and underachievement. It has even helped children with hyperactivity (ADHD) or behavioral problems.

Perhaps this interesting nutrient's best bonus, though, is its effect on mood. Doctors and psychiatrists report that patients on DMAE are more affable, develop a more outgoing personality, and show greater insight.

Pantothenic acid

Your body can't make acetylcholine for intelligent thinking without using pantothenic acid, also known as vitamin B5 (see page 95), for its assembly from choline. So if you're taking lecithin, choline, or DMAE, you need to make sure you have a source of pantothenic acid as well. Because it is essential for making steroid hormones, including natural cortisone, pantothenic acid is also a stamina-enhancer, which is particularly important when you're under stress.

Pyroglutamate

As people age, their memory tends to decline. This may be connected with a reduced ability to make certain substances, such as acetylcholine. When older people with age-related memory losses were given pyroglutamate, an amino acid, their verbal memory improved. Another research trial, with people suffering from poor memory as a result of alcohol use, found that pyroglutamate significantly improved short- and long-term memory retrieval and also helped storage and consolidation of memory.

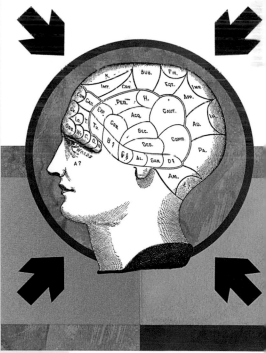

Pyroglutamate is a more potent relative of glutamine, the amino acid that can improve reduced mental performance (see page 120). It is found in large quantities in the brain, cerebrospinal fluid, and the blood, and is also present in vegetables and other foods. In Italy, a form of the nutrient called arginine pyroglutamate is used to treat senility, mental retardation, and alcoholism. Arginine pyroglutamate is also used as a growth hormone to build body muscle and burn fat.

Niacin

Niacin, or vitamin B3 (see page 95), has been shown to enhance memory. When young and middle-aged subjects were given either niacin or a placebo, the ones who got the niacin managed between 10 percent and 40 percent improvement on memory tests.

depression

Psychiatry has a long history of bad ideas for treating depression. Lobotomy, poking a scalpel or similar though the roof of the eye socket and cutting away at the brain cells beyond, was used till the 1950s for serious cases. SSRIs (selective serotonin reuptake inhibitors), which increase the amount of the feel-good neurochemical serotonin, have been prescribed for millions for mild to serious blues more recently, although studies now show that they can be addictive, may increase the risk of suicide and on average are only slightly more effective than a placebo. But the biggest mistake of all may be the assumption that depression involves only the mind and the brain; that nothing physical – what you eat or how much exercise you take – affects your psychological state. When did any doctor you talked to about depression ever ask how much sugar you ate, or test the level of B vitamins in your blood?

And yet both clearly influence your mood. Ever binged on chocolate, felt boosted up for a little and then edgy and uncomfortable? Of course you have. Doctors learn in medical school that depression and irritability are side-effects of B vitamin deficiency, then instantly forget it when faced with the blandishments of the drug companies. More and more people are being diagnosed with depression: overall the figure has risen ten-fold since the 1950s, while the number of depressed young people has doubled in the last 12 years. In the UK, approximately 15 per cent of people are now labelled clinically depressed. So if you want to avoid pills, and the waiting list for psychological help is impossibly long, could food and supplements help to cheer you up?

There is nothing woolly or magical about treating depression with supplements. The reason you are given an SSRI is to increase the amount of serotonin in your brain; the nutritional approach aims at giving you more of an amino acid found in food that serotonin is made from called 5-hydroxytryptophan (5-HTP). In its turn, 5-HTP is made from another amino acid, tryptophan. Both can be found in food: many protein-rich foods such as meat, fish, beans and eggs contain tryptophan, while the richest source of 5-HTP is the African griffonia bean. Not getting enough tryptophan is likely to make you depressed.

But, and this is the part where the nutritional approach gets interesting, unlike the drug approach, which uses a single purified molecule, food and supplements never work on their own. Instead the nutritional approach uses a variety of substances, all of which work together, just as chemicals do in the body. So in order for 5-HTP or tyrosine to work, they need the catalysts that turn them into neurotransmitters. These include the B vitamins, magnesium, zinc and something called trimethylglycine (TMG).

The benefits of the supplements don't stop there. The B vitamins are also vital for another of the transformations that affect depression, which involves an amino acid known as homocysteine. Too little of the B vitamins or too much homocysteine and you are more likely to be depressed.

And there is more. In the last year a number of studies have reported that giving omega-3 fats, especially one called EPA, are vital for psychological well-being. Not only do they also act as catalysts, but they are also needed to build the receptors – the docking ports in brain cells that serotonin and the other neurotransmitters attach themselves to. Omega-3 fats are found especially in oily fish, such as salmon, mackerel and herring. One big study found that the more fish the population of a country eats, the lower their incidence of depression.

Finally, the whole system needs a constant and stable supply of energy, which is why blood sugar levels matter. Eating lots of sugar is going to give you sudden peaks of glucose in the blood, when you feel briefly energetic, followed by a rapid drop. Do that for year after year and the drop will come to be linked with fatigue, irritability, dizziness, insomnia, poor concentration, forgetfulness, and crying spells – all markers for depression.

There is an added bonus to all this. Making sure you get a good supply of B vitamins, omega 3 and a stable blood sugar level will not only go a long way to helping with depression, it will also lower your chances of getting diabetes or heart attacks.

Herbs to help with depression

One of the most famous herbs traditionally known for its efficacy in treating mild to moderate depression is St. John's wort. In many studies it appears to work in more than 70 per cent of cases, which makes it as effective as prescription drugs but without the inherent risks and side-effects of the latter.

Kava-kava is a wonderful natural remedy for promoting a feel good factor. It has been shown in scientific studies that this herb helps improve mental functioning and memory and that it can help alleviate the anxiety that depression often provokes. Sadly, over-regulation and greed means you can no longer buy this herb over the counter in the UK. Happily, the freedom to do so still remains intact in the USA, but for how long?

Oats too have a very calming effect on us. A nourishing and soothing food all in one, oats are a great tonic for the nervous system and are good at combating stress and fatigue too. Ginkgo biloba improves nerve-cell function because it increases the blood supply to the brain, while vervain can have a balancing effect on the entire nervous system and help detoxify the liver at the same time. Along with milk thistle, vervain provides very good support for people who are battling alcohol and drug addiction.

GOT THE PICTURE?

Our prefrontal cortex is the part of the brain associated with perceiving the whole picture, planning ahead, and using our creative imaginations. Interestingly enough, studies have shown that people with clinical depression have an overactive prefrontal cortex.

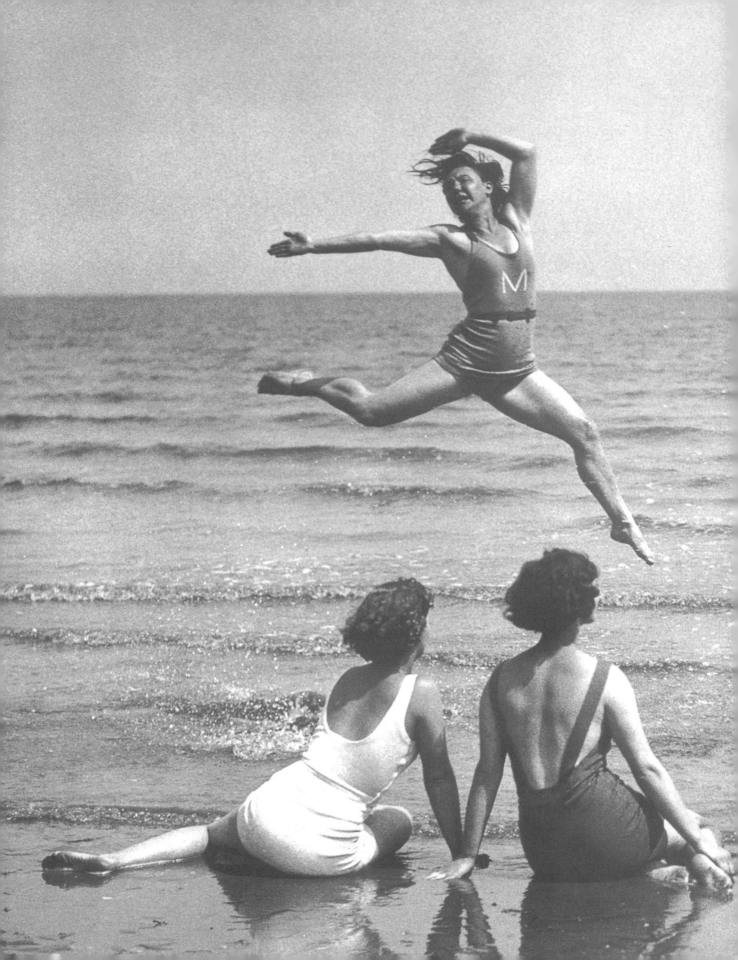

healthy mind, healthy body

The deep, interconnected, and dynamic relationship between the mind and the body is rarely disputed these days. Science and mysticism have found a meeting place in measuring the effect meditation has on brain waves. By slowing down brain-wave patterns, the rest of the body seems to follow suit; the respiratory system, heart rate, etc., all calm down. However, you don't have to meditate to observe or experience the mind/body relationship. Just pay attention to your own physical responses when you are very happy, sad, or angry. Have you ever noticed how tired you feel or how sensitive to physical pain you are when you are depressed? It's a real "chicken and egg" situation— which comes first? What we do know is that the mind has a dramatic effect on the body, just as the body affects the mind. This is why holistic medicine makes so much sense, and why treating the whole individual holds the key to a practical, balanced, natural health-care plan—one that each of us must create to meet our own unique needs and body.

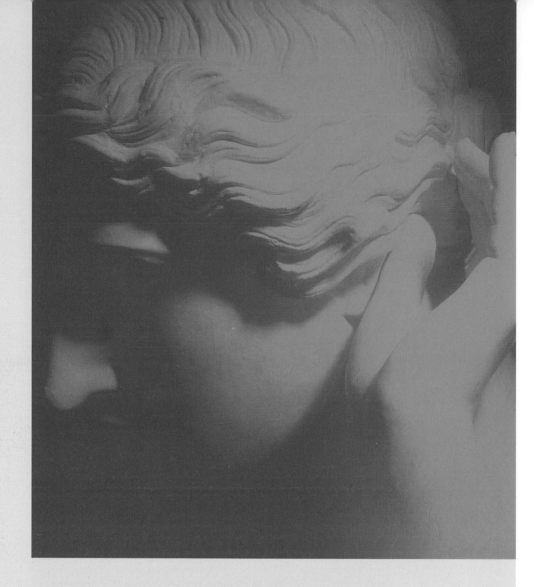

The connection between mind and body is, without a doubt, the most exciting area of modern research into the causes of illness and disease and the maintenance of good health. It is now a proven fact that when you are depressed, your immune system is too. More and more areas of science and medicine are being forced to give serious consideration to the mind-body relationship and its implication in your overall mental and physical health.

your body speaks your mind

An important new science, psychoneuroimmunology, is the in-depth study of mind-body relationships and looks at the interaction between psychology (the mind with all its thoughts and emotions) and the central nervous, immune, and endocrine or hormone systems. Studies all over the world seem to bear out what most complementary therapists and holistic practitioners have always maintained—the whole person is much greater than the sum of all their parts. When looking at creating enduring optimum health, the interconnection of all the mind-body systems holds the vital key to continued wellbeing.

The research and work of Dr. Dean Ornish, founder of the Preventative Medicine Research Institute in Sausalito, California, certainly support these findings. In a landmark study of heart disease, Dr. Ornish proved for the first time that the clogging of the arteries—which can lead to heart attack and stroke—can be reversed without the use of drugs or surgery, and that love was the key factor in this reversal. He concluded that a sad and broken heart was as damaging and dangerous to health as bad dietary habits or lack of exercise.

Dr. Ornish believes that one of the main causes of heart problems is the profound isolation that growing numbers of people are experiencing in modern society. We are not, by nature, solitary creatures. Our roots take us back to extended families, the community, and the "tribe." However, our lifestyles have changed dramatically in a relatively short span of time, and the end result is increasing numbers of people living alone, or living far away from either their family or a social network that can offer support and comfort when it is needed. A weakened, inadequate immune system is often the result of an inadequate social support system. One indicator of the immune response is the natural killer cell activity, levels of which are more likely to be lower in people who are lonely. As Dr. Ornish says, "Looking out for No. 1 isn't enlightened self-interest. It's just lonely, and loneliness kills." Recent research has shown that people who are usually lonely and isolated suffer more poor health and are much more susceptible to all kinds of illness and disease.

In her excellent book, *Your Body Speaks Your Mind*, Debbie Shapiro reports on "the link between psychological stress and physical problems as illustrated by research, cited by Dr. Larry Dossey in *Healing Breakthroughs*, which states that more heart attacks occur on a Monday than on any other day of the week—and not only on a Monday, but most often at 9 o'clock in the morning. No other animal suffers death more consistently on a particular day of the week. If we believe that there is no connection between the mind and the body, then what causes so many heart attacks to take place just as the first work of the week is about to begin? Certainly there are physiological reasons why death might be more likely in the morning than in the afternoon, such as higher heart rates or blood pressure, or adrenaline surging in preparation for the day ahead. There is, however, no reason why more deaths should take place on a Monday rather than any other day."

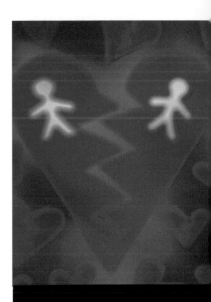

The *Journal of the American Medical Association* published evidence which showed that emotional risk factors for heart attacks might be more important than the physical: "anger and deprivation of love might overshadow the contribution of serum cholesterol to the likelihood of a coronary." Therefore, it is important to learn how to express and resolve emotional issues and conflicts.

There is a growing body of research in recent decades that demonstrates the close mind-body relationship. This mounting pile of evidence is stimulating increasing scientific inquiry into psychoneuroimmunology (PNI). Even earlier studies have shown fascinating results. Between 1948 and 1964, researchers followed the health of around 1,300 medical students who graduated from Johns Hopkins University in Baltimore, Maryland: "While in medical school, some of the students claimed to be emotionally removed from one or both parents. After 30 years, the investigators found these same people suffered an unusually high incidence of mental illness, suicide, and death from cancer."

It is medical fact that stress has a big effect on our general and specific health and on our sense of wellbeing. If the mental and emotional pressures that build up inside us cannot be expressed and resolved, they are likely to find a way out through the body, usually through the weakest point—whether it is the nerves, the digestive system, the immune system, or our sleeping patterns. Debbie Shapiro says, of stress, "Pushed down, it becomes illness, depression, addiction, or anxiety; projected outwards, it becomes hostility, crime, prejudice, or aggression."

"It is everyday stress that affects us most deeply, by slowly grinding away at our inner reserves. The fight-or-flight response enables us to respond to danger, but it is not just major life-threatening situations that stimulate this response. Fearful or anxious thoughts do it too—the car not starting, being late for an appointment, unpaid bills, arguments with your partner, your children, or your boss—all these can create a stress response."

Debbie says that Joan Borysenko, author of *Guilt is the Teacher, Love is the Lesson*, puts it well: "The fight-or-flight response is like the overdrive on a car. It comes in handy to get us out of occasional tight spots, but if we keep the car in overdrive all the time, the wear and tear on its parts will cause a variety of mechanical problems. In people, these problems are commonly called stress or anxiety-related disorders."

Taking the mind-body relationship another step, the "mind over matter" school of thought has a large body of evidence and testimony to support it. Here the belief is that you can *think* yourself well or young. How well we feel—and even how we age— is intimately linked with our state of mind, according to celebrity Ayurvedic doctor,

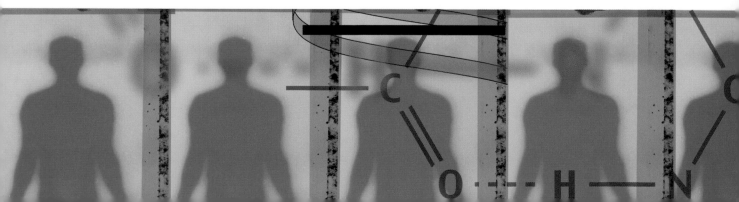

THE "FIGHT OR FLIGHT" RESPONSE

The adrenal glands, located above the kidneys, produce the "fight or flight" hormone, adrenaline. Adrenaline is completely vital to our survival; it stimulates all the body's systems, getting us prepared to flee from danger, or if this is not possible, to confront and overwhelm, or to fight off, that which is a threat to us.

Adrenaline is released in response to situations that we perceive as life-threatening—whether or not they actually are life-threatening. The body immediately responds to everyday stress and tension as a threat and increases the release of adrenaline that will speed up instinctive life-saving functions.

The fact that we are not actually having to run or fight physically suggests this hormone is pumping through the body unused, and unchanneled, except for the undesired effect of producing a heightened sense of anxiety and stress. The body then has to work harder to eliminate the by-products of this unused adrenaline, which can lead to overtaxed and exhausted adrenals.

Deepak Chopra. In his book *Ageless Body, Timeless Mind*, he says many people lose vitality and decline in old age simply because they expect to do so. He believes that by programming the mind to have different expectations, you can retain youthful abilities and outlook. He likes to quote one of his 80-year-old patients: "People don't grow old. When they stop growing, they become old." Teaching his patients how to restore all body rhythms to their intended functioning, how to calm rapid heartbeats, conquer asthmatic wheezing, and stave off degenerative conditions is paramount to Chopra's approach and, according to him, has huge implications for aging.

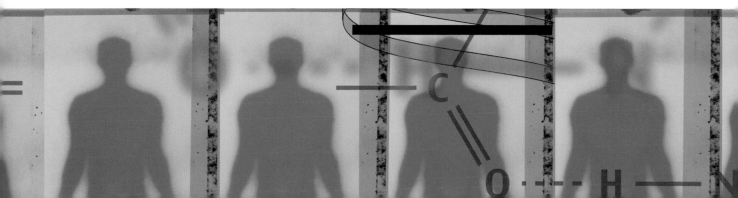

laughter and chocolate

One of the most interesting developments in the natural health field is the research into the beneficial effects of pleasure and happiness on health. Scientists all over the world are studying the effects of enjoyable experiences on the pleasure centers of the brain, and it is now a proven scientific fact—pleasure is good for you!

Happiness and humor increase our sense of wellbeing and help us live longer. Indulging (in moderation) in things that you enjoy—like chocolate—and having fun in general have been proven to boost the immune system by increasing the production of immunoglobin A, which protects us against many infections, including colds and flu. When we're having fun, we also relax more, our cholesterol levels drop, and our brain waves change to the more calming alpha form. Another piece of folk wisdom is validated—a little of what you like does you good.

Laughter is one of life's great pleasures and a primary signal of friendship. Laughing expresses our humor and playfulness. Laughing together is a way of strengthening family and social bonds, facilitating and providing the human contact we need to survive. Laughing has many other important physical and psychological benefits. The old adage "laughter is the best medicine" has some factual basis. A study by Dr. William Fry of the Stanford University School of Medicine, California, clearly demonstrated that laughter boosts the cardiovascular, respiratory, muscular, hormonal, central nervous, and immune systems. When laughing, we draw more air in and out of our lungs than during normal breathing, and in doing so we push more oxygen into the bloodstream, which, in turn, stimulates the circulation.

If just the act of smiling can produce demonstrably lower levels of "stress hormones," and as laughter has been clinically proven to increase the "feel good" hormones in the brain and the "fighting fit" hormones in the immune system, then we should all laugh a lot more. British psychologist Robert Holden organized "laughter clinics" and workshops around the world for many years. His clinic in Birmingham is renowned worldwide and he has managed to organize free laughter clinics for patients under the National Health Service.

The awareness of the power of laughter to enhance and help maintain our wellbeing is increasing, and is supported by clinical studies. These show how our heart rate usually rises when we are laughing. Studies of blood samples taken from people while they were laughing show high levels of the "arousal" hormones, adrenaline and noradrenaline. We are more physically aroused during a good session of laughter and, as a result, we are mentally sharper and more alert afterwards.

Laughter helps us relieve the burden of mounting daily stresses and tensions. When we laugh, there is a burst of energy—physical and mental activity—followed by a cycle of relaxation, when the muscles are less tense than they were before. These alternating cycles can help prevent us becoming too stressed out about our daily problems. Laughter promotes a healthier, more positive attitude, which, in turn, seems to attract more positive energy, people, and events to our lives.

Use it or lose it—a good sense of humor is like a muscle. The more it is used, the more developed and toned it becomes. A sense of humor is an important way of dealing with day-to-day problems. Seeing the funny side of a problem can help us manage it with ease and helps diffuse the tensions between people personally and professionally. People with a well-developed sense of fun often have fewer emotional problems than those who find it difficult to laugh—particularly at themselves.

In their book *Ultra Age*, Mary Spillane and Victoria McKee observe how "the sense of humor is one of the first things that disappears from depressed people, and is a precious commodity to cultivate. It will not desert you with age, like your looks eventually will, and may be a truly saving grace. The ability to laugh at yourself, and even at the tragic events that touch you, can help to get you through the toughest times intact."

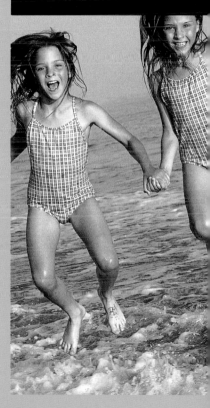

Professor David Warburton, founder of ARISE (Associates for Research into the Science of Enjoyment) observes how "a child of six laughs 300 times a day, while the average adult has 50 laughs and a depressed person less than 6."

One of the most popular "mood foods" is sweet, creamy, mouthwatering chocolate. The pleasure of eating chocolate may be rooted in physiological fact as well as in the psychological "naughty but nice" syndrome that eating chocolate provokes. If eating chocolate pleases you, allow yourself the indulgence without guilt—the guilt is counterproductive and provokes anxiety and stress. It is important to keep your pleasures pleasurable and, therefore, guilt-free. Give yourself permission to eat good-quality dark chocolate in the knowledge that it is good for you, it is a source of protein, iron, magnesium, and valuable B vitamins, and, like laughter, it often triggers the release of the feel-good endorphins, the body's natural opiates.

Another reason why humans crave chocolate may be because cocoa contains tiny traces of cannabis-like compounds called endocannabinoids, and although these are not nearly powerful enough to reach "cannabis-like intoxication," according to Italian researchers, this may help explain the enduring appeal of chocolate. For some, eating chocolate may seem like an addiction. This may be because chocolate contains theobromine, a psychoactive stimulant of the central nervous system, which may also cause you to experience enhanced performance after eating chocolate.

However, do watch out for addiction signals—a cycle of craving can result in overeating chocolate because of the release of endorphins it stimulates. Relax and enjoy the pure sensuous delight of eating chocolate—regularly but moderately. Try to avoid overly sweet confections; instead, choose organic quality milk or dark chocolate made from more than 70 percent cocoa solids.

A huge study of the life spans of more than 7,000 people was carried out by researchers at the Harvard School of Public Health in Boston. It concluded that regular candy-eaters outlived abstainers by around a year.

affirmations

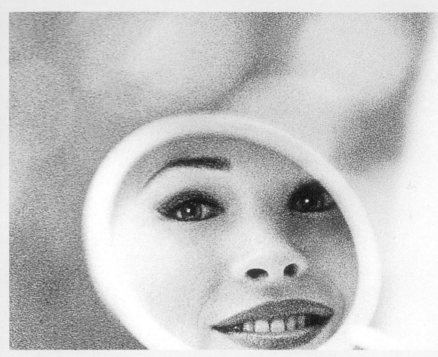

Affirmation—the repetition of a thought over and over again to embed it in the mind—is one of the principal tools of learning. There are two types of affirmations—positive and negative. Negative affirmations can start very young, even in babyhood. A baby or young child responds more openly to love than it does to anger. However, the stresses and strains of current daily life can often prohibit parents, siblings, and teachers from always acting "with love."

Part of learning to heal and take responsibility for ourselves starts with positive thinking. We must start by learning to love ourselves. It may feel strange, perhaps, or even intimidating to some, to admit openly their love for themselves, but it works. The power of positive thought cannot be overestimated.

How many times a day do you feel you have a negative thought? Countless times, possibly. "I'll never get that done in time," "I'm not capable of doing that," "I'm useless,' to name just a few possible everyday thoughts. Try switching the thoughts around: "I am capable of achieving all that I want to," "There is always enough time," "I'm able." Add "I am loving and loved—I love and approve of myself" and you are on the way to changing those instilled thought patterns.

One of the most popular affirmations to offset the negative is to say, "I love myself"—not just once a day, but a hundred times or even more every day! Eventually you will feel the power of this statement. Keep it up. Check yourself. Notice any changes in your attitude as your belief in yourself starts to improve. Catch yourself when you are feeling negative, write down what you are thinking or

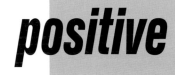

positive

positive	negative
I can	I can't
I am worthy	I am unworthy
I have a right to be here	I don't belong here
I am loved	I am unloved
I am loving	I am unable to love
I am in the right place at the right time	I am never in the right place at the right time
I achieve all I need and want to achieve	I am a loser
I know my skills and talents are valuable	I am no good to anybody
There is always enough time	There's never enough time
I draw into my life exactly what is right	I can never attract what is worthwhile for me
I love myself exactly as I am right now	I want to change everything about myself

feeling, and then write down the affirmative statement. How does it feel to change "I am lazy" into "I am productive and use my time well for me"?

You have to do a lot of positive affirmation to combat all the negativity that usually clouds the pattern of thinking "I'm not good enough," "I can't do that," "That's not for me," "I'm too fat... too thin... too old," "Oh, I would never do anything like that," or those negative affirmations thrown at you by others, such as, "You're no good," "You never do anything," "You'd be better if you had money... got that degree... had that job."

Unwittingly we can be programmed to believe the "truth" of these negative messages we receive very early on in life. They can be very damaging to us and can form the root of a failure to love ourselves, which projects deeply into our teen, adult, and elderly years. If we switch the negatives into positives—into the affirmative—we begin to heal ourselves and our lives of all the negative energy we have amassed. Such energy is useless, wasted, and needs to be released. Feel the anger, resentment, fear, bitterness, and guilt, and let it start to dissipate with constant affirmations.

Much of the illness and stress we experience are brought on by negative thought patterns. Changing your negative thoughts into positive ones can literally improve your health and have a knock-on effect on all those who come into contact with you. A person who truly loves themselves, unconditionally, will express this love and optimism in all they do.

Getting positive

Can you look in the mirror and say "I love you"? Try it. This can feel very strange, but it is certainly one of the most empowering ways of making a positive affirmation. Try to do it at least once every day, perhaps when you first wake up. Hear yourself say the words "I love you." How do you sound? Genuine? Embarrassed? Insincere? As you practice the affirmation day by day, make a note to yourself about how it feels to say those words. It will become easier.

Try creating your own affirmations. What feels comfortable for you to say? You may need to create new affirmations every day, according to your physical and emotional needs at that moment. The events of a day may prompt you to create new affirmations in the evening to recite before you go to bed. Perhaps you are feeling stressed after a hard day. Take some time out, just a few minutes if that's all you have, to breathe deeply and focus on where in your body you are feeling that stress. Perhaps your body is giving you signals that may previously have been ignored. Create an affirmation around the stress, remembering to make sure it is a positive statement!

Be mindful to be kind, gentle, and patient with yourself while beginning to change your negative thought patterns. If you "forget" one day, then begin again the next day. After many years of negative programming, it may take some time to adopt this new way of being. Encourage and praise yourself as much as you can, and enjoy feeling positive about yourself and those around you.

Positive pointers

Positively affirm yourself throughout the day. Congratulate yourself when you feel you have achieved something. Encourage yourself. Avoid panic and negative, derogatory thoughts about yourself or your associates. Thinking positively requires so much less energy and enhances your own feelings of wellbeing. Smiling to yourself and at others is so much more positive than frowning and worrying.

If you have fears and worries, acknowledge them. Don't try to suppress them with stimulants, such as alcohol or cigarettes, or by stuffing yourself with comfort food. If they are very pressing then try to find a support group, therapist, or natural therapy that really appeals to you to help you through the crisis. Do not be afraid to call on those you love to help you in times of need. It is better to ask for help than to try to handle all that life doles out to you in isolation. Perhaps you, in turn, will then be able to help someone you love in their time of crisis.

Show love and appreciation to others and expect to receive it back. It works wonders for your own self-esteem and is a beautiful way of creating harmonious relationships with those around you.

visualization

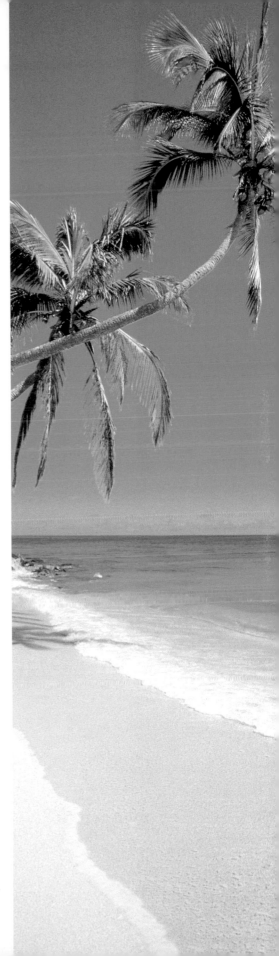

As discussed at the beginning of this chapter, an increasing number of doctors and scientists worldwide are acknowledging the existence of a strong mind-body connection. Today, even the most conservative practitioners accept that the mind has the power to heal, and that mental pictures are powerful tools which can dramatically enhance or depress our sense of wellbeing.

Just as laughter has been proven to stimulate the immune function (see page 206), we can use our imagination to visualize a particular image and invoke a particular response. By focusing with your inner eye on an image that symbolizes calm serenity, you can lower your blood pressure, slow your breathing, and generally reduce a stress response.

Mind control techniques—such as creative visualization, biofeedback, meditation, and hypnosis—are some of the therapeutic relaxation methods used to reduce stress levels and redress the mind-body balance. The techniques help the body eliminate stress before it can accumulate and cause physical or mental disorders. All of us have, within our grasp, a profound and simple tool that enhances the ability to stimulate self-healing, increase energy, and create a state of inner peace.

Practicing creative visualization

All you need to do is make yourself comfortable, concentrate on your breathing to help you deeply relax, and let go, leaving all thoughts behind you. Then think of something that represents a peaceful calm scene; some image that evokes a deep sense of serenity. It may be a place you have visited, or an imaginary utopia.

Many professional athletes use creative visualization or "imaging" to improve their performance. They see themselves winning or beating their own best time and often create positive outcomes with their confident beliefs. This mental rehearsal is sometimes called the "inner game" by athletes, and is part of "psyching up" for the performance. Not just physical performance, but also bodily responses can be regulated by mental imagery. Your immune system can be improved and stabilized by imaging techniques. Many people with HIV and AIDS have had remarkable success in visualizing and befriending their few remaining T cells and encouraging them to fight back, as have cancer patients who visualize killing off their wayward cells.

the relaxed mind

We are much more creative and intuitive when the mind is relaxed, rather than tense, overworked, and exhausted. Relaxation and mind control go hand in hand, and relaxing the mind and body releases our creative and intellectual powers.

Most people agree that relaxation is an integral ingredient of a balanced, healthy lifestyle, yet fail to incorporate enough of it into their daily routines. However you define it, relaxation is the antidote to stress in our lives and we need it for our survival, let alone our wellbeing. It is only while you are sleeping or relaxing that your body can repair and heal the damage incurred while rushing through your days. No matter what your circumstances, you owe it to yourself to take time out of your daily life for activities that relax you and help you unwind.

Learning to relax

Fortunately, the art of relaxation can be learned, and there is more than one path to achieving it. Relaxing is a simple habit, but, like anything else, it needs to be practiced regularly to get it right. Don't wait until you get near breaking point before you start. In addition to bringing you a calmer mind, a daily relaxation program can relieve physical symptoms, such as aches and pains, and even lower your blood pressure.

Relaxation means different things to different people: a walk in the woods, a swim, or a hot shower may relax you, while a friend may unwind by listening to music or playing a game of basketball. For some people relaxing outside with a good book and a mug of coffee is the answer; for someone else, it might be weeding, planting roses, or redecorating the house. A vacation on a hot sandy beach may be your idea of relaxation, while skiing down an icy mountain could be your best friend's antidote to stress. Discover what truly relaxes you and make regular time to listen to your needs.

It does not matter what your personal preferences are. What matters is that you make or create the time to indulge in your whims and your personal needs for relaxation, fun, and creative expression. The important thing is to take time out to do the things that make you feel good and help you to relax. It's a simple message, but your life—as well as your wellbeing—may depend on it.

When you add up the waking hours of the day you spend doing things that please you—that enhance your life and your sense of wellbeing, and just make you feel happy, engaged, and fulfilled—what percentage of the day do they fill? Maybe it is 5 percent, 10, 20, 50 percent? Or are you one of the rare lucky ones who fills more than half their days with pleasurable pursuits? Most of us, unless we are nourished by our work life (like an artist or an athlete), really can't expect that, so 20 to 30 percent would be a reasonable expectation. If your percentage is seriously below that, make it your goal to double it over a period of a few months.

A relaxed mind is a healthy mind that encourages greater self-awareness and, therefore, greater self-care. By listening to yourself, your mind and your body, you will become much more in tune with what your real needs are. Do you need to exercise? Eat more fruit? Drink more water? Sleep more? Make sure you have quiet time to yourself, instead of filling every waking moment so that spare time becomes an elusive commodity—if it exists at all?

Daily practice of some form of relaxation of the mind, whether it is simple deep breathing or an unhurried walk around the block, at a time that suits you, will enhance all this and more. Even coping with life's great pains, such as the loss of loved ones or financial pressures, becomes easier to handle with a peaceful mind.

Next to deep breathing and intelligent eating, one of your best defenses against the destructiveness of excess stress is making time for yourself. Just consider what these four words mean to you. They entail listening to your needs and giving them priority in your long list of "to do"s. Identifying the pastimes that you really enjoy is tantamount to naming the tools for your mental and physical survival.

The relaxed mind finds it easier to organize, prioritize, and manage an otherwise hectic lifestyle. In fact, ironically, the more effort you make to "make time for yourself," the more likely you are to have time! Taking time to notice how you are breathing, shallowly or deeply, and correcting your breathing needs to take only a few seconds, but can have wonderful results. If panic sets in when you hit rush-hour traffic or are up against a deadline, deep breathing will help to waylay your fears. Panicking will not make the traffic move more quickly or help you work harder; it will merely increase your heart rate and cause you stress.

If your mind is constantly rattled with thoughts and plans or reliving discussions on the telephone or the movie you saw yesterday, take time to quieten and empty out those thoughts. A clear mind is a calm, relaxed mind that is more easily able to focus on the tasks in the day ahead. When the mind is peaceful, there is more room for creative, inspired thoughts and for ideas to surface. Intuition is enhanced because you are more in tune with your body and environment. After addressing your own needs adequately, you are better placed to address the needs of others.

Spending time with people you genuinely love and who love you in return will enhance your self-esteem and relax you. Take the time to tell those people that you love them. Show that you care: buy flowers, gifts, make time, listen, and share. Children naturally express themselves, in the moment, whether happy, sad, angry, or tired. We can learn so much from observing the behavior of the children around us. They often reflect our own moods back to us. Tension can breed tension, and children will respond as they see you respond. Likewise, a calm and peaceful state will induce the same state in those around us… "the ripple effect."

TIPS FOR TIME MANAGEMENT

One of the most important things you can do to maximize relaxation is structure your day's activities, being realistic about what can and can't be done, and prioritize.

- At home, organize your meals, your housework, etc., to avoid being overstimulated by a noisy vacuum cleaner at midnight or a washing machine at 3 a.m.
- At work make sure you take time out for lunch. At least get away from your desk into another environment. If the weather is good, try to find a pretty spot outside to enjoy the sunshine or fresh air.
- Take time for exercise.
- Take time for eating.
- Take time for play/socializing.
- Take time for support (healing treatments, counselling sessions).
- Take time for study.
- Take time for family and friends.

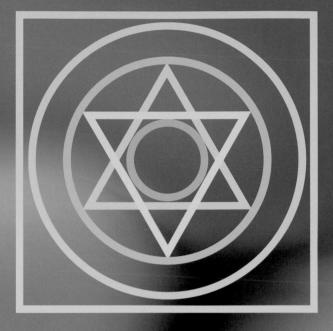

the meditative mind

If someone was to tell you that there was an incredible new drug that could not only make vaccines work more effectively and speed up healing of a nasty skin complain by 400 per cent but could also change the brainwave patterns of people suffering from psychiatric problems, you might look rather sceptical. In fact there is something that can do all those things and more — but it isn't a drug. It's old fashioned meditation, a technique for focusing the mind that dates back thousands of years and that been used by most of the world's religions in some form or other.

With the aid of high-resolution scanners, scientists have been peering into the brains of meditators as they turn their mind inwards, and they have found that meditation can produce lasting changes in particular areas of the brain, such as those linked with happiness.

This research shows that meditating for just a few minutes every day can have all sorts of health benefits, from lowering your risk of heart disease to boosting your immune system and helping to control binge eating. Simple, free and effective, meditation looks like as though it could become as essential a part of everyone's healthy living regime as exercise.

> **Mindfulness can help with psychological problems as well. Research at Cambridge in the UK, for instance, found that groups who were getting standard cognitive behaviour therapy (CBT) for depression were 50 per cent less likely to relapse if they practised meditation as well.**

Another term for meditation is 'mindfulness'. In other words, it's paying attention to what you are experiencing right at this moment without drifting off into thoughts about the past, wondering about the future or having opinions about either. Researchers questioned 1,500 people and found that those who were rated as being more 'mindful' also had better moods, were more optimistic and reported greater satisfaction with life.

What has been getting the scientists excited, though, has been the research showing that these reports of what it feels like to meditate fit perfectly with the effect it has on the brain. For instance, a recent study found that that 25 people who had been meditating for two months nearly all had much more activity in an area of the brain associated with happiness and optimism, which is the left side of the frontal lobe (just behind the left eye).

But that wasn't the only benefit. When the meditators got a 'flu jab at the end of course, they produced 25 per cent more antibodies – immune cells to fight the 'flu virus – than a non-meditating group. Equally impressive was the finding that people suffering from the scaly red skin of psoriasis healed four times faster when meditation was combined with standard ultraviolet light treatment, than when the light was used on its own.

Scientific research into meditation dates back 30 years, when Dr Herbert Benson of Harvard University found it induces a calm state that is the opposite of the hyped-up stress response, known as 'fight or flight', that we have when we are anxious or angry. 'It is simply a doorway that clears the mind', says Benson.

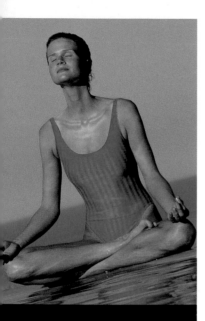

Few of us ever experience the full immensity of the mind's extraordinary capabilities. We are curious, intrigued, excited, and drawn to further exploration of what we call normal consciousness. How fascinating to realize that we normally live only on the edge of a mostly unexplored territory, which is as vast as the universe itself, and beyond.

What is meditation and why is it so good for you?

Meditation is primarily an experience of stillness. When thoughts drop away and there is no thinking, you enter into a quiet space. We often experience this naturally when walking in nature or sitting on a beach, looking out to sea. Meditation helps us connect to this natural state purposefully—to enter fully into the present moment.

The act of meditation is defined in a number of ways: "to think over, consider, reflect, contemplate" or "to fix the mind upon" are just a few. Meditation is about learning "mindfulness," about entering into the present moment by observing the mind's activity. To work *with* your mind, to watch your thoughts come and go without becoming attached to them, is the most fundamental aspect of personal free will. Meditation helps us develop constructive mental habits that enhance mental and physical wellbeing. It teaches us how to let go of our thoughts—our "busyness"—and just "be," to experience our "beingness" without thinking about anything in particular. This is what really relaxes the mind. Meditation is the quiet space between thoughts.

Debbie Shapiro has these thoughts to share on the power of meditation: "Throughout the ages, meditation has been used to enter within and explore the wonders that are there. True meditation is a fully conscious natural awareness, a mind that is clear and free. Through relaxation and meditation, we unfold the vast inner world that lies hidden at the core of our being. Meditation is a process of stilling the mind and developing a completely calm mental state. Its joy is in its simplicity, in the flow of thoughts through the mind, in being in the moment."

Clinical trials have shown that meditating regularly reduces stress. The pulse and respiratory rate slow down. If your blood pressure is too high, meditation will lower it. Your body consumes less oxygen because cell metabolism slows down. The brain's alpha waves (those associated with relaxation) increase. Meditation and yoga practice are based on learning to focus your attention and observe your thoughts. If you can master this practice, you can master anything.

How to meditate

Meditation is taught to millions of overstressed Westerners as a way of reaching a tranquil state of mind. It can relax and refresh your body and mind. If practiced properly and regularly, it will do away with the need for drugs or alcohol to cope with life. That's how powerful a tool it can be. Meditation is simple, safe, and free. It can be done anywhere, any time, but it is most easily practiced in peaceful surroundings. Dress comfortably, without shoes (wear socks or soft slippers if the weather is chilly).

The mind moves in cycles of concentration and relaxation. Meditation is about being in the moment—you just need to be still and sitting comfortably with a straight, but not tense, spine. It is good to have a quiet place in your home for meditation, where you can build up the atmosphere of peace and serenity away from the distractions of your daily life... a little corner for contemplating your wellbeing.

steps to meditation

1 To get the best out of meditation, set aside space and time every day for practice. An ideal start is 5 minutes twice a day, gradually working up to at least 15 to 20 minutes once or twice a day. Take the time to be quiet, to be still, and to be mindful of yourself in the present. Don't worry if your mind seems to leap around in endless turmoil; just being still wiill encourage a deeper silence.

2 Find a comfortable, quiet spot away from distraction, where you feel safe and warm, even if you are only meditating for 5 or 10 minutes to start with. After you have learned to meditate, you will be more adept at watching the flow of your thoughts and being fully present in the moment. You may even be able to meditate in motion, while walking along a country lane, for example.

3 The next step is to find a position for meditation, in which you can sit and relax without straining the back or legs. It doesn't have be in lotus position or cross-legged, if these positions are uncomfortable. A chair, or on the floor with your back against the wall for support, is fine. In any pose, your back should be straight and upright, without being fixed and rigid. This helps you maintain your concentration and steady your mind. A good way of keeping a straight back is to imagine a string pulling you gently up through the crown of your head (see also the "inner dialogue" in the Alexander Technique, pages 260–61).

4 Now begin to release any inner tension by relaxing all your muscles and internal organs. Many people find it helpful to imagine each part of the body contracting and relaxing in turn, starting with the head and ending with the tips of the toes.

5 The next step is to steady your breath by allowing your natural deep-flowing and gentle breath to emerge without force and without judgement. By first doing a relaxation exercise, you should have little or no problem finding your lowered respiratory rate reflected in slower, deeper breathing. Flowing, even breathing reflects a calm, meditative inner state.

6 Do the "following the breath" exercise: to begin with, just sit still and become aware of your complete breathing cycles. Following your breath with your consciousness/attention as you inhale and exhale is a good meditation practice. The "following the breath" exercise will help you get used to being still and focused. Because we are so used to being busy all the time, we no longer find it a simple task just to "be." As the great mystic philosopher and author J. Krishnamurti said, "Most of us want to have our minds continually occupied so that we are prevented from seeing ourselves as we actually are. We are afraid to be empty. We are afraid to look at our fears."

---

1 Find a regular time.
2 Find a comfortable space.
3 Find a comfortable position, checking that your posture is straight and upright.
4 Allow your muscles and organs to relax to help you focus the mind.
5 Practice a gentle breathing exercise to slow down the mind and body.
6 Follow your deep, but gentle inhalations and exhalations.

By observing your mind's activity you can learn to *be*. Meditation is not the same as concentration. The purpose of meditation is to let go of all your worries, to free you to experience the infinite peace, both within and around you. Concentration, on the other hand, frees your attention from all objects and thoughts, allowing you to focus your mind on one thing at a time.

To start, you need to set aside some time to practice "being without doing," just to be with your inner reflections. To watch, observe your thoughts, and then learn to detach from them and let them go, along with all distractions. There are many approaches to meditation, but they all have the same goal. Each technique is a means to calm and quieten the mind by focusing attention inward. Meditation helps us understand our mind. It doesn't always come easily at first, so practice and perseverance are important.

Do some breathing and relaxation exercises to help you before you begin, particularly if you are setting aside time for your meditation practice at the end of the day. It may then take a little bit more time and effort to clear away the day's events, but once you have, you will emerge from your meditations much more refreshed and recharged. Breathing is the key to meditation. Breathing exercises and generally paying attention to your breath are the easiest and most natural ways to learn meditation. As soon as you start watching your breath, you are taken into your body.

Try this simple exercise: Breathe in to the count of one, breathe out to the count of one; breathe in to the count of two, breathe out to the count of two; breathe in to the count of three, and so on up to ten, then start at one again. Without strain, do this as long as it feels comfortable. This exercise helps you to focus on your breathing and to really be in the moment without distraction. Be gentle with yourself; it takes time to learn and there is no right or wrong, or only one way to meditate.

At first you may find steadying the mind difficult enough, let alone stilling it. Don't worry—everyone experiences the "playful monkey of the mind" and the frustration that goes with these visits! The next most important tool you must develop, after relaxation and steady natural breathing, is patience. This quality will help you learn meditation more than any other.

When learning how to "sit and do nothing," beginners should keep in mind a few basic pointers. The three major areas of attention are body, breath, and mind; that is, the "Three Treasures" of essence, energy, and spirit. An ancient Tao text states: "Shut off the three external treasures of hearing, sight, and speech in order to cultivate the three internal treasures of essence, energy, and spirit." You must acquire the art of being still before you can meditate. You may be surprised just how difficult that is for many people, so do not be alarmed or dismayed if you are one of them. With patience and practice, you will learn how to meditate and, before long, experience the benefits of this ancient technique.

Concentration exercise

Another excellent meditation exercise is concentrating and softening your gaze on an external object, such as a candle flame. This is a good way to learn how to focus and empty your mind, helping you develop powers of relaxation, concentration, and "one-pointedness."

There are many different ways to meditate, both "inner" and "outer." Everyone approaches meditation in their own unique way: some use a mantra to focus and empty the mind; others use mandalas, sacred art that suggests a meditative state; and some people just close their eyes and go into a relaxed state that is meditation.

Transcendental meditation

Over the last thirty years, transcendental meditation (TM) has become one of the most popular meditation systems in the West. Many people in the business world are attracted to TM because it teaches you how to reduce stress levels and promote a sense of wellbeing that can greatly enhance personal and professional lives.

Deepak Chopra took transcendental meditation to a new level of popularity after his book *Ageless Body, Timeless Mind* became such a hit in the 1990s. He helped people understand TM and how silently repeating a specific Sanskrit mantra or word can help the mind snap out of its normal patterns and move into the silent space beyond thought. Chopra said that a mantra is a way of getting a direct message to the nervous system, and that mantras have been a part of meditation practices in India for thousands of years. To learn TM properly, you should receive personal instruction from a trained teacher.

Chanting

Chanting is a meditation technique that focuses the mind on a sound which sets up resonance in the mind–body. Mantras are repetitive sounds that you can chant over and over because of the vibration and concentration they stimulate. You become centered and serene by means of the power of the chanted word.

To begin with, certain vowel sounds are used as mantras because they have great healing value. One of the most important and common of these is the sacred sound "Om" or "Aum." The chanting of "Om" for a few minutes at the end of your meditation will have a very uplifting effect. Take a deep inhalation through your nose and begin to chant "Om" as you exhale, chanting over and over with great resonance for as long as one breath will allow. Start with the mouth open and gradually close it until you are making a low humming sound through gently closed lips. Repeat three or more times. Mantras should be spoken slowly or quietly chanted with utmost concentration. Repetitively chanting the "Om" or "Aum" ("O-ooo-mmm" or "ah-ooo-mmm") often follows a Hatha yoga session or ends a meditation. "Om" represents the "universal vibration of absolute consciousness, the sound of infinity of which we cannot fathom."

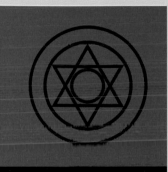

Some of the popular sounds for chanting are "Ra," "Ma," "Ram," "Om," or combinations of these sounds, like "Aum-ra-ma-om" or "Om-na-ma-ha-shi-va-ya." You can practice more than three sounds at a time if it feels good to you, but start slowly and work your way up as you gain more confidence in meditation practice.

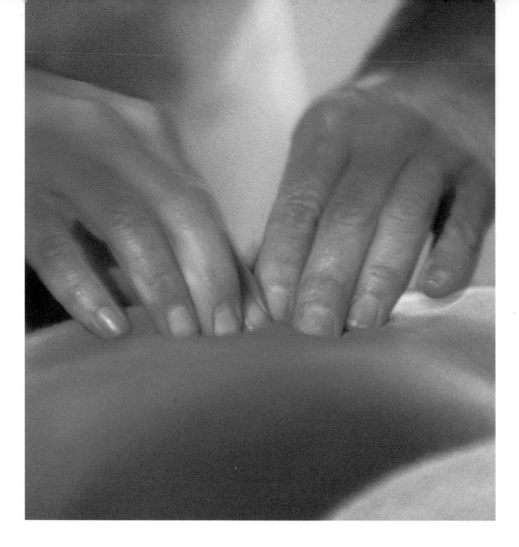

the magic of massage

Massage is a beautiful healing art enjoyed by many today who recognize its value in de-stressing and clearing away day-to-day anxieties. Treating yourself to regular massage helps to reduce stress levels and goes some way toward preventing the development of illnesses that are often stress-related.

In addition to being a wonderful de-stresser and a relaxing therapy, massage is very powerful and can also be extremely provocative. During or after a massage, you may experience emotional changes—either in a very subtle way or in a striking and powerful manner—and the changes may stay with you for some time. This is because massage has an excellent ability to uncover emotional issues held deep in the body's tissues, either from the near past or from many years ago. This is one of the strengths of massage: its ability to aid in the healing of emotional issues.

Massage imbues a feeling of being gently nurtured, which allows us to feel in tune with our bodies in a way that, perhaps, many of us are no longer used to. If we are past the age when mom and dad give us daily hugs, where do we receive that comforting touch? Massage is a wonderful way of making sure that we continue to be nurtured in adult life, and it serves as a reminder to our bodies of those early years when we were taken care of by those who loved us.

Various forms of massage have been practiced down through the centuries and are now widely followed around the world. Much of the holistic massage practiced today in the West, for example, finds its origins in Eastern techniques combined with Swedish approaches. Many civilizations used massage as a curative therapy and preventative treatment. In China, the massage practiced there is renowned for curing all kinds of ailments, from the common cold to irritable bowel syndrome (IBS). In fact, any condition is believed to be a manifestation of blockage in *chi* along the body's meridians and so, by using massage to create a free flow of *chi* throughout all the meridians, good health is believed to be ensured.

Massage holds many possibilities for us as givers and receivers—it is communication without words. The practitioner will receive as much, if not more, information from the client during the treatment as they will in the discussions before and after. The body speaks its truth, and the practitioner will detect areas of tension, if sadness is being held, if overexcitability is causing a rushing heartbeat, or if pain—both physical and emotional—is being experienced. The practitioner will tune into the client and allow their hands and their intuition to guide them.

If you are aware of carrying unresolved issues (things that you have not dealt with) that may cause disturbance for you emotionally, such as bereavement, body/image issues (ranging from eating disorders to even abuse), abandonment, etc., these may resurface when you are massaged. This is naturally a part of your own healing process. If issues do come up, it is a sign that you are ready to deal with them. Massage is not simply a luxurious, sensuous, hedonistic pleasure. It is important and essential for all of us to receive a nurturing, caring touch. If we have not experienced this for many years, since childhood—or maybe not even then, receiving nurturing touch could bring up great waves of emotion. We may hold deep, unrecognized sadness at not having received a loving touch in our early lives; if touch has been aggressive for us, then this may, in turn, bring up other issues.

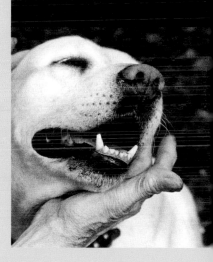

Massage is for everyone, with very few contraindications, even for pets. How wonderful does it feel for us to pet a purring cat or a devoted dog? Children adore stroking the soft fur of their pets, and at any age we can reap great benefits ourselves from this experience. A pet is a loving companion that gives as well as receives.

COMMONLY USED STROKES INCLUDE:

EFFLEURAGE Long strokes, using the flat of the hand, which connect different areas of the body and allow the therapist to sweep up or down the legs, for example, and which also help to induce relaxation in the client. It is also a way of "connecting" for the therapist. During the stroke, the therapist will learn a lot about what is really going on in the client's body and any areas that may need deeper work, such as petrissage (see below), to iron out those tension knots.

PETRISSAGE Small thumb circles for intensive work in such areas as the shoulders or joints.

TAPOTEMENT Very light percussion or tapping action with the tips of the fingers, which may be used on the face, for example.

CUPPING Making cup shapes with the hands, trapping air inside the "cup" to form suction, generally on fleshy areas, like the backs of thighs and the buttocks. Cupping is done quickly and firmly to encourage circulation.

HACKING This is the famous technique often seen in the movies! Performed with loose wrists, the sides of alternating hands are rapidly brought down in a chopping motion over large, fleshy areas to encourage circulation and disbursal of fat.

After a massage session, you may feel tired because the process of moving through deeply held emotions can be very draining. It is important to continue with ways of nurturing yourself. Drink plenty of water or herb teas and rest until you are replenished. Give yourself space and time to consider any issues that may have come up. If necessary, seek the help of a therapist or counsellor. Even just being with a loving partner or good friend, who will give you time and space to talk and feel your feelings, can be a wonderful complement to your healing therapy. (See also Relaxation Techniques, page 252.)

The person being massaged will drift into a state of what is best described as "near sleep," similar to the moments before actually going into real sleep, or like a meditative state. Fully allowing another person to work on your body and to feel the trust, respect, and healing that is shared between the giver and receiver goes some way towards explaining the feeling of wholeness that massage gives. As you become more accustomed to receiving massage, you will find it easier to let go and allow the processes to take their natural course.

Massage is a way of taking care of people, and of taking care of yourself. It is such a simple way to give, it seems inconceivable that it holds so much power. Massage is much more than a relaxant and giver of health. Those who enjoy regular massage cannot fail to recognize the healing qualities that massage possesses. Massage can act as a cleanser for the entire body, mind and spirit, and once cleansing is in place, positive energy has room and space to flow into all the systems. Healing takes place on all levels, and conditions of which the client may not even be aware can be positively affected by this gentle therapy.

Strokes and movements

Holistic massage, Swedish massage, aromatherapy massage, and any other types of massage that are based on any of these three forms utilize a wide range of strokes, depending on the training the therapist has received and also on the varying needs of the client.

different types and styles of massage

Aromatherapy massage

This is generally a lymphatic drainage form of massage (see right), using long, gentle, sweeping strokes over the entire body. The main aim is to introduce essential oils (see pages 228–29), blended with a very light vegetable oil, into the recipient's body through the capillaries. (For more details, see pages 226–29.)

Chinese massage therapy

Chinese massage therapy is becoming more widely utilized in the West. Chinese practitioners spend at least three years in training at specialist centers. The treatment is both preventative and curative, and well worth experiencing. The system focuses on the movement of negative energy out of the meridians, so positive *chi* can flow freely to create balance throughout the body. The various methods of creating this balance include: thumb-and-finger techniques, like acupressure; firm pushing-out-of-energy strokes; and invigorating, light, frisking movements, on the head, for example, to release stress and wake you up! (See also t'ai chi and massage, page 225.)

Holistic massage

"Holistic" is a term used to describe considering the person as a whole, rather than as a range of conditions. All aspects of the client are weighed and examined, including any emotional upsets and physical ailments. Holistic massage will generally follow a format that starts with the back and the back of legs and ends with the client lying on their back, receiving long strokes from head to foot in order to aid relaxation, grounding, and a sense of being back in the world after the treatment. The strokes themselves are adapted to suit the needs of the individual, whether by deepening or lightening the stroking movements, for example, or spending more time on healing, holding, or gentle rocking. The massage involves many long, connective strokes between the body parts, and a treatment usually lasts about an hour.

Hot stone massage

Heated smooth stones (usually basalt, which absorbs and retains deep heat naturally) are placed along the spine and other areas of the back and shoulders, and, sometimes, too, on the hands and feet. This soothes and relaxes in preparation for a Holistic or Swedish-type massage. The heat helps tight muscles relax, but cold stones may be used if there is inflammation or muscle injury. Invented in 1993 by Mary Hannigan of Tucson, Arizona, hot stone massage has been trademarked as La Stone Therapy. Now, there are many versions practised in spas and natural health clinics all over the world.

Indian head massage

This treatments places its emphasis on stimulating the muscles and lymphatic drainage system. It helps alleviate such problems as anxiety and depression, migraines, and sinus conditions, to name just a few. The massage has been around for thousands of years and uses a variety of circular movements and rubbing motions around the hairline, making clients feel as if they are floating.

Kahi loa and Kahuna (Hawaiian massage)

These wonderful hands-on therapies are becoming very popular. They have a deeply spiritual side, making them totally holistic and healing.

Kahi loa was created by Hawaii's Master Healers and is based on the ancient Hawaiian philosophy of healing through connecting with nature. After a discussion with the therapist regarding the reason for seeking treatment, the client receives a gentle massage, fully clothed, while the therapist guides them in a visualization of nature where healing can take place.

Kahuna body work originated in the ancient temples of Hawaii, where it featured as a part of a rite of passage. The movements are derived from an ancient Hawaiian martial art and dance. It has now been adapted to suit Western criteria of acceptability and palatability, but is still basically a transitional experience for people wanting to overcome emotional problems. The fundamental idea is that stimulating the body permits a physical, emotional, and spiritual release. Sessions usually last two hours, and you do remove your clothing for the treatment. The therapist uses his or her whole arm in the massage, as opposed to primarily just the hands used in Western forms.

Manual lymph drainage (MLD)

Specialized training is required to master this extremely light, hands-on massage treatment, which moves the skin across and along the lymph pathways in specific directions. Although extremely gentle, it is an amazingly powerful treatment, and good for anyone congested by a bad diet, a sedentary lifestyle, and exposure to pollutants. It increases the movement of the lymphatic system of the body, throwing its powers of cleansing, regeneration, and healing into top gear. It also affects the nervous system by instigating a change from the normal stressed "daytime" (sympathetic system) state to the "nighttime" (parasympathetic system) state we use when asleep. This has the effect of strengthening the immune system, and because it stimulates the lymph system, it relaxes and refreshes you.

MLD is an excellent preventative and natural nonintrusive treatment that will increase resistance to colds, infections, and flu. It can also firm and improve the look of the skin—it has become a very popular beauty treatment as a "natural face-lift"—and can treat and prevent water retention anywhere in the body—cellulite and swollen ankles, legs, and eyes can be successfully treated, as can premenstrual swelling and discomfort. MLD also works on the skeletal muscles, which is helpful for those who often feel stiff after exercise. It can also lead to the fast removal of the lactic acids that form in the muscle tissue, causing a rapid and pain-free regeneration of the muscle fibers.

On-site massage

This form is becoming more and more popular as a way to experience the benefits of massage without removing any clothing and without having to devote more than 15 to 20 minutes of time. The technique can be received at home or in the office and is based around acupressure points, focusing on the head, neck, shoulders, spine, lower back, and arms. It induces deep relaxation and relief from stress, and culminates with a brusque set of movements to perk you up so you are ready to return to work relaxed but invigorated.

Reichian massage

This was developed by Wilhelm Reich, a follower of Freud. Reich discovered that when he used a variety of physical contact techniques on his patients, they were able to release energetic blocks and the emotions held within those blocks. This belief system has been developed and is now more commonly known as "bioenergetic therapy." It is most often utilized by those who are also qualified therapists, as they are best suited to dealing with the strong emotions that surface in the client.

Rolfing

Also known as "structural integration," this is a method of deep massage that was developed by Dr. Ida Rolf, a biochemist with a background in osteopathy and yoga. Its purpose is to realign the muscular and connective tissue, and it is achieved by the application of extremely heavy and concentrated pressure for several seconds at a time with one knuckle, elbow, or sometimes even the knuckles of a fist, often on a single point on a subject's body. The results can be startling, completely reshaping the body's physical posture.

Being rolfed is quite different from receiving a relaxing holistic massage. The sensations can be very strong, with momentary pain and exhilaration being experienced simultaneously. The "pain" will only last as long as the pressure is applied, about two or three seconds, and immense relief is felt instantly when the rolfer's hand is moved away. Strong emotions are often felt and people have been known to experience amazing psychological changes, too. More energy is felt when the body is correctly aligned, since the release from physical tension held in the body is eliminated.

Self-massage

Although nothing can really take the place of a full-body massage given by a qualified professional, in times of need we can do a lot for ourselves. Learning the basic strokes of holistic or Swedish massage is very useful, but specific techniques—often employed with stretches—can go a long way toward reducing stress and helping you to develop a better relationship with yourself by putting the gift of nurturing in your own hands. There are many good books on this subject.

Shiatsu

This is a Japanese massage therapy practiced widely in the East and growing steadily in popularity in the West. The word "shiatsu" means "finger pressure," and the therapy was, at one time, practiced almost entirely with the balls of the thumbs, applying pressure to any or all the hundreds of points located along the meridians (energy pathways) for several seconds at a time.

Shiatsu is a form of acupuncture without needles, stimulating pressure points with the fingertips and even the elbows. There are also general strokes over parts of the body to stimulate a harmonious flow of energy. The practitioner may also use gentle manipulation to stretch the meridians and to loosen joints to encourage healthy flow of energy. This helps tone up the body's energy, releasing lots of stress and tension and helping alleviate countless symptoms and prevent many conditions.

Sports massage

With the increased interest in exercise, sports massage has become an ingredient of many avid exercisers' health programs. It differs from physiotherapy in that it incorporates many of the techniques of Swedish and holistic massage and aims to induce relaxation. The differences will become apparent when an injury is present, such as with torn hamstrings due to overexercising or incorrect exercising. In such cases, specific techniques are performed to enhance healing in the injured areas, and exercises may be given for strengthening the surrounding areas or to reduce the risk of loss of mobility from lack of movement while healing.

Swedish massage

In this type of therapy, talcum powder is often used instead of oil, as a firmer grip is required. The practitioner will follow a specific routine, using invigorating movements, such as cupping and hacking, and rotation stretches—on the shoulders and hip joints, for example. It is more exhilarating than holistic massage and, although relaxing and equally beneficial, it is less meditation-enhancing.

T'ai chi and massage

In China massage is considered a high art and the massage practitioner must learn the practice of t'ai chi (see page 182) as an integral part of his massage training. T'ai chi is a form of moving meditation, and the movements are based on those of animals. The emphasis lies in clearing the meridians of any blockages or imbalances, and making sure that *chi* flows correctly and yin and yang are balanced where appropriate. The *chi* is the same quality of energy found in yoga practice, called *prana* (see page 168).

With so much attention given to balance, gravity, and grace, it is easy to see how t'ai chi becomes a relevant and integral part of massage training. It is vital that a massage practitioner is grounded, centered, and free to allow the flow of *chi* from heaven and earth through them into their client—in doing so, creating a two-way movement of energy. This flow of energy is like the dance that is t'ai chi: the receiver is also the giver and vice versa, rather than a process of submissive receiving or focused giving.

Although it is not vital for a massage practitioner to be experienced in t'ai chi, the basic ideas are undoubtedly useful. They help protect the therapist from picking up negative energy from the client by providing an inner stillness and a shield, so only clear and positive energy is drawn into the therapist and then channeled back to the client.

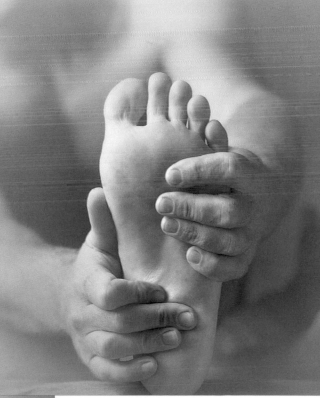

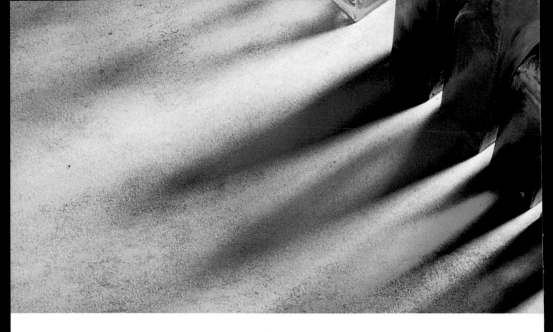

AROMATHERAPY DOS AND DON'TS

- Carefully read all labels and the manufacturer's instructions when buying essential oils and products.
- Look for essential oils that are as pure as possible. Only buy high-quality essential oils.
- Pure, undiluted essential oils should never be applied directly to the skin, with the exception of lavender and tea tree oils, which can be applied to insect bites and other wounds; for example, lavender oil is excellent for burns.
- Aromatherapy oils may already be diluted essences in a carrier oil, ready for application to the skin. Do not dilute the oil until you check the instructions.

the art of aromatherapy massage

Therapeutic massage can be made into an even more powerful tool by using it in combination with aromatherapy (see page 261). In fact, massage is probably among the most efficient means of administering aromatherapy treatment.

When essential oils are used with massage, small quantities are absorbed through the skin, and the oil's healing effect then goes straight into the system. For massage, essential oils are diluted in a carrier oil, such as almond, cold-pressed soy, or wheatgerm oil. Pure essential oils are too strong to use neat unless under the guidance of a qualified aromatherapist. Oils are highly potent and should be used with care. Use around eight drops mixed with every tablespoon of carrier oil, or up to ten drops in a teaspoon of salt or milk powder (to help the oil dissolve) when adding oils to a warm bath.

The form of massage used with aromatherapy oils is generally manual lymphatic drainage (see page 223), using long, gentle, sweeping strokes over the entire body. The main aim is to introduce the essential oils (see page 228–29), blended with a very light vegetable oil, into the client's body through the capillaries. As in Swedish and holistic massages, a basic structure is followed, starting with the back.

A detailed personal medical history may be taken, beginning with a reflexology diagnosis on the feet to determine particular physical problems and a discussion about any current or past emotional problems. The oils will be chosen in a holistic way, with the aim of balancing the whole mind, body, and spirit in the therapy.

WHAT ARE THE BENEFITS OF AROMATHERAPY MASSAGE?

- The power of touch is so comforting and calming that distressed hospital and psychiatric patients respond positively to aromatherapy treatments. An increasing number of nurses are taking extra training in aromatherapy to complement the orthodox medical treatment of their patients, in order to help stimulate their patients' own healing processes. These nurses are in the best possible position to witness the effectiveness of this marvelous treatment.

- Aromatherapy massage is undeniably one of the most powerful treatments available to help combat illness and stress and to maintain balance in the mind-body-spirit.

- Aromatherapy massage is especially suitable for anyone suffering from tension, stress and anxiety, and nervous disorders. If you are the type that gets all tied up in knots, aromatherapy (more than any other complementary therapy) helps you ease out of your tension, releasing pent-up energy that is needed elsewhere to soothe away disturbances and help alleviate your state of stress.

- Aromatherapy has been used for enhancing beauty for centuries. It is said, in fact, that Cleopatra was not really beautiful, but the power of the oils she used seduced her many suitors into believing in her beauty! Today an aromatherapy facial is an effective and luxurious treatment to ease signs of stress from the face and can help to soften wrinkles. Essential oils are found in many beauty products and cosmetics.

- This is one of the most immediate, effective treatments for stress. Tensions melt away under the experienced touch of a qualified aromatherapist.

- The lymph system is stimulated, which helps your body move on and expel the accumulated toxins or "stress crystals" that build up in the body's tissues.

some popular essential oils and their effects

BASIL
Helps breathing and digestion, mental fatigue, stress and depression, and is a nerve tonic and antispasmodic. Aids concentration and a positive attitude.

BLACK PEPPER
A warming, pungent oil, effective for catarrh, headaches, food poisoning and digestive pain, rheumatism, and toothache. Improves circulation and is a diuretic.

CLARY SAGE
A balancing oil that can lift depression. It is calmative, nervine, treats PMT and period pain, restores tranquillity, and can lower blood pressure.

EUCALYPTUS
An antiseptic, it protects against colds and flu, can help in the treatment of wounds, relieves PMT and period pain, headaches, and general muscular aches. Eucalyptus aids concentration, bronchitis, and rheumatism. It is a natural insect-repellent and bactericide.

FRANKINCENSE
The oil of the ancient Egyptians and burned in churches, frankincense has an uplifting and relaxing effect on the spirit. Alleviates depression and helps to treat stress and skin problems. Increases immunoglobin levels, so it is excellent for the immune system and even for cystitis.

JUNIPER
Juniper and clary sage are the aromatherapists' "clearers," used to dispel negative energy from clients. Use in an oil burner or rub a drop or two into the palms and inhale. As a balancer, it can relax you while stimulating your mind and body. Treats cellulite, sleeplessness, cystitis, arthritis, and is an antiseptic, diuretic, emmenagogue, and a good general tonic.

LAVENDER
A pharmacy in an oil. This very special and therapeutic oil is useful as an antiseptic, it uplifts and soothes while relieving stress, and has a balancing effect on the nerves. Excellent for treating burns and helps prevent scarring when used in a compress (under your aromatherapist's guidance). Those with rheumatism benefit from massage using the oil.

MAKING YOUR OWN SIMPLE MASSAGE OILS IS EASY

For a body massage oil: mix 2 or 3 drops of your chosen essential oil with a tablespoon of carrier oil (such as almond, cold-pressed soy, or wheatgerm oils).

For a face oil: add 1 drop of your chosen essential oil to a teaspoon of carrier oil, as above.

LEMON

An excellent essential oil for treating oily skin, acne, sluggish circulation, and digestive disorders. It is emotionally uplifting, with a zingy, fresh scent. Used to treat insomnia and nightmares. It is a diuretic and can be used in a spray as a disinfectant.

ORANGE BLOSSOM

Orange blossom is a soothing relaxant with spectacular effects on acute anxiety attacks and stress. This beautifully fragrant oil also treats depression and insomnia, helping to release worry.

PATCHOULI

With its heady, instantly recognizable aroma, patchouli is effective in treating and preventing depression. Burnt in a room, it will lift despair and balance moods. It is antiseptic, and can be used to treat dry skin and cellulite when blended with cypress, rosemary, and juniper. Helps healthy circulation and is a natural insect-repellent.

PEPPERMINT

Often used in confectionery, this is a powerful oil with a familiar minty aroma. Extremely effective in treating digestive disorders, ranging from flatulence, nausea, and indigestion to heartburn and overacidity. A natural painkiller, peppermint can help treat headaches and general muscular aches. It also helps relieve morning sickness.

ROSEMARY

A wonderful energizer, a drop or two of rosemary rubbed into the palms and inhaled deeply will clear a burdened mind. Relieves mental fatigue, poor memory, and is good for students because it aids concentration. It is useful for chest and lung problems, and for colds, sinusitis, mucus and catarrh build-up, and cystitis.

TEA TREE

A powerful antiseptic, use tea tree around the home or burn it in a bedroom when you are sick for an antiviral effect. Treats athlete's foot and other fungal conditions, such as ringworm, helps insect bites, and can be used to clean wounds (under guidance). Treats thrush when combined with lavender: two drops of each in a bath may relieve symptoms. Add a few drops to household cleaning products for extra protection from germs.

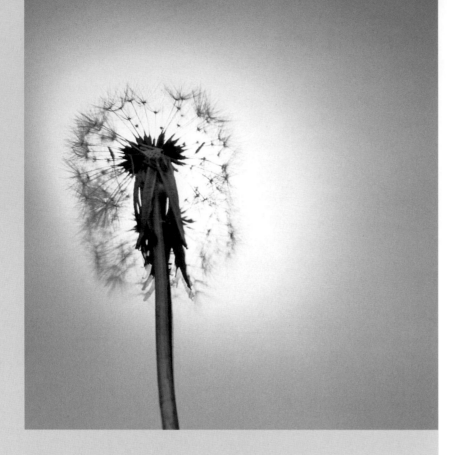

natural pleasures

Ahhh, the bliss of being able to... ? Whatever word springs to mind when you read that sentence, stop and think: Is it possible for you to do it? What's stopping you from being able to do just that? "My busy life!" is usually the answer. More often than not, the reason we can't have a little of what we want revolves around our busy schedules rather than the needs of the small voice in the back of our heads saying, "What about me?!" If that voice is piping up louder and louder every day, it could be time to take matters away from the appointment diary and back into your own hands.

In spite of our busy schedules, we are all sensual creatures who need the support and peace that "time out" provides. And a little bit of what we want… well, we all know that, in theory, it does us good. Of course, it's one thing to know that you need a break, but what if you're working to deadlines or you really can't take time out at the moment? Maybe you can allow yourself a small, token pleasure right now. Or write an IOU to yourself, promising a special treat when your project is finished.

If the projects and deadlines in your life appear ongoing, it could be time to take an honest look at what your needs are and why you are not allowing them to be expressed and heard on a regular basis. Delving deeper into finding out the "why not" factor can be a precursor to making sure that, next time, you allow for more pleasures in your life alongside the commitments.

If, however, it really is that this particular week you simply don't have time to head out to the golf course or go to the movies, then see if you can book a few minutes by yourself with a mug of coffee and a good book, listening to music and doing nothing else, or just to breathe deeply and find your peace in the middle of all the confusion. You are the only one who can make an active commitment to your sanity. Once you do this, though, it doesn't need to be a lonely road. Asking for the support of friends and family can ensure that you remember to take the time to meet your needs. Sharing in this way reminds family and friends that their own pleasure bank needs to be filled on a regular basis, too. Enlisting the support of others means that honoring the needs of your soul doesn't need to be limited to just one trip to the golf course or only one session of meditation.

Relaxation, like happiness, works within a complex and interrelated framework of interdependent beliefs and emotions. Believing that we are worthy of taking that break (or that trip to the art gallery, for example), is the first step in making sure that we actually do it. Once we have agreed with ourselves that we are worthy of being able to take important time to nurture ourselves, then finding the time is the next step.

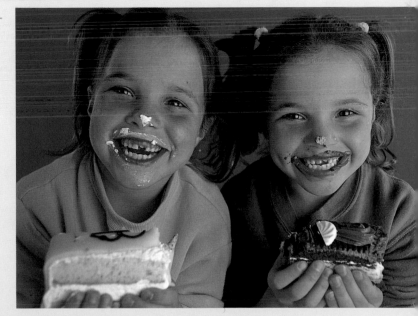

If this feels too challenging for you, or there simply aren't enough hours in the day to get all you need to accomplished, then pretend that you have promised your time to a small child who would be devastated if you didn't show up. In the quest for natural pleasures, it is also important that you recognize you are not simply committing to another task in a possibly mounting pile of things to do—and avoid negating the pleasure with guilt!

Most of us want to be happy, or happier, and are forever seeking the elusive elixir of happiness. The search for happiness and fulfillment is universal; what is unique is what makes us experience feeling happy and fulfilled. Happiness is so individual, subjective, and relative. Freud believed the two elements of happiness were to be found in love and work. Many studies would support that view. It is well documented that extroverts with loving family and friends are happier than introverts, who have more difficulty connecting with others and who often describe themselves as unhappy, lonely, or depressed. True happiness is tied up in a sense of purpose, a raison d'être, and feeling valued for your contribution, deeply interested in what you do, and satisfied with the choices you've made.

We are often misguided into believing that happiness will come to us when we have achieved such and such, or acquired a certain amount of material security, or fame, only to discover that once we are surrounded by these comforts and pleasures

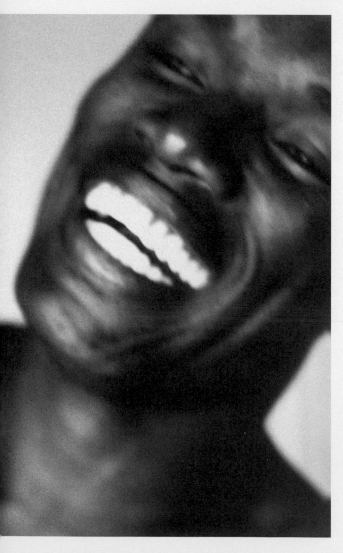

that there is still something missing, and that happiness is, indeed, the elusive treasure so many seek, but so few find.

Spiritual teachers might suggest we are missing the point, creating increasingly more complex lives and then looking for, or expecting to "find," happiness at the end of the rainbow, along with the pot of gold. We fail to find something that is not lost—so how can it be found? Perhaps in seeking to find happiness "somewhere," we are overlooking where happiness is. We are always looking outside ourselves when, in fact, real happiness can only be found within.

positive psychology

A few years ago, Martin Seligman, a psychologist from the University of Pennsylvania, organized a meeting with a group of professional peers to put forward a new agenda. He wanted to shift the emphasis of psychology away from pathology and toward functionality, resilience, and well-being. He used the term "positive psychology" to describe the study of happiness in a scientific frame work. Interest in this field is now spreading like a wildfire in the USA.

Happiness and the exercise factor

An approach to working with happiness in our ongoing lives is to treat happiness as if it was a muscle in need of exercise. If happiness was a muscle that needed to be toned regularly, we might take more care of it by getting it to the gym or out for a walk. So if the practice of adding happiness into your life is sorely needed, then try the "exercise" approach. Be willing regularly to "work out" with what makes you happy. Add it to part of your routine, make it a habit, and you will find your experience of what makes you happy expanding.

Ingredients for cultivating personal happiness

While everyone's secret recipe for happiness is different, finding something to be passionate about is absolutely key. Get enthused about something and cultivate that enthusiasm by learning as much as possible about that subject. Make yourself into an expert about something you really love.

Seeking happiness

Be less of a critic when it comes to looking at what is "wrong with your life" and more open to the improvements offered by what could happen if you become willing to allow more happiness in. Literally "lightening up" helps take away the load of what is standing between you and a natural state of being.

Auditing your happiness quotient

Are you spending too much time doing things that make you miserable because you feel you should? Be honest about what it is you actually need to get done today; try to spend less time caught up in the errands of the day's activities and allow more time for the joys of the day's fun.

Experiencing happiness

Are you surrounded by grumpy faces? If you've been there recently, you'll remember that sour looks can rub off on you as easily as a smile does. If long faces are part of your current landscape, and you are serious about expanding your happiness horizons, then find different company where there is more laughter and fewer grievances. Surrounding yourself with those who value you and respect your worth is another crucial key in the happiness combination.

And when all else fails...

Just act yourself into the part. Sometimes the "fake it till you make it" approach really works. If your own sense of the blues finds you living life closer to the indigo hues than the sunny yellows, then acting the part for an hour or so could give you the lift you need to begin appreciating life again.

self-acceptance

Why is it that some people seem to sail through difficult situations with dizzying levels of self-confidence, achieving the seemingly impossible, while others stumble along the same path just barely scraping by? Self-confidence is the reason why, and self-acceptance is crucially linked to self-confidence. But how do you get the desired "package deal" operating successfully together?

Difficult as it may be to do, accepting yourself exactly as you are at the moment is the most fundamental tool at your fingertips, if you desire to move forward with an expanded sense of self-confidence. When you are brave enough to be totally honest with, and about, yourself, then you automatically free up an enormous amount of energy. If you have been wearing a mask to help you make it through the day, then much of your vital force is being depleted by the energy and concentration it takes to present this image of yourself to the outside world.

If you are operating with a chronically low sense of self-esteem, it can crucially withhold the vitality of your life force. The capacity for real intimacy with a partner or friends also deepens when you are willing to accept yourself as you are. This approach to seeing yourself provides the catalyst for moving forward and bringing into your life what you actually want more of. The crucial trick is that you must first acknowledge that you are "fine exactly as you are."

This type of self-acceptance provides the incentive and courage to delve deeper into personal relationships, whether they are with family, friends, or with an intimate partner. Allowing a more positive sense of self-esteem is vital to uncovering deeper layers of the personal peace and contentment that you desire.

Mirror work

If a confidence-building regime is what you need, then self-acceptance exercises are the place to start. These can be as lighthearted or as deeply felt as you are willing to allow at any given moment. The simple act of looking in a mirror can bring up many feelings of frustration, coupled with an all-too-real vision of what we dislike about ourselves. We often see ourselves with critical eyes, looking for the flaws and the things we want to change, rather than acknowledging the brilliance that is already there, albeit perhaps lying dormant or unfulfilled.

Stay looking at your image as you breathe deeply in and out. Allow yourself to feel love for the real image you see reflected in the mirror. Seeing yourself exactly as you are now, and not as you want to be perceived, can be daunting at first, but well worth it if you are willing to persevere.

Self-acceptance and affirmations

Affirmations (see page 208), such as "I am now willing to accept myself exactly as I am," when used with mirror work, can provide the spark for moving forward in life with a new and renewed enthusiasm. However, don't be surprised if a deluge

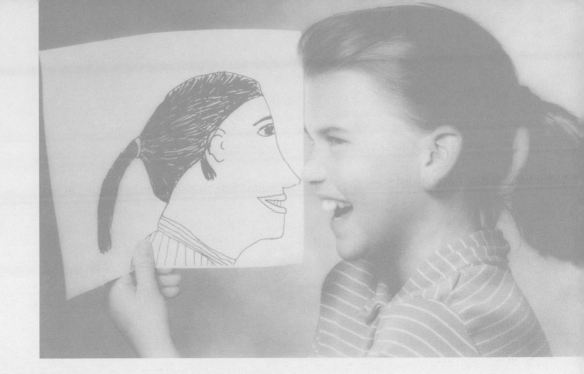

of emotions and doubts come flying to the surface first. Perseverance with this work is key, and yields golden results as you move through layers of perception to finding a real and vital you.

Labeling and unlabeling

Set aside some time to allow yourself to go through your "labels." Take a pen and paper and go through the big "labels" in your life, the tokens by which you identify yourself. Start with the obvious ones, like gender, age, race, religion, parents, etc., and then acknowledge the labels the outside world uses to identify who you are.

Next make a note of all your mental and emotional beliefs through which you experience yourself: what do you feel about things? What are you passionate about? What are your thoughts and emotional beliefs about who you are?

Now have a look at what the masks are that you use in presenting yourself to the outside world. Do you wish to be perceived as in control? At peace? Funny? Carefree? What kind of work does it take to present this image to the outside world? Relax for a minute and see if you can go to what lies beyond the projected image. In that state of honesty, and breathing deeply and gently, pick up a hand mirror and see if you now appear any different. Is there a more honest side of you that you've just uncovered? Is this something the outside world (and you yourself) could see more of?

Now that you have established your sense of safety with this open, and possibly vulnerable, state, take a deep breath in and relax gently as you exhale. Move now into meditation (see pages 216–17), and see if you can keep that sense of openness available to you throughout the meditation. As you come out of it, see if your face has retained some of that openness and honest reflection of the true you. Is it something you can carry with you more often?

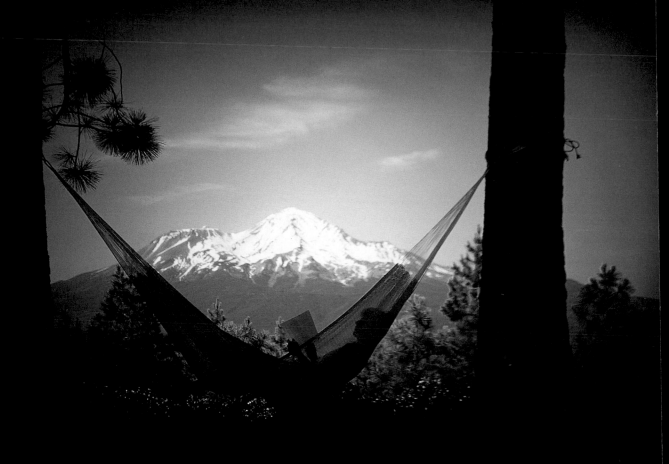

rest & sleep

It takes up about a third of our lives and if we don't do it we feel terrible, but what is sleep for? That's the great sleep mystery, but supporting the immune system seems crucial. Rats deprived of sleep will die after about a week, following the collapse of their immune system, while human volunteers kept awake until 3 o'clock in the morning for just a couple of nights show a drop in immune hormones, making them more vulnerable to infections. Shift workers, who generally get less sleep, are 3 times as likely to suffer from heart disease. Poor sleeping habits may also lead to colds, depression, diabetes, obesity and cancer.

So it's probably not good news that, in general, we are getting less sleep than we used to. The average night's sleep decreased from about 9 hours in 1910 to 7.5 hours in 1975 and millions of shift workers average less than 5 hours per working day. About 1 in 4 Britons are thought to suffer from chronic lack of sleep and the effects of this are just beginning to be explored. 'The effect of a widespread lack of sleep is of the same magnitude as poor nutrition', says one expert, 'yet it has barely been recognised'.

And as if this wasn't bad enough, insomnia affects anywhere between 10 per cent and 30 per cent of the adult population at some time, with women being particularly vulnerable. Sleeping pills are the medical standby but they should be taken for only a few days in a crisis. Anxiety is a major cause of insomnia, which is why sleeping pills are never a long-term solution; they are also addictive and make you drowsy in the daytime. Far better is a form of psychotherapy known as Cognitive Behaviour Therapy (CBT), which encourages you to acknowledge the stress that's preventing you from sleeping and then helps you to handle it better. You'll learn to identify negative or unhelpful thoughts – for example, 'I just can't sleep without my pills' – and change them.

The right food can help to keep stress hormones down, too. Keep your blood-glucose levels stable – stay off sugar and refined carbohydrates – because constantly high levels trigger the stress hormones. Raised levels of the stress hormone cortisol at night doesn't just make it hard to fall asleep, it also lowers production of the growth hormone needed for cell repair.

Many herbs are said to have sleep-inducing properties. Best known is valerian; others include chamomile, passion flower, lavender, hops, lemon balm and bitter orange. One double blind study of 60mg of valerian 30 minutes before bed time for 28 days found it to be as effective as oxazepam, a drug normally used to treat anxiety.

There is also no shortage of imaginative products on the market to help you sleep well, including mattresses and pillows containing static magnets, which have long been popular sleep aids in China and Japan (http://www.nikken.com). Alternatively, you could fill your bedroom with soothing sounds – rushing air, surf or a country evening complete with owls – from a device called the 'Sound Conditioner' (www.justnaturalstuff.co.uk).

SLEEP STRATEGIES

If anxiety is keeping you awake then the more you fail to fall asleep, the more anxious you will become. So create a sleep-promoting regime.

Keep the bedroom quiet and dark, wear comfortable clothing, don't have a big meal before bed, avoid coffee and alcohol, and exercise regularly but not within three hours of bedtime. Be aware that certain prescription medications, such as steroids, bronchodilators (used for asthma) and diuretics, can cause insomnia.

Most importantly, make sure that your bed is associated only with successful sleeping. Go to bed only when you are sleepy. If you don't fall asleep within 20 minutes, get up and do something relaxing till you feel drowsy and then try again. Repeat until you fall asleep.

watery delights

All of life depends on the presence of water, so we should not be surprised at how valuable water is as a therapeutic medium. Two-thirds of our body tissues are water, and water transports most of our body's waste products. On a daily basis, our sweat glands excrete a certain amount of water and waste matter, and one of the main benefits of hydrotherapy (water therapy) is the increased action and efficiency of the sweat glands.

Water has long been recognized as possessing therapeutic and healing qualities. The popularity of the early Roman and Turkish baths has not diminished in modern times. People have been "taking the waters" for a cure throughout history, and water and spa treatments, in many and varied forms, are sought for health and beauty reasons.

The three basic baths in hydrotherapy are cold, hot, and alternating cold and hot. Cold baths are invigorating and have a tonic effect, causing the small blood vessels to contract and then the small arteries of the skin to dilate. These baths should not be taken for too long or be too cold, usually not less than 60 degrees Fahrenheit. Young children, old people, and those with any serious illness, such as heart disease, anemia, and nervous conditions, should avoid cold baths.

Hot baths increase the activity and the efficiency of the sweat glands and have a relaxing effect. The increased perspiration promotes inner and outer cleansing, since the opened pores of the skin facilitate the elimination of toxins. By adding various herbal or other preparations, the healing action of a hot bath can be increased. Sea salt, Epsom salts, seaweed, herbs, or essential oils can all be added to a hot bath to enhance its healing properties. Poor circulation, arthritis, rheumatism, muscle pains, and nervous complaints all respond well to medicinal hot baths.

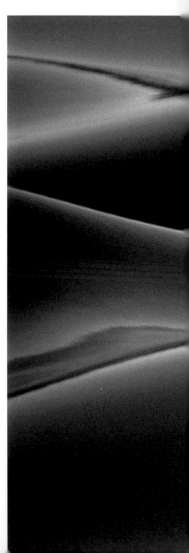

Alternating hot and cold baths or showers act like an artificial pump to stimulate blood flow and lymphatic and venous drainage. This kind of bath can quickly reduce inflammation and increase circulation, and it is excellent after an injury, like a sprained ankle or pulled muscle. As a general rule, you should spend two to three minutes in hot water, followed by half a minute in cold water, repeating this three or four times and finishing with cold water.

Relaxing or lying in a bath is very different from actually taking a bath. The difference with lying in a bath is that you are supposed to do nothing but relax. This is not the bath you take to scrub your body or wash your hair; this is bathing at its most therapeutic and relaxing. In the quiet privacy of your own bathroom, create an atmosphere and ambience of peace and serenity. Calm

HINTS FOR SELF-PAMPERING

1 Warm your towels and bathrobe.
2 Turn off the lights. Use candles, or a bowl of floating candles for light.
3 Add a few drops of a favorite essential oil to your bath, especially one of the stress-reducing oils, like lavender.

your emotions, soothe and smooth your stresses, and watch your woes float away in a hot bath (see also Hydrotherapy, pages 270–71).

Whirlpool baths

Whirlpools, Jacuzzis, and hot tubs use small electric agitators to produce an underwater massage effect. These baths are therapeutic for treating all kinds of ailments, from insomnia and tension to damaged nerves, joints, and connective tissue, and also provide an enjoyable way to release the tensions of the day.

Sitz baths

These are two baths in one, designed so that the upper part of the body, hips, and abdomen can be immersed in water at a different temperature to the feet. The upper part of the bath is usually filled with warm water, while the feet are in cold or cooler water. This kind of bath is useful for treating intestinal, urinary, and genital problems, as well as for disorders of the reproductive system.

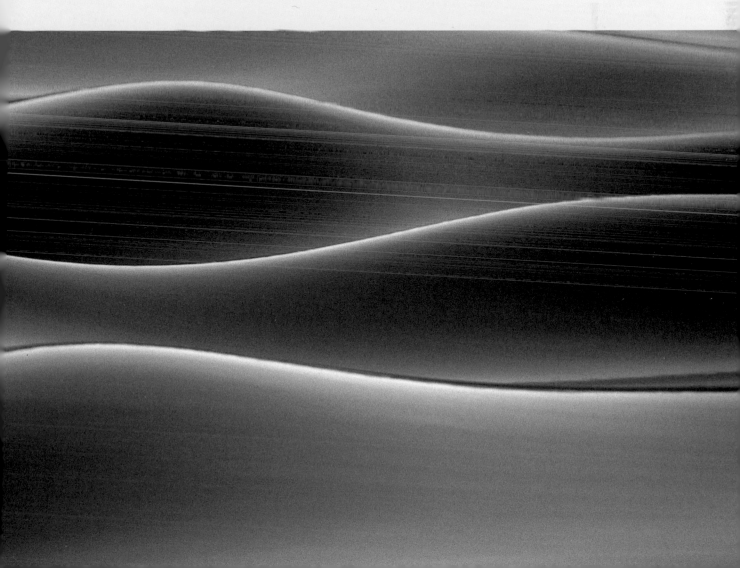

sensory delights

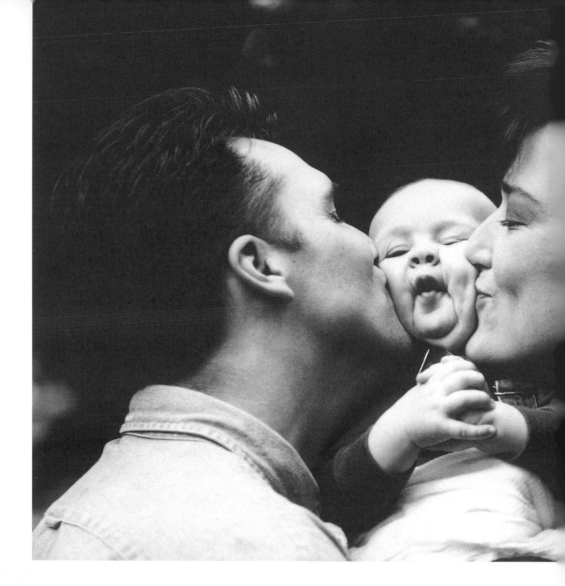

Touch

One of the greatest gifts we give ourselves and each other is the gift of touch. More than just the delight of sensuality and sensation, touch is a language that crosses all barriers, carries messages of love, of friendship and tenderness, of healing and hope. Most of us have experienced the comfort of a hug, a kiss, a hand touching our back— all which show how deeply nourishing and necessary touch is to our wellbeing.

Touch is not only about comfort and communicating love, it is also vital to the healthy function of our immune system. Touch is such a primal need and primary force that it is part of what sustains us and ensures our survival. Without touch, many living creatures wither, withdraw into depression, and, in some cases, die.

All of us need touch, and deprivation can be damaging. Research carried out on baby monkeys showed that the monkeys became withdrawn and unable to relate to other monkeys if deprived of touch. At worst, they became psychotic. Humans who are not touched enough as children may find integration into society difficult, mixing with other people traumatic, and can even become frightened of touch—unable to

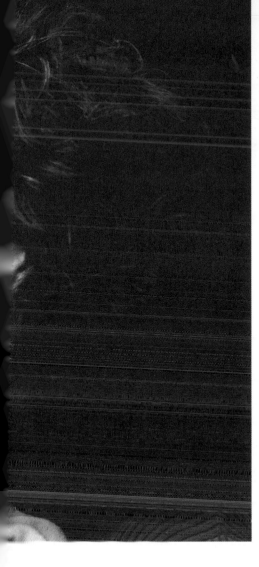

give or receive from others. Through the large numbers of orphans created by wars, such as the recent conflicts in Africa and Eastern Europe, it has been shown that those young children and babies removed from the family by the ravages of war, and not having received touch, became very depressed and unable to develop normal social skills and language, some even losing their will to survive. The global problem of AIDS/HIV has not only left children without parents, but has also bred a fear of touching and normal human contact.

Touch is now recognized as a powerful tool for stimulating healing, encouraging a positive immune response. For this reason, some hospitals and health care facilities have welcomed "animal assisted therapy." National Pet Assisted Therapy organizations regularly visit people who are terminally ill, disabled, depressed, or elderly to bring the comfort of touch, which brightens the mood, along with lowering the blood pressure. Young children learn easily about love, responsibility, and care-giving when small pets are put in their charge. Petting and nurturing pets is healing and therapeutic for anyone, and the pets love it too!

Different cultures respond to touch in different ways. In the warmer Mediterranean countries, it is acceptable for men to kiss on greeting, for women to hold hands and clasp arms while walking, and for touch during conversation to be effortless, warm, and natural. In some cultures, public displays of touch are frowned upon between opposite sexes, but often these cultures are vastly more tactile when in appropriate settings than we are in the West.

For centuries people have recognized how soothing, relaxing, and life-affirming massage can be. How wonderful to share this experience with someone you love, your children, your partner, or your friends. If touch is unfamiliar to you and makes you feel uncomfortable, start with yourself. When massaging oils or creams into your skin, notice how it feels. Massage your scalp when shampooing your hair. This can be relaxing and stimulating at the same time.

Allow yourself to enjoy touching other people. When speaking with friends, place a hand gently on their forearm or their back. Touch can bring people closer together in a way that words never can. Experiment with touch on loved ones. Children who are massaged or touched frequently, or have their hair stroked and feet and back rubbed, respond more lovingly than those who do not receive frequent loving touches. The same rules apply for grown-ups. Take time out to touch your partner. It doesn't have to be sexual unless you want it to be. Let go and enjoy how it feels to give as well as to receive.

sensual delights

We've all felt the sensual pleasure of slipping into a warm bath, of bare feet padding through wet grass, or the feel of sand between our toes as we run across a hot beach to a cool and waiting ocean. In an ideal world, indulgences such as these would be a part of our daily activities, but in our busy lives it is not always easy to find the time. Of course, it's easy to appreciate how blue the sky or the ocean is while on a vacation because we have traveled beyond our sensual "familiar territory." However, it is equally easy to fall back into the dullness of routine when we get home and reexperience life within the limited sensuality of what we know is "safe."

Since our five senses are the tools we use to navigate our way through daily life, it can be easy to tune out the offers of spontaneous and unexpected pleasures they can give. Fortunately, working to expand and heighten your sensuality beyond the realm of the usual can make the "limited ordinary" into the utterly extraordinary, with just a simple shift of focus.

Reexperiencing a completeness of sensuality can hold intimate and rewarding links with reactivating childhood imagination and creativity. The therapeutic effects of playfully using senses can not only help reduce stress but can also actively enhance a personal sense of wellbeing.

The tangibility of touch

Our sense of touch is not limited to what we experience with our hands, or at the hands of an experienced bodyworker. Whether you are stuck in a rut or stuck in traffic, try to expand your sensation of what encompasses touch by regularly moving your awareness around your body. Notice the everyday way you touch yourself and things around you. The feel of your feet in shoes, sandals, or socks is just as valid a sensual experience as the obvious pleasure of letting velvet slip through your fingers, or the sensation of a long-awaited cup of coffee nestling in your hands.

Exercise: If you decide to spend a day working with expanding your consciousness through your sense of touch, check whatever touches your skin, as and when you remember throughout the day. What is its texture? Its temperature? Can you enhance the experience by closing your eyes and breathing into the feeling?

Scent-ual secrets

At one time or another, we have all been reminded of a lover by smelling their signature perfume or cologne or of a mother by the hint of her powder in the air. Scents can carry emotional charges—memories waiting to be unlocked by our reexperiencing a scent we associate with them. The therapeutic effects of aromatherapy (see pages 226–27) are well documented. It can be an equally sensual pleasure to let the play of memories we associate with a particular scent parade before our consciousness.

Exercise: Decide one day to work at heightening your sense of smell. Try not to limit yourself, out of habit, to experiencing only the enjoyable smells: really experiencing what you think is unpleasant can sometimes be as rewarding as avoiding it. If you come across a repellent smell, ask yourself what, about that scent, is particularly distasteful to you. Does it hold memories of someone or something that you are now willing to let go of?

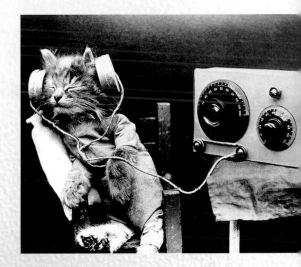

Reveling in sound

Sound is an equally fascinating sense to play with, beyond the obvious enjoyment of listening to tuneful music. If this is your favorite sense, or "sense of the day," what can you do right now to enhance its effect in your life?

Exercise: Even in silence, what can you hear? What sounds are outside the house, out in the yard or in the street? Do objects have a sound? Let your imagination experience what an object would sound like (see also Sound therapy, page 280).

Color therapy

The visual effects of color on stimulating the activity within the brain are well documented. For example, restaurateurs have been known to cover the walls of their establishments in luxurious reds because red is known to excite the appetite. Other, less extreme, associations with the healing or stimulating effects of color are all around us. Allowing your eyes to travel to a leafy tree in a moment of panic or tension can significantly reduce the effect of stress on your body; not just through the enjoyment of the tree's natural beauty, but also by an active association with the healing color of green.

Exercise: As you move through the day, try to discover how, and if, certain colors affect your mood. Wear a color you're not usually drawn to in order to see the effect it has on your mood and on the way others perceive and relate to you.

Tasting the unusual through the usual

Forget about the joys of taste being limited to the gourmet's kitchen or those lucky enough to eat out at the top restaurants. Allow yourself to experience the delights of fresh, raw, or organic food, and be adventurous enough to look for the wonderful tastes in your mother-in-law's Sunday lunch!

Exercise: What does your mouth taste like at this moment—when it's empty? Even "apparently nothing" has a taste: revel in it and see what it has to offer.

the natural home & office

Feng Shui is a sufficiently popular part of our "East meets West" culture to warrant countless magazine and newspaper articles. There are also many books and television programs dedicated to the design and placement of rooms in order to sanctify and reflect spirit, and channel the most positive energies possible for good health, wealth, relationships, emotional and mental growth, and general wellbeing.

The basic idea behind the ancient art of Feng Shui is that every part of life is connected to, and affected by, our physical surroundings. Our general wellbeing, health, wealth, family, and relationships are influenced by the way we arrange our rooms, our space. The orientation and placement of furniture and ornaments, water, light, and space can enhance and promote "positive energies," improving lifestyle and wellbeing.

Many people are reporting real and positive changes by paying attention to the principles of Feng Shui. Professional consultants of this ancient Eastern practice are almost as plentiful as interior designers, and are considered a priority for many people setting out to buy or renovate a home or professional space.

If you are feeling weighed down with lots of negative energy, you might want to have a look at a few of Feng Shui's golden rules.

Clutter is a big issue, according to Feng Shui practitioners, and the sooner we eradicate it from the home and office environment, the better. A cluttered environment confuses and can create chaotic energy. Clearing out that mess really helps if you need to "pick-up" energy because you are tired and frustrated much of the time. Clutter in the office and house can create blocked fields of energy, so throw out or store away all that "stuff" lying around that you do not need.

FENG SHUI TIPS

- Unclutter your space at work and at at home. Keep space clean and tidy to discourage a build-up of negative energy.

- The front door (the mouth of the house) must be kept clear of debris, and clean and free from dust, to encourage positive energy to flow freely into your home. The same applies to any back door you have.

- A pond full of fish in the garden or a fish tank and other water features in the house can bring good luck.

- Mirrors increase the energy of a room, but they must be placed in their optimum position. Two mirrors should not be placed facing each other. It is also best to avoid mirrors in the bedroom; if you must, limit numbers and don't have any facing the bed!

- House plants can absorb toxic energy from electrical equipment. Spider plants are notable for this effect. House plants with rounded leaves are especially beneficial.

Color

Color is an important aspect of Feng Shui. It is common knowledge that colors have a direct effect on mood and, in many cases, even on the body's nervous system. More and more people are paying attention to the colors they choose to paint offices, hospitals, prisons, and public and government buildings, and the harmony of the soft furnishings they provide in such interiors. In Feng Shui, colors are associated with the five elements: red signifying fire; black or dark blue corresponding to water; green related to wood; white or gold, metal; and yellow or brown, earth.

Color guidelines

The blue and green end of the spectrum are the healing colors. They are soothing and calming, making them good colors for an area or room in which you want to relax. If you tend to be a hyper type of person, always on the go, and find it quite difficult to relax, then try wearing blue or decorating your living room in blue to aid relaxation.

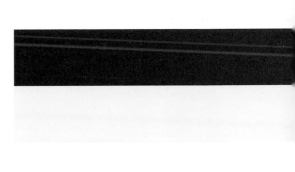

The yellows, oranges, and warmer colors are wonderful for keeping heat and passion alive in the bedroom. They are also good for kitchens, and orange especially will aid digestion. The deeper reds and purples work for some people, since both are warm and sultry.

For those of us who tend to err on the side of laziness and generally seem to lack motivation, warm, peppery, vibrant colors are amazingly beneficial in adding spice to life and energy to our days.

Try to avoid overloading an environment with one color—make use of a color wheel, with its complementary colors. Complementary color combinations include: blue and yellow, violet and yellow, pink and green, magenta and green, red and turquoise, orange and blue, and yellow and gray (see right).

Orange and blue is a very effective combination for an interior. Pink and green work well together, especially in a bedroom, to create an environment that is both loving and harmonic. Another variation of this color scheme is magenta and green, which creates a much more striking and even bolder color combination.

Despite all these rules, it is really important to find colors that appeal to you and which are appropriate for the space they are intended to enliven. Where coloring your home is concerned, your own intuition is the greatest tool. However, taking advice from Feng Shui experts or color therapists is useful and can help you make your own informed choices.

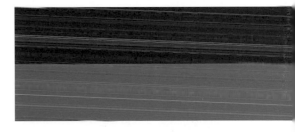

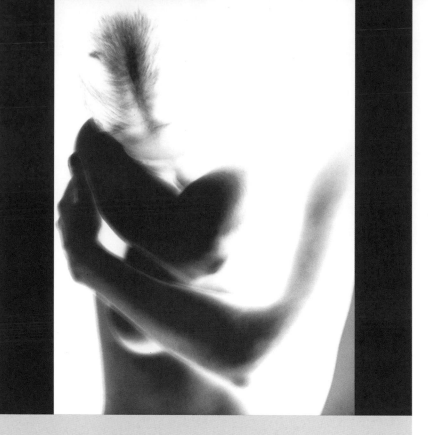

crisis management

The quickening pace of life today seems relentless, and almost every adult is aware of the rapid changes gripping most communities, cultures, and countries. At the turn of the last century, people rarely moved far from family and friends, and got around by horse-and-buggy. Clothing was modest and just about covered up the entire body. Sex and biological functions were never talked about, and certainly not in mixed company. A mere hundred years later, the brave new world of the 21st century finds us moving helter-skelter across the globe at the speed of sound, sending messages at the speed of light, while satellites thousands of miles above the earth measure our movements and our weather.

Today we are swamped with gadgets and technology that tease and test us and change our lives irreversibly. The PC—in fact, the microchip and all the resulting information technology—has revolutionized our world, and we are all caught up in a wave of electronic, digital wonder as we integrate ever more amazing gadgets into our daily lives. All these devices are designed to make our life easier, but they sometimes seem to create a whole new level of anxiety and stress. Think of all the time it takes, every day, to consult your personal organizer, reply to all your e-mail messages and cell phone text messages, deal with your Internet website, or interactive television?

Where does it stop? And how many of our human interactions—and therefore our relationships and intimacy—are compromised by the continual electronic demands on our time? If this wonderful life in the fast lane of the global village is so good for us, why do the seams of society appear so frayed? What are the ramifications of all the time spent alone, using the Internet for work and play? Can the estimate that a quarter of under-4-year-olds in the USA have their own TV set really be accurate? And is it really true that these children watch three to four hours of television a day, on average? Is it possible that this can really help children develop their creative, communication, and social skills? And, if it is not good for the development and growth of our children, how can it be good for us?

Life's crisis points

If you live long enough in this world, you will undoubtedly face crises and have to work and live through them. At some time in life we all have to confront crisis and cope with major life changes that shift our perceptions of reality and cause us to question our choices.

Bereavement, divorce, job loss, loss of home or identity, ill health, an accident, acts of crime or violence—these can all trigger a state of crisis that finds us at the bottom of a pit of despair, which, at that time, seems impossible to climb our way out of. We can slip into a crisis state when more than one stressful situation occurs at the same time, for example a bereavement and a job loss, or a divorce and moving house, the same week. Everybody has their own unique way of coping, but we may all eventually reach rock-bottom at some point when our usually dependable inner strength and resourcefulness disappears.

Negative or challenging life events may provoke people, but it is usually one new item in the loss department that can set a personal crisis in motion. Sometimes it can even be a good event combined with a personal loss that tips the scales—like a job promotion that brings increased responsibilities at the same time as the death of a parent. Whatever the particular combination of factors that provoke crisis mode in your mind and body, it is important to admit to yourself, and to close family and friends, that you are in crisis.

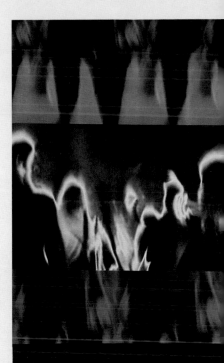

DEALING WITH SHOCK

If you have experienced a shock and are feeling faint, sit with your head between your knees. Otherwise, sit quietly or lie down if necessary. Don't forget to breathe: let the breath out and breathe deeply but avoid hyperventilation.

To help someone else in shock, guide their breathing, keep them warm and gently rub their hands, feet or upper back to restore calm. Administer rescue remedy (page 264), 4 drops on the tongue or a drop on each temple and 2 drops on lips.

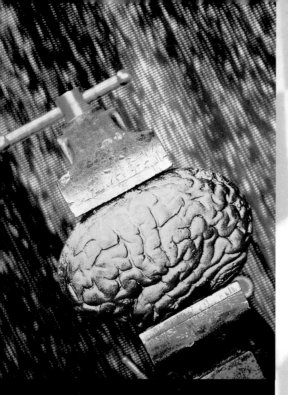

RULES TO APPLY DAILY TO LIGHTEN YOUR STRESS LOAD

- Pay attention to your breathing; notice if it is shallow. If so, practise deep breathing. While doing this, visualize positively any "difficult" situations in the day ahead.
- Eat and drink healthy, nutritious food and liquids.
- State boundaries; be aware of what you can and cannot do.
- Sleep well, allowing enough time for recuperative, healing sleep.
- Plan ahead; if you will be out socializing one night, make up for it the next.
- Check in with yourself privately throughout the day; e.g. how are you feeling after lunch? Notice this and give yourself even just five minutes to become centered if you are stressed or frantic.

A crisis can take a big toll on your mental and physical health, and the problem needs to be addressed and confronted, rather than ignored and denied, in order for wholeness and equilibrium to have a chance of reinstatement somewhere down the line. An important healthy self-view is an honest and courageous assessment of your state of mind and wholeness. No one knows better than yourself when you are in trouble and need to seek help outside yourself to restore a balanced state.

When giving yourself positive feedback and self-counseling is not enough, a positive counseling encounter with a therapist can offer insight from another viewpoint. Too many of us keep going, ignoring our needs, symptoms, and stresses until we reach a real crunch point, and a state of crisis is revealed. There are times when it is important to seek help. In the same way that you visit the doctor if you display symptoms of serious illness, consider visiting a professional counselor or therapist if you find yourself in an emotional/mental crisis.

If you are experiencing a crisis because of the death of a loved one, there are many places you can go for help. Look for a bereavement support group or counselor in your area to help you get over the trauma and back to your old self again. Quite often, you only need to retreat from the world for a few days—to reflect and mourn in solitude—to overcome a "mini-crisis," or have a talk with an old friend or others sharing your grief. But don't be afraid to ask for professional help if the crisis seems too big to cope with alone. It takes courage to overcome the problems we encounter in life, but it requires even greater inner strength to admit that we need help. Reach out for and demand help from one of the many sources available to you, however and whenever you need it.

stress management

Stress that is allowed to get out of control can induce a debilitating and enduring state of anxiety that destroys your peace of mind and erodes physical health and wellbeing. It is a well-known fact that stress contributes to several very serious health conditions if it is allowed to develop unchecked.

How to take the stress out of your day

Letting go of stressful habits and replacing them with de-stressing habits is a positive step toward creating a personal program to reduce stress levels during the day. At this stage of your overall stress-management scheme, it is important to make an honest assessment of the habits in your life that are creating, rather than reducing, your daily stresses.

First look at the obvious ones. Do you overcommit, stretch yourself too thinly? Do you drink too much coffee and alcohol, or smoke excessively? Do you consume unnutritious fast food between appointments, not leaving yourself enough time to eat slowly and digest your food? If you can answer "yes" to more than one of the above, you have some real work (or play, depending on how you look at it) to do. De-stressing your day won't be so easy until you amend or moderate your more dangerous habits.

You can stop drinking large quantities of coffee or carbonated sodas a day. Cut down to, perhaps, two cups of coffee or two sodas, and replace the rest with herb teas, water, and natural fruit juices. You can make the choice to be more disciplined concerning your negative stress-producing habits. Do you really need that extra salt and sugar with your food? Can you choose healthy salads or sandwiches instead of junk food? Can you give up one commitment to allow more time for yourself and your family? Where your stress is concerned, a little moderation goes a long way.

Think about your daily routine and compile a list of any stress-inducing habits or activities. In a second list, outline how you can start to change those habits or limit your involvement in stressful activities—be realistic and patient and, above all, try to avoid even more stress by setting targets that are unrealistic and hard to achieve. Don't expect instant results, because it takes time to undo the habits of a lifetime. Take things one step at a time, replacing one bad habit with a good one, then moving onto the next when you feel happy with your progress. Try to have fun giving up unhealthy routines for healthy ones—after all, you'll feel so much better making the changes.

DE-STRESSING WITH YOGA

Yoga's powerful system of mind/body exercises can be an excellent de-stresser because it works on the nervous system as well as on the muscles, bones, and joints. Yoga postures, called "asanas" (see page 168), are designed to stretch, tone, and refresh the body, while calming the mind. Pranayama (see yoga breathing exercises, page 181) are an integral part of yoga practice, which is one reason why it is useful for reducing and managing stress. Among the best asanas for stress are the Padahastasana pose (see page 173), which is excellent for warming up, opening the lungs, expanding the chest, stretching the back of the legs and spine, and "letting go" of tensions, and the Corpse pose (see page 180) for deep relaxation.

THE COMPLETE BREATH EXERCISE

This quick, seated exercise can be done anywhere, any time: at home, at work, or on the move.

Sit in a chair, with your back straight but not rigid, using the chair back for support, if necessary. Relax the shoulders and place your palms on either side of the abdomen. Inhale slowly though your nose, drawing your breath first into the abdomen to fill and expand it, and then up though your middle, and finally to expand the chest. When exhaling, contract your abdomen first, and then your middle and chest. Repeat two to three times.

This is a powerful exercise and should be done in moderation at first. Done regularly over time, it can enhance your vitality and help reduce your stress levels for good.

The yoga exercises known as the Horse position or "Calming Inhalation and Calming Exhalation" (see page 172) are also very useful.

the importance of breathing properly

One of the main keys to successful stress management is your breathing. Breathing is such a primary function for survival that we constantly take its power for granted and overlook this amazing tool, with which we can regulate and stimulate our own good health.

Your automatic nervous system is responsible for your breathing process, which is why you do not need to think about it—you will breathe anyway! By understanding the very direct relationship between your breath and your brain and nervous system, you have a useful vehicle to help you achieve and maintain a more balanced, positive, stress-free inner and outer life. After all, if you are feeling calm and centered, then your ability to solve problems, think more creatively, and cope with the world is enhanced.

Breathing and relaxation are powerful tools in the daily challenge of coping and overcoming stress. Notice how your breath is fast, short, and shallow when you are angry, fearful, or just under pressure, and how you naturally take deeper, slower, and longer breaths when you are in a peaceful and relaxed state.

The chest expands when we breathe deeply, helping the release of inner tensions as we exhale. By changing breathing patterns and consciously breathing deeply into the abdomen, you can create a calm, relaxed state out of a fraught one. Deep breathing calms body and mind by slowing down heart rate and easing the nervous system.

The fact is, the act of breathing is not necessarily the same as the art of breathing. Many people rush around, shallow-breathing their way through life, and then wonder why they always feel stressed, unwell, and out of breath. Learning to let go of stressful symptoms, feelings, and thoughts, by doing deep breathing and using your exhalations as channels of release, can do yourself some real short- and long-term good. Take a deep breath, inhaling through the nose, and, when you exhale, imagine you're blowing out a candle, exhaling firmly through the mouth. Other variations on the same theme are using the "S" sounds or a wide open-mouthed "AH" sound when you exhale. Repeat the exhalations two or three times.

It may seem too simple to be true, but your breathing holds the key that can unlock the stranglehold of stress and teach you invaluable lessons on how to cope. Through breath awareness and conscious relaxation, you can take control of all aspects of your health and enhance your ability to cope with the pace of life. The importance of understanding how useful your breath is in stress control, of how to breathe well and breathe deeply, cannot be overemphasized. Deep breathing also enhances concentration, releases tension, and can be used to ease pain.

By learning simple breathing exercises and by becoming more aware of the art, as well as the act, of breathing, you can bring powerful changes to your mind and body. Try steady, deep breathing three or six times, while you give yourself the inner direction to "LET IT ALL GO," and then return to your own rhythm of calm, quiet breathing (through the nose with the mouth closed).

Breathing and brain waves

The developing technology of biofeedback and electroencephalograph machines has demonstrated the direct relationship between breath and brain. An electroencephalograph measures brain waves and biofeedback machines allow the monitoring of the state of the mind. There are four major types of brain waves: alpha, beta, delta, and theta, each associated with a different level of mental activity.

Alpha When you are awake and in a very relaxed state, listening to music or just closing your eyes, your brain emits alpha waves. Breathing is slow and easy. This state can be induced by meditation or hypnosis, and makes you highly receptive.

Beta When you are awake and attentive, your brain remains in beta mode during periods of intense concentration or anxiety, even if your eyes are closed. When you are alert, busy, walking, talking, writing a letter, reading a book, or operating under pressure, all theses activities require beta-type brain waves.

Delta Slower than the other waves, delta waves are usually generated during sleep or coma. Some neuroscientists believe delta waves act as the brain's defense mechanism. The brain often emits delta waves when endangered by disease or injury.

Theta When a yogi is able to lie comfortably on a bed of nails or can walk on fire without feeling pain or heat, his brain is in theta-wave emission. Theta waves usually suggest a deep trance, a state when sensations of pain are dulled. Their slow frequency is associated with drowsiness or dreaming. Slow theta waves also occur during periods of creative thinking.

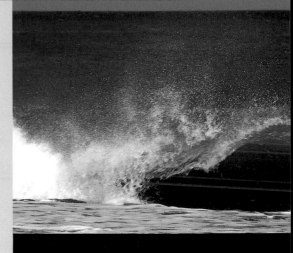

IONIZERS

Have you ever noticed how invigorating it is to breathe mountain and sea air? How clean and fresh the air is after a thunderstorm? How well you feel after a walk in brisk air? This is because the air is charged with negative ions, which are refreshing and stimulating.

Fresh air is rich in negative particles; whereas, city or industrial air contains little or none. The conditions in modern houses and offices, and the electrical gadgets we surround ourselves with, destroy negative charges and account for the rising rate of asthma, chronic respiratory infections, and allergic reactions.

If these situations are relevant to you, an ionizing machine may be helpful. Ionizers are electrical devices that produce a steady stream of negative ions. They help restore the balance of positive and negative ions in the air around you. Small machines are economically priced, and can be found in electrical goods stores, pharmacies, and department stores.

RELAXATION TIPS

When you feel tension mounting, do 3 sets of complete deep breathing, remembering to inhale and exhale through the nose and listen to your breath as it journeys through you.

Take a hot bath by candlelight, with soothing music in the background. Add bath salts or aromatherapy oils, like lavender and camomile.

Take a sauna, Jacuzzi, or whirlpool bath after a swimming or exercise session. Pamper, relax, and rejuvenate yourself. Book an appointment with a qualified aromatherapist.

Lie down with a special cooling eye pack, listening to gentle music, for 15 to 20 minutes.

Learn to "catnap." Just closing your eyes for 10 to 15 minutes can really refresh you, whether in the office, on the train, or sitting in your favorite armchair at home. Just close your eyes, let go, and relax. Turn off to everything while you rest.

Have a foot, head, neck, and face massage.

Take a walk in a favorite place, perhaps the woods or beach that you love. Or just close your eyes and imagine you are there, taking in fresh, invigorating air with every inhalation.

relaxation techniques

In spite of how essential relaxation is to wellbeing, many people do not really know how to relax (for a fuller treatment of the subject, see pages 212–13). The following yoga-based exercises will help you learn some of the subtleties of true relaxation.

This first relaxation exercise is very good for releasing some of your physical and mental tensions. Lie down on your back, with feet shoulder-width apart, arms relaxed, a little away from your body, and palms turned up. Close your eyes and take a few deep breaths, following your breath's journey with your conscious attention as you inhale and exhale through the nose. Make sure some of those breaths get into your belly, and, while you are exhaling, imagine all your tensions flowing out of your body with each outgoing breath. You can also do a version of this sitting at your desk or in a traffic jam.

Another excellent relaxation exercise to do while lying down with your eyes closed uses creative visualization and affirmations (see also pages 208–11) to relax you completely. First do at least three sets of steady deep breathing through the nose, and then just move naturally into a calmer, natural breathing rhythm of your own, observing, with your inner awareness, your breath's journey. Listen to your breath. Become aware of your head and neck, maybe gently moving your head from side to side a few times and then relaxing back into the center. Inhale deeply and then, as you exhale, give yourself the inner direction to release all tension you are holding in your head and neck. Feel the tensions flow out and away from you.

Next move your awareness into your shoulders, arms, hands, and fingers. Perhaps flex or tense them a few times and let go, and then breathe into them. As you exhale, imagine all the tension you hold in hat region flowing away. Move your attention down through your chest, middle, and abdomen, breathing into these areas and releasing all tension as you exhale. You may need two or three sets in each area to let go of all the held tension. Continue down the body, through the pelvis, hips, and buttocks, thighs, knees, legs, feet, and toes.

By learning the art of relaxation you can do more to ensure your future good health and wellbeing than any other remedy. Reducing stress levels is something only you can do for yourself, and it is the most important contribution you can make to a healthy future.

antistress lifestyle program

On waking, greet the day and thank the night

- Drink water.
- Do gentle stretching exercises (qigong, yoga, or simple stretches).
- Eat a cleansing and substantial breakfast.
- Take time to consider the day ahead. Make lists or plan movements: create a realistic structure within which to work, allowing flexibility.

Cleanse the body

- Take stimulating showers or relaxing baths.

Create a harmonious environment at home and work

- Be aware of lighting—harsh, hot lights can cause headaches.
- Try to take time to be in natural light every day.
- Be aware of your comfort levels: If you are seated most of the day, is your body (particularly your back) well supported? Be aware of your posture—hunching over a keyboard can cause stress in the back and poor circulation in the hips and legs.
- Try to walk or stretch away from your desk for a few minutes every half hour.

Traveling

- If driving in frustrating traffic jams causes you stress, can you take the train?
- Always allow plenty of time.
- Read, focus on deep breathing, or meditate while traveling by train or air (it is possible, even on a crushed commuter train!).
- Listen to healing music at low volume.
- Walk to the station or to work, if possible.
- Breathe in fresh air every day, and notice nature and the cycle of the seasons.

State your boundaries

- Can you really work every day until 7:00 p.m. or later, when you have a comfortable home to go to? Be realistic about what you can and cannot do.
- We all deserve consideration, and it is important to treat each other respectfully. Kind words of encouragement or praise enhance self-esteem and create a pleasant ambience in the workplace. Too much criticism and rudeness only serve to create disharmony and increase stress in the individual and others. Constructive criticism works wonders when given politely and with positive advice.

Work and social life

- Most people enjoy socializing with their work colleagues. Offer to organize, or encourage your employer to arrange, in-office athletic facilities or natural health therapists to come in and treat staff during lunchtime hours.

- Encourage get-togethers with your coworkers for relaxation and letting off steam, such as company ball games, picnics, and parties.

Social and family life

- Make time to socialize with yourself! You deserve some time alone. What do you enjoy doing? It may be reading, walking, thinking, or working out in the gym. Whatever it is, you deserve it.
- Make time to be with those you love and who love you—family and good friends. A few hours spent in the company of loved ones works wonders for boosting morale. Laughter and shared experiences are all "money in the bank" for your own health.
- Look at your diary. Do you have NO TIME? Reassess, and try to make time for yourself, family, and friends. It is worth the effort and you are worth the effort. Positive experiences boost the immune system and your general health, and that of those around you.

Time management

- Structure your day's work and be realistic regarding what can and cannot be achieved. Prioritize.
- At home, organize meals and housework to avoid overstimulation in the evening hours. Don't take on tasks too late at night, such as working away busily on a personal computer at 3:00 a.m.
- Schedule time for *you*. Work will be enhanced the more you take care of yourself. You will get more done in less time if you create harmony where there was chaos.
- At work, make sure you take time for lunch. At least get away from your desk into another environment. If the weather is good, try to find a pretty spot outside to enjoy the sunshine and fresh air.

Exercise

- Try to exercise at least three times a week. Choose a sport or physical activity that you really enjoy (see pages 126–83).
- Stretch daily to retain flexibility.

Breathe deliberately (see pages 16–19 and 250–51)

Enjoy eating

- Have meals with your family. Sit down to relax and enjoy food. Don't grab a snack on the run.
- Eat healthy, nutritious food, allowing indulgences when you feel the urge!
- Even if you are eating alone, pleasure yourself. Chew slowly, continuing to breathe, and make the process of preparation and eating a sensuous pleasure. It is!

Support yourself when in need

- Consider your need for good mental health. In times of crisis, seek help. Counseling, psychotherapy, support groups, or time spent talking to your friends and family—find what suits you and your needs, and allow yourself the space and time to be well.
- Try a complementary therapy or hands-on treatment. Massage and aromatherapy are notably useful therapies for dealing with the stresses of everyday living. Treat yourself… you're worth it!
- For specific physical problems, find the treatment that will help the problem, whether it is osteopathy, homeopathy, conventional medicine, acupuncture, or any of the wonderful natural therapies listed on pages 258–81.

Rest and sleep

- Sleep is an essential ingredient for a stress-free lifestyle. A good eight hours, or whatever your particular requirement for peaceful and healing sleep is, will work wonders in helping to keep stress levels lowered in the day that follows.
- Make sure you give yourself enough time to "wind down," an hour or so at least, before bedtime.
- Avoid any stimulants, like coffee, cheese, spicy foods, or anything that may keep your mind alert and awake.
- Don't watch television, especially anything that will make your mind work overtime, in the last hour before bed.

Thoughts

- Practice positively affirmations throughout the day (see pages 208–10). Thinking positively requires much less energy than negative thinking.
- Congratulate and encourage yourself when you feel you have achieved something.
- Avoid panic and negative, derogatory thoughts about yourself or your associates. Smiling to yourself and at others is so much more positive than frowning.
- If you have fears and worries, acknowledge them to yourself and, where possible, to another. It is true that a problem shared is a problem halved. Another person witnessing your worries helps prevent the worry from getting out of hand and driving you out of your mind!
- Do not be afraid to call on those you love to help you in times of need. Better to ask for help than to try and handle problems in isolation.
- Don't suppress your fears with stimulants and comforters, like alcohol, cigarettes, or comfort food. If those fears are very pressing, then try to find a support group or therapist, or a natural therapy, to help you.
- Show love and appreciation to others and expect to receive it back. This helps your self-esteem and creates harmonious relationships.

why therapy?

At one time, living more than a few miles from closest family and friends was unusual. People often ended up living their entire lives in close familiar groups, turning to an elder in the family or close community for advice and counsel during periods of personal difficulty. Now we're lucky if we live in the same state—let alone city—as our nearest and dearest. The post-technological revolution of the last century has given rise to the mobile society—people seeking a living on the other side of the country or across the globe, rather than just down the street.

The rise of more fractured family units, expanding urban cultures, and, in many cases, increased social isolation, may account for the growing use of counseling or psychotherapeutic support during periods of intense emotional strain in our lives.

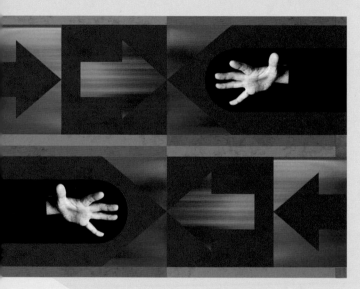

Where once we may have turned to the church or a family member for support, we now seek help from the map-readers of the maze of existence we call "modern life." Talking therapies have replaced the tribal hearth. A new language has developed in the last century: a language that depicts the twists and turns of an individual psyche as it journeys from birth to death and endeavors to explain the many experiences and levels of consciousness. In addition to coping with changing circumstances or catalyzing turning points in our lives, another underlying motivation for therapy is the quest for meaning while facing and coming to terms with our own mortality and limited "tenure of being." (See more on various types of psychological therapy on pages 275–77.)

Counseling

Counseling is often more short-term than therapy and will be focused on one area—bereavement or career, for example. Counseling provides a space for the client to be heard, which may otherwise be lacking. Counseling aims to assist the client in releasing pain, dealing with difficulties associated with life stresses, learning to know themselves better and be more self-loving, and so more outwardly loving.

What is humanistic counseling?

The humanistic approach to counseling, developed in the years just before World War II, had become a widely recognized therapeutic approach by the 1950s and '60s. Carl Rogers, one of the "fathers" of humanistic counseling, was very familiar and experienced with the development of analytical therapy (see page 276). In humanistic counseling, great emphasis is placed on getting more and more in touch with, and honest about, feelings and emotions. The counselor needs to be working on his/herself as well as working with the client; in doing so, utilizing his/her own unique collage of skills, techniques, feelings, and knowledge to empower the client to make the sometimes difficult and scary journey within. The humanistic counselor listens, reflects, mirrors, empathizes, respects, and nurtures. By establishing a safe, caring environment, the client may be encouraged to explore, unravel, discover, have hope, and dig deeper within to find those inner resources that will lead to understanding, resolution, and transformation.

This form of counseling empowers the client because the counselor communicates genuine care and respect, and empathy and a nonjudgmental attitude create an environment in which the client can feel safe and understood. Carl Rogers refined his approach and view of a more humanistic psychology by observing his own evolution, stating: "in my early professional years I was asking the question 'How can I treat, or cure, or change this person?' Now I would phrase the question in this way, 'How can I provide a relationship which this person may use for his own personal growth?'"

Family counseling

The importance of the family in our development as whole and healthy individuals is recognized as a basic truth by family counselors, therapists, and analytical psychotherapists. That is not to say that strong blooms only blossom from a loving and nurturing early environment. It is possible that some individuals are so strong and evolved that they can survive the worst possible starts in life. In most cases, however, a disturbed and distressed client will have some difficult challenging relationships within his or her family, and these will need to be explored and addressed if the client is to discover and create relief and resolution of their problem.

Transpersonal psychotherapy

Transpersonal psychotherapy takes a holistic approach and represents a reintegration of mainstream psychological theory with spiritual inquiry and research into the mind/body relationship. It incorporates many principles of accepted psychological streams, but aims to provide a more spiritual perspective. The client is encouraged to develop trust in their instinct and intuitive powers, and in their power to self-heal. Transpersonal psychotherapy is especially good for those searching for an ongoing process of self-awareness, and who may feel that the structure of a typical Freudian psychotherapy session, for example, is too rigid. Meditation is commonly used by transpersonal psychotherapists to clear and create "sacred space" in the all-important therapeutic relationship. Clients who are struggling with the integration of spiritual and material values benefit from this particular branch of psychotherapy.

natural

Over the past twenty-five years, a revolution in attitudes toward health has been taking place. We have realized that modern "orthodox" medicine does not necessarily hold the only key to perfect health and that hospitals are not always sanctuaries of healing. While most people accept that current advances in medical and surgical skills are staggering, they are not always without side-effects, risk, and failures. At the same time, the increasing exposure to, and interest in, cultures from all over the world, introduces us to a wider, more diverse approach to healthcare. Its not just Eastern philosophies that have captured Western imaginations; healthcare practices from the East are also growing in popularity. Yoga and Ayurvedic medicine from India and traditional Chinese medicine, combining acupuncture and Chinese herbalism, help millions of people worldwide every day. The ancient temples of Greece and Egypt used essential oils and massage to help restore balance and well-being to the body and mind. Today aromatherapy, as it is now called, is practised in spas and natural health centres worldwide.

therapies

In the light of all this, it has dawned on large numbers of the populations of "first world" industrialized nations that, perhaps, it is foolish to abnegate all responsibility for your own health and wellbeing, when all around us we see casualties of bad health habits—or even bad luck—that the best in modern medicine can't cure. The general public has become increasingly educated, aware, and concerned about the effects of orthodox medicine on them, their children, and even their pets. Many have become disenchanted with the medical profession or their doctors, with regard to the treatment of common ailments with antibiotics and other strong drugs that often create a whole set of other symptoms while curing or alleviating a particular complaint.

At no other point in history have our immune systems been so taxed. The modern world isn't necessarily a safer or healthier place, in spite of our amazing scientific and technological feats. We understand how important a healthy immune system and nervous system are to our health, and that we can't possibly keep physically fit unless these systems are in good working order. We also now understand that "prevention is better than cure," and that no one is better placed to ensure our good health and continued wellbeing than ourselves. Each of us is in the front line when it comes to our own health—the way we treat our bodies on a day to day basis determines our state of health and wellbeing in both the short- and long-term.

Perhaps this is why there has been such a tremendous increase of interest in alternative medicine and natural therapies. From nutrition and herbalism to homeopathy and aromatherapy, people are flocking in droves to practitioners of these "holistic therapies," who do not just simply treat the symptoms but who try to determine the cause and endeavor to treat the "whole" person.

When using any of the natural therapies listed on the following pages, always consult a fully qualified practitioner recommended by the society or institute holding a register of qualified practitioners in each field. Always follow instructions carefully when self-administering natural medicine.

manual lymphatic drainage
naturopathy
negative ion therapy
nutritional therapy
osteopathy
polarity therapy
pyschological therapies
radionics
rebirthing
reflexology
reiki
self-hypnosis
shiatsu
sound therapy
thai massage
therapeutic massage
tissue salts
tui na
yoga therapy
zero balancing

Acupressure

Acupressure is a combination of finger pressure and acupuncture, and considered by some to be the forerunner to acupuncture. Acupressure comes from China and from Japan, and it is used by practitioners and families who have trained in this technique. See also Acupuncture and Shiatsu.

Acupuncture

Acupuncture is an integral and highly respected part of traditional Chinese medicine, with a history spanning the last 4,500 years. The theory behind acupuncture embraces the concept of *chi*, the life force in your body, in the air you breathe, or in the water you drink—an invisible but all-powerful, all-sustaining energy, the unseen force all around and within us. This is a basic tenet in the system of thought that created one of the most powerful natural medicine therapies in the world.

According to acupuncture theory, dual flows of energy exist in the body; which the Chinese call *yin* and *yang*. Duality, the manifestation of opposites—opposing but complementary forces—is reflected everywhere in life: positive and negative, masculine and feminine, creative and receptive, day and night, sun and moon, for example. The first in all these pairs is considered yang and the second yin. The Chinese believe that balancing the opposing energies is the path to good health, wellbeing, and wholeness throughout life.

They teach that vital energy—*chi*—circulates along "meridians" throughout the body. There are fourteen main meridians, paths or channels of vital energy. The acupuncturist assesses the condition of your internal energy grid by feeling two radial pulses on the arm near your wrist, by checking your tongue and many other visual clues, and listening carefully to what you have to say, as well as considering your entire health history. In this way the practitioner can assess the condition of the meridians and detect any disturbances or serious imbalances in your body. There are dozens of different variations in the pulses and an experienced acupuncturist can distinguish all the differences and assess why they are there.

After the therapist locates the specific meridian that needs rebalancing, and then chooses the actual points—there are hundreds of acupoints along the meridians—a needle is inserted in that point to stimulate or soothe the energy in order to redress the balance of *chi*. The acupuncturist usually places needles in a few points, leaving them for various lengths of time or twirling them, depending on your symptoms and condition. This is not nearly as painful a procedure as it sounds. In fact, at its worst, it is only mildly uncomfortable. Acupuncture produces very immediate, dramatic results in some cases, and in others it may be a gradual movement back to balance and wellbeing.

The use of acupuncture for pain relief is renowned. In many Chinese hospitals general anesthesia is replaced with acupuncture anesthesia for numerous major and minor operations. The needles placed in specific points, many in the ear, enable patients to endure surgery while fully conscious without the dangers or side-effects of general anesthetic and without pain. It is also well documented that drug addicts do not experience any physical craving for their drug while under the influence of acupuncture anesthesia. Increasingly, acupuncture is recognized as an invaluable, important diagnostic and therapeutic treatment.

Some conditions that acupuncture has been demonstrated to treat effectively are: anxiety, arthritis, asthma, bronchitis, colds and flu, depression, dermatitis, diabetes, digestive problems, eczema, headaches, high blood pressure, infertility, impotence, lumbago, migraine, psoriasis, respiratory conditions and infections, and stress.

Alexander technique

The Alexander technique was created at the turn of the century by an Australian actor, Frederick Mathias Alexander, who had chronic voice problems and endeavored to find out why in order to save his career. Alexander sought medical help, but to no avail. He continued to lose his voice on stage, and recover it when resting. He realized that he had to discover why, so he studied himself in the mirror, acting out a stage role, and noticed how the position of his head changed, as did his breathing, while he delivered his lines.

Alexander felt how his throat tightened and his head lowered as he prepared to project his lines. He became aware of the effects of stress on his neck, throat, and vocal cords, and began to make conscious corrections and observations to support his radical new "view" that mind and body are connected and interdependent, always affecting each other. He eventually evolved a whole new language for the body/mind relationship—a new way of looking at the effects of negative patterns and bad habits on the whole person.

Look at yourself now. How are you sitting? Are your legs crossed? Are you collapsed back in your chair? Lower back unsupported? Do you throw your head back when talking, like Alexander, or forward when walking? By studying himself in the mirror, Alexander had discovered the importance of a balanced, open, relaxed, and full approach to body/mind health. By correcting negative, compensating patterns of attitude and movement, we too can treat and prevent all kinds of conditions.

Alexander realized that, unless you discovered the root cause of the unconscious bad habit behind your ailment, treatments would only alleviate the symptoms temporarily. All his experiences and observations seemed to confirm that most of common health problems are caused or exacerbated by a lifetime's accumulation of bad habits. The Alexander technique teaches you how to improve your health and prevent disabling conditions through practicing conscious movement, stillness, and better posture.

An Alexander teacher or practitioner would describe what they do as "an educative process with preventative and therapeutic consequences." It is one of the most subtle and gentle of the manipulative body therapies. It retrains you to become more aware of your body and shows you how to use it in a healthy and balanced way. In practicing the technique, you experience an awareness of the alignment of your skeleton on a whole new level and achieve an "inner dialogue" with it that allows optimum relaxation and equilibrium in the bones, muscles, and the mind. Release is achieved by gentle suggestion and persuasion.

The technique can teach you how to recondition your body/mind responses, how to unlearn bad habits through observation, and achieve self-empowerment through suggestion, allowing yourself to be wholly conscious of how you use and treat your body. Simple movements are relearned, like getting in and out of a car, getting up from a sofa, or sitting down in a chair—movements we do all the time, some with more ease and grace than others, but all usually with little conscious thought about how we are moving and using our body.

Bad habits, like crossing your legs or slouching with your weight on one leg more than the other, are so long-standing and unconscious that they feel absolutely natural and easy to you. The Alexander teacher gently guides you through very subtle adjustments and positions, whether standing, sitting, or lying down, to encourage correct coordination, posture, poise, and alignment. You simply learn how to change harmful positions into healthy ones, and how to use your muscles with maximum effect and minimum effort and strain. If you or anyone close to you suffers rounded shoulders or an overarched back, the Alexander technique will help improve your spine and skeletal/muscular system through this gently manipulative treatment.

The Alexander technique is widely recognized today and its teachers are employed in many prestigious institutions of the arts, because the therapy has such a beneficial effect on posture, voice, breathing function, and the ability to manage stress and tension. The Alexander technique gives you the opportunity to learn some very simple, yet powerful, health secrets. The importance of posture and deportment should not be underestimated in health. The Alexander technique teaches you how to release the body's power through balance and equipoise of posture.

The technique is an effective treatment for all postural problems, such as rounded shoulders, stoops, and an overarched back, as well as for backache, a shortened or tight neck, a tight throat, headache, repetitive strain injury (RSI), breathing and respiratory conditions, voice problems, stress-related conditions, and arthritis.

Aromatherapy

In modern terms, this touch therapy, which combines soothing strokes, lymphatic drainage massage, and gentle, deep muscle massage using essential oils of plants and flowers, is only a little over half a century old. Yet there is irrefutable evidence that, many thousands of years ago, oils were regularly used in the ancient temples of Egypt, Greece, and Rome for their healing and comforting qualities.

The more recent history of this therapy leads to France before World War II, when a cosmetic chemist called Rene Maurice Gattefosse discovered the positive effect on the skin of a number of essential oils with which he was working. This led him to research the efficacy of essential oils for treating medical skin conditions. He also noticed the antiseptic and antibacterial qualities of some essential oils, and he is credited with the term we use to describe this healing tradition, aromatherapy.

Today, we have rediscovered the beneficial effects that can be induced by inhaling the potent fragrances of plants and flowers, or applying them to the skin. Research is currently being carried out by many major universities on the effects of essential oils on serious medical conditions, such as inflammation, infection, depression, and dementia, as well as on alleviating symptoms and side-effects, such as those resulting from radiation treatment.

Aromatherapy, as practiced today, is a combination of creating highly concentrated essential oils (potent plant extracts that contain the "essence" of the plant) and applying the appropriate oils, generally by massage techniques, which can be either relaxing or stimulating, depending on your needs (see also pages 226–29).

It is highly likely that the system of aromatherapy developed in response to the recognition of the therapeutic and mood-altering powers of fragrances. Cells in the nose send rapid messages to the brain when they detect a smell, which relays the information around the body, depending on the type of fragrance detected. Each essential oil possesses varying properties (see pages 228–29); furthermore, one plant can even produce more than one type of oil. For instance, neroli oil comes from the flowers of the orange tree and orange essential oil from the peel of the fruit.

Blending oils plays an important part in an aromatherapy treatment, and for use at home, too. Oils can be divided into three main categories: uplifting, balancing, and calming. An aromatherapist will try to create a blend that is pleasing in aroma to the client; if the client doesn't like the blend, then the oils are the wrong ones. Blending can be surprising, even startling, with mixtures like lavender with ginger for a warming, relaxing, circulation-improving winter mix.

Aromatherapy is one of the most important components of a health program, and regular treatments will help encourage an experience of sublime wellbeing in a way few other therapies can.

Warning: essential oils are for external use only and should not be taken internally. There are a very few oils that may be prescribed by a doctor or aromatherapist for internal use; in any case, never treat yourself internally with the oils.

Autogenic training

Extensive research into a simple exercise system called autogenic training (AT) has demonstrated that this relaxation technique can help banish stress forever!

Autogenics training has proven to be an effective catalyst for the whole healing process. Its biggest plus point is that people immediately feel better, calmer, and able to cope. AT helps the body cure itself by eliminating the effects of excessive stress that are so threatening to wellbeing.

Autogenics was developed by a German neurologist, Dr. Johannes Schultz, in the 1920s in Berlin. It grew out of his observations and use of hypnotism in his own practice. The technique's reputation quickly spread around the world and today it is established as one of the most brilliantly effective, simple, harmless techniques available to the seeker of a truly stress-free life.

AT can significantly relieve tension, pain, and insomnia, and lessen anxiety. It helps prevent heart attacks by lowering both blood cholesterol and blood pressure. It has been used in the treatment of all kinds of ailments—sufferers from asthma, diabetes, infertility and migraine have all been helped by learning this simple exercise technique. It is now recognized by many doctors and nurses, in addition to holistic natural medicine practitioners, and by many in the business world too—indeed, some airlines use AT to help their staff combat sleep problems and jet lag.

AT teaches you how to focus your attention through a simple series of mental exercises. No wonder many professionals use it to reduce stress and improve concentration, communication, and decision-making skills.

The three basic components of AT are:
1 The art of passive concentration, quietly allowing your mind to focus on your body and learning how just to watch your breath.
2 Repeating words or phrases to target certain parts of your body, inducing feelings of relaxation, such as heaviness or warmth.
3 Using one of three basic postures that help you relax and let go of the outside world while you do passive concentration or repetition exercises. First, the reclining position, where you lie on the floor or a bed in a totally relaxed position (like the Corpse pose in yoga, see page 180). Second, you can sit comfortably in a chair, preferably an armchair, with your arms resting on the chair or on the thighs. Finally, you can do it on the edge of a hard chair, with your back, neck, and head hanging forward in a kind of slump position.

Eventually, you don't need to do all the steps; you just need to think of the exercises to suggest and evoke the stress-release response. However, you do need to learn the technique from a qualified therapist. It usually takes about eight sessions to master the technique and acquire a treasured tool for a healthier life. There are wellbeing clinics and courses specializing in AT, and many universities offer courses as part of a degree or as a noncredited course. Some psychologists and psychotherapists use AT in their work.

Ayurveda
Ayurveda is the oldest system of natural medicine in the world and has been practiced in India for over 5,000 years. It is a holistic system that seeks to treat the whole person by examining lifestyle, ways in which you express yourself, and your nature, as well as hereditary and environmental factors. Ayurveda strongly emphasizes the connection between the individual and nature; not only does it aim to treat disease and improve your general quality of life, but also to bring you into harmony with nature. Ayurvedic treatment methods include diet and nutritional changes, herbal remedies, exercise, meditation, aromatherapy, internal cleansing and detoxifying, among others, all of which can help restore your wellbeing by promoting balance and harmony. Because your path to good health and optimum wellbeing is highly personal, your unique needs and individuality are always considered in any Ayurvedic treatment.

Ayurveda is still the main form of medicine in India and has gained a great deal of recognition in the Western world in recent years. A Sanskrit word, ayurveda has two roots: *ayur*, which means "life" or "daily living," and *veda*, which means "knowledge" and can be interpreted as "science of life." It is a medical system which emphasizes that all beings come out of nature; if we are all integral parts of the universe, we therefore have a responsibility to our source. Living a balanced life in accordance with the laws of nature lets us fulfill this primal responsibility.

Ayurveda evolved at the same time as yoga and meditation, and is connected to both of these in many of its treatments and programs. It seeks to create harmony by balancing the five elements—earth, water, fire, air, and the ether (from which the entire material world is composed)—in the *doshas*, or bodily "humors." There are three forms of dosha: Vata, Pitta, and Kapha. Each person has their own unique doshic mix (known as *prakruti*), although most of us have one or two dominant doshas. Internal and external change may throw your doshas off balance and restoring this balance is the aim of Ayurveda (see also pages 11–15).

The Vata dosha is a combination of the ether and air elements. People with the Vata physique tend to have dry hair and skin, a light frame, little body fat (they are often underweight), and an active metabolism. They may have bad circulation and prefer warm weather. Vata people are quick-witted and creative with lots of ideas. They are often restless. When out of balance they tend toward irritability and, in extreme cases, nervous exhaustion.

The Pitta dosha is a combination of the fire and water elements. The Pitta person has a medium frame, soft, warm, and often fair, pink or red freckly skin. They have a strong appetite and possess a sharp mind and a quick wit. They are busy and like to achieve a lot. They are clear, sharp, and precise. When out of balance, they can be angry, judgmental, and fiery. They are usually very intelligent and love knowledge and reading.

Kapha represents the earth and water elements. A Kapha person has a tendency to gain weight due to a slow metabolism and digestive system combined with a strong appetite. They often have a pale or white complexion, lustrous hair, big eyes, and walk and talk at a slow, steady pace. Kaphas can often be slow to grasp an idea, but have an excellent long-term memory and are loyal and caring. When out of balance, they can be greedy and possessive.

The degree to which a person possesses different proportions of energies accounts for individual diversity. Despite this variation, however, doshas tend to collect in certain areas, causing illness: Vata energy accumulates in the colon and nervous system; Pitta in the intestines, skin, eyes, and liver; and Kapha in the stomach, joints, and mucus membranes. When a severe blockage of energy occurs, the affected area can become weakened, and susceptible to bacteria and viruses.

There are a number of possible causes of energy imbalance, including heredity, environmental factors, and bad habits. Behavior, however, is the biggest determinant; in other words, how you choose to live your life directly affects your wellbeing. Ayurveda describes behavior by classifying human temperament into three constitutions, which describe an individual's basic qualities and the way they react to their environment: the first, *satva*, represents purity and clarity of perception; *rajas* denotes overexcitement, ambition, and aggression; finally, *tamas* indicates inertia, sloth, and materialism. A Kapha person with tamasic tendencies, for example, takes little exercise and overeats, and their health will suffer accordingly.

By examining the patient and questioning them about their medical and family history and behavior patterns, by feeling the skin and key parts of the body and listening to the heart, lungs, and intestines, the Ayurvedic practitioner makes a personalized diagnosis based on the needs of the individual. Tongue diagnosis is a highly specialized practice used in Ayurveda: areas of the tongue are thought to correspond with other body parts, so examining and touching the tongue provides an extra perspective on possible health problems.

A practitioner will recommend a combination of treatments to rectify a dosha imbalance—perhaps lifestyle and nutritional changes specific to the condition, herbal remedies, and detoxifying and cleansing rituals (*panchakarma*). Meditation and yoga may also be suggested, or even marma therapy, which is Ayurvedic acupuncture.

According to Indian Ayurvedic doctors, marma points are the 107 "junction boxes," where nerves and muscles meet, around the body. While marmas are clear and balanced, you remain in good health and are strong enough to prevent illness. If, however, your marmas become unbalanced or clogged, your health and state of mind start to suffer. The job of the Ayurvedic practitioner is to bring a person's constitution back into balance.

Bach flower remedies

An English doctor of medicine and bacteriologist, Dr. Edward Bach, developed a series of 38 flower treatment preparations made from a wide variety of plants and wild flowers—not to treat our physical ailments directly, but our mental attitudes instead, as he thought this would have a direct bearing on our ability to heal our body's problems and imbalances.

Dr. Bach trained at University College, London, at the beginning of the 20th century, later gaining a diploma of public health at Cambridge in 1913. He began his career in London's Harley Street in 1915, where he practiced homeopathy in addition to orthodox medicine. Dr. Bach strongly believed there was a natural cure for every known ailment. Even during his medical training, Dr. Bach recognized the importance of a positive state of mind in the healing process. He noticed how patients with a fearful, worried, depressed mental state made slow progress when recovering from serious illness; whereas those of a more cheerful, hopeful, and determined, positive mental state seemed to recover much more quickly.

Dr. Bach believed a practical approach to helping the sufferer overcome a negative attitude was the course to pursue when treating the cause of ill health. Negative thinking was the root of most physical and emotional problems, as far as Dr. Bach was concerned. After pursuing a number of branches of conventional medicine, and conducting research in bacteriology, he discovered the work of Dr. Hahnemann, father of homeopathy (see page 270). Dr. Bach became a homeopath and successfully developed remedies for temperament types, achieving excellent results in treating emotional problems.

His approach was totally holistic and ahead of its time, like that of Hahnemann. The basic principle he embraced was to "treat the patient and not the disease." Bach then decided to seek a more direct approach to treating the whole person. He wanted to find a harmless cure that could restore hope and peace of mind to sufferers. He believed that trees, plants, and flowers must hold the natural key for anything that ails us. He retreated to the country in 1930 to seek the information he needed.

He became highly attuned to nature and quickly developed a keen intuition about the healing qualities of different flowering plants. Over a seven-year period, Dr. Bach identified 38 harmless tree, plant, and wildflower remedies that he prescribed to treat a patient's state of mind—from emotional upset and anxiety to despair—and not a particular physical ailment.

He divided his 38 remedies into seven groups to treat despair, fear, insufficient interest in life, loneliness, overconcern for the welfare of others, oversensitivity to influences and ideas, and uncertainty.

The Bach flower remedies are still prepared at the Bach Centre in Mount Vernon, England, using the original methods devised by Dr. Bach. Perfect flowerheads are used and instantly placed into bowls of spring water, in which they are left for three hours in bright sunshine. This process is considered to "potentize" the water, meaning that the water takes on the elements of the flowers placed within it. The potentized water is mixed with equal parts of brandy for preservation.

The Flower Essence Services (FES) creates similar flower extracts using North American species of plants. These essences are for more specific conditions than the Bach remedies. Both FES and Bach flower remedies are available from nutrition and health food stores and wellbeing centers.

The following are some Bach remedies and the states of mind they treat:

Agrimony Suffers a lot internally, but keeps it hidden
Aspen Fear of unknown things
Beech Arrogant, critical, and intolerant
Centaury Weak-willed, subservient, and easily used
Cerato Lack of self-confidence, asks advice
Cherry plum Fear of going crazy, losing control, or causing harm, violent temper
Chestnut bud Fails to learn by experience, repeats mistakes
Chicory Overpossessive, selfish, and attention-seeking
Clematis Absentminded, dreamy, and mentally escapist
Crab apple Self-dislike, feels unclean
Elm Temporary inadequacy
Gentian Depression with known cause, easily discouraged
Gorse Depression, all seems pointless
Heather Obsessed with own problems
Holly Jealousy, suspicion, revenge, hate
Honeysuckle Living in the past
Hornbeam Procrastinators
Impatiens Impatient
Larch Depression, inferiority, expects to fail
Mimulus Fear of known things
Mustard Severe depression with no known cause
Oak Brave, plodders, determined
Olive Mental and physical exhaustion
Pine Guilt, self-blame
Red chestnut Fear for others
Rescue Remedy A combination of cherry plum, clematis, impatiens, rock rose, and star of Bethlehem used for shock, trauma, and external and internal first aid
Rock rose Terror, panic
Rock water Self-demanding, self-denial
Scleranthus Indecision, mood swings
Star of Bethlehem Shock
Sweet chestnut Despair, no hope left
Vervain Fanatical, tense, overenthusiastic
Vine Ambitious, tyrannical, demanding, unbending, power-seeking
Walnut "Link" breaker, for times of change
Water violet Reserve, pride, reliability
White chestnut Persistent thoughts and mental chatter
Wild oat Helps define goals
Wild rose Apathetic slackers, unambitious
Willow Bitter, resentful

Bioenergetics

Bioenergetics works directly with the dynamic link and interaction between our body and mind. Physical and psychological techniques, combined with bodywork exercises, help to locate the physical resonance of a stored trauma within the body. Bioenergetic work allows for these conditions or memories of trauma to be brought safely to the forefront of the consciousness. Not only does bioenergetic work safely access these traumatic states, but it assists in successfully reintegrating and healing them.

Wilhelm Reich, an Austrian associate of Freud, identified the energetic and kinetic force in the body as being sexual in nature. Reich labeled this energy "orgone." His work formed the basis for Alexander Lowen's system of bioenergetics, which emerged fully in the 1960s.

Bioenergetic work helps you become aware of how your habitual stances are the effect of negative attitudes and emotional states. Extreme states, such as anger and fear, have a direct effect on posture, as well as on the way you move and breathe.

The first consultation with a bioenergetic practitioner is on a one-to-one basis. After this, the work is done in group sessions. Exercises can include work in grounding, animal games, and breathing exercises.

Grounding In bioenergetics, how you stand, and what your relationship with the earth is like, is of vital importance. Group participants are encouraged to find different ways of interacting with the ground, from stamping to tiptoeing. Feedback on each participant's response is shared within the group.

Animal games By choosing a favorite animal to identify with, and mimicking its stance and behavior patterns, important information about how a person operates within his or her relationships can be revealed. This work, done in groups, provides stimulus for acting and reacting to each participant's animal choices.

Breathing How we function within emotional states directly affects our breathing patterns. Learning to breathe efficiently helps stabilize the body's energy flow, so participants are shown how to breathe correctly. This may seem very basic, but is crucial in dealing with a variety of emotional states.

Bowen technique

The Bowen technique is a gentle hands-on therapy that promotes healing where long-term muscular pain has been inhibiting a client's lifestyle. Although it involves active bodywork, Bowen work is not a massage.

The treatment comprises a specific series of vibrational movements applied to muscles, tendons, and connective tissue, performed in a fixed sequence. The aim of this is to disturb the muscles and soft tissue, as well as the energetic field surrounding the physical body. After three or four of these movements, the client is left in peace to process the last section and allow for the body to be receptive to the next sequence.

The treatment was developed by Tom Bowen, an Australian, who established it as a recognized therapy between the 1950s and the 1970s. Now practiced worldwide, the Bowen technique is useful in treating cases of chronic or acute musculoskeletal pain, and in the healing and regeneration of tissue as a result of sports injuries.

A Bowen technique treatment lasts for approximately 45 minutes and is performed with the client wearing light clothing.

Chinese Oriental medicine

Chinese medicine, like Ayurvedic medicine (see page 262–63), is an ancient form of healing. There are several aspects to it, two of which have become popular in the West: Chinese herbal medicine and acupuncture/ acupressure. Traditionally Chinese medical practice has been one of prevention. You saw a doctor and, as long as you lived by his guidelines, you paid him to keep you well. If you got sick, it was his problem—he had to fix it and you stopped paying.

Chinese herbal medicine stems, as all ancient and traditional herbal medical practice, from the gradual evolution of knowledge over millennia about the effects of plants on human health. Unlike in the West, where older forms of treatment are considered by most modern doctors to be outdated and irrelevant to the 21st century, in China great reverence is expressed for the treatments that have evolved over thousands of years.

Not only is Chinese herbal medicine an ancient and historical form of medical treatment, it is also the dominant form of prescription therapy today in China. There are now more than 4,000 herbs that have been studied and that are used, singly or more often in combination, in Chinese medicine. In addition, Chinese doctors will prescribe foods that should be eaten and foods that should be avoided, activities which should be done and those to avoid. They are concerned, to a far greater extent than Western doctors, about the total wellbeing of the person, involving both therapy and lifestyle.

Chinese doctors study the writings and teachings of medical practitioners going back to the earliest documents. The literature contain details of acupuncture procedures and the principles of Chinese medicine, and although written several thousand years ago, they are still relevant today. As a result, knowledge of the action of herbs is detailed, extensive, and precise, and the practice is essentially devoid of unwanted side-effects. This approach is in sharp contrast to Western medicine, in

which the unfortunate tendency to deride the old methods goes hand-in-hand with acclaim for the modern, new, and often unproven drugs, many of which have adverse side-effects—effects that are considered worth the perceived benefit of the main action of the drug.

The Chinese consider that each person has their own individual balance of the yin and yang energies (see Acupuncture, page 260) and the five elements of earth, water, wood, fire, and air/metal. If these balances are disturbed, ill health will result. It is the job of the traditional Chinese practitioner to maintain the balance and to restore it when it has been lost and poor health has resulted. Each element is associated with specific characteristics, like color, smell, flavor, sound, and so on.

Chinese herbal medicine has grown in popularity in the West, starting in the 1980s and increasing in the '90s and on into the new century. There are now many people practicing Chinese herbal medicine. However, unless they have been fully trained over many years within the Chinese system and fully enter into and appreciate the Chinese philosophy, it is probable that they are only practicing a part of this therapy. (See more on pages 109–13.)

Taoism states that we, as humans, are a microcosm representing the macrocosm, and that everything, and every small part of everything, contains within in it a reflection of the whole. With this tenet in mind, Chinese practitioners believe that they can come to an understanding of the whole of you by studying a part of you. This is exemplified in the West by reflexology, in which information can be gleaned about the whole body by studying the feet and their pressure points (see page 278).

For this reason a session with a Traditional Chinese Medicine (TCM) practitioner may involve a study of parts of your body seemingly unrelated to your presenting problem. They may look closely at your face, mouth, and tongue, your skin, nails, and hair. They may listen to your voice, your breathing, and to other sounds

you make, such as those stemming from the digestive system. The nature of urine and stool are important. You will also be asked many questions, almost certainly more than when seeing a Western doctor, and many of the questions may seem strange and unrelated to your problem as you see it.

A major part of a diagnostic work-up in TCM is the taking of pulses. You may think you have only one pulse, but TCM practitioners identify a large number of pulses and will almost certainly take three pulses (shallow, medium, and deep) at three points on each wrist. After observing, asking questions and listening, and feeling the pulses, they will then put all this information together and determine your balance of yin and yang, of the five elements, and of the *chi*, or energy flowing in your body. Finally, they will decide on the appropriate form of treatment. This will almost certainly involve lifestyle modifications and herbal remedies, but may also involve acupuncture treatment. Your prescription, taken to a Chinese herbal pharmacy, will be prescribed as weights of a variety of dried herbs. These will be combined and you would be told to infuse and drink them as a tea. Usually the flavor is not too good.

Chiropractic

Chiropractic is arguably one of the "oldest" of the modern alternative therapies, having been founded in 1895 by Daniel David Palmer, a "magnetic healer." Daniel David Palmer's first patient was his office cleaner, who had become deaf after a back problem. He discovered that some of the small bones in the cleaner's spine were misaligned. After manipulation, the cleaner's hearing was successfully restored.

Palmer then went on to found the Palmer School of Chiropractic, the word "chiropractic" coming from the Greek *kheir*, meaning "hand," and *praktikos*, meaning "practical." "Displacement of any part of the skeletal frame," he said, "may press against nerves, which are the channels of communication, intensifying or decreasing their carrying capacity, creating either too much or not enough functioning, an aberration known as disease."

Chiropractors aim to correct any disorders of the joints and muscles—especially the spine—primarily by joint manipulation. By working on the muscles, joints, ligaments, and tendons, and focusing on spinal function, the chiropractor can treat a range of conditions. Relieving pain by joint manipulation is their main goal.

Chiropractic differs from osteopathy in that osteopathy works on a joint indirectly by working on the surrounding muscles, ligaments, and fascia, whereas chiropractic treats the problem joint directly, often using high-velocity thrusts. Treatments vary according to the needs of the client.

The treatment includes an in-depth discussion about medical details, lifestyle, and symptoms, and an assessment of your posture will take place. Any pain you are feeling will be talked about, and you will discuss how this affects your movement. Pulse and blood pressure are usually taken and reflexes checked. Your spine will be studied in detail and, while sitting, it will be palpated to test the muscles, bones, joints, and connective tissue.

The treatment used may include, for example, manipulation of a painful lower lumbar joint, while the patient lies on one side. The chiropractor will then manually rotate the upper spine one way and the lower spine in the opposite direction. This movement will partially lock the joint that needs adjusting. Often the patient's upper leg will be flexed to assist the locking. The chiropractor will then feel the vertebra, either above or below the joint. At this point the chiropractor will apply slight pressure and it is this, combined with the patient's position, that frees the joint to resume its normal position.

The chiropractor will then make a very rapid thrust to the vertebra which will move the joint just a little beyond its usual range. This will allow normal movement in the joint and a sudden relaxing of the surrounding muscles, which helps the deep spinal muscles to relax around the affected joint. Four or five treatments are usually necessary to make sure the joints maintain their correct positions. Advice will be given on correct posture to aid in the recovery process and to avoid further misalignment where possible.

Chiropractic, like osteopathy (see page 274), is highly regarded by complementary and orthodox practitioners, including many medical doctors. Chiropractors may use X-rays to help with diagnosis. The therapy is used to treat musculoskeletal problems, neck, shoulder, and back pain, RSI (repetitive strain injury), sports injuries, indigestion, sciatica, lumbago, slipped disc, asthma, arthritis, catarrh, constipation, migraine, period problems, and stress.

Colonic irrigation

Colonic irrigation is an extremely effective way of cleansing the colon. The colonic irrigation equipment is far more elaborate than an enema, although it is based on the same hygienic principles.

Purified water, at the same temperature as the body, is flushed into the colon through the rectum. The water then flows out again through a two-way tube. The water reaches up through the descending colon to the transverse and ascending colon, areas that are not within the reach of normal defecation. Repeatedly washing this water in and out allows for a deeper cleansing, loosening fecal matter stored in all areas of the ascending, transverse, and descending colon.

A colonic irrigation treatment usually lasts about 45 minutes. Treatments are often combined with a dietary cleansing regime and/or a fast. Problems that can be effectively treated by colonic irrigation include bloating, constipation, flatulence, fatigue, headaches, PMT, skin problems, and circulatory disturbances.

Color therapy

The entire material world is a symphony of color, and our bodies are not separate from this experience. From the subtle to the overt, colors—and the vibrations with which they resonate—make up our world. Following this line of thought, the body can then be brought back to a state of wholeness by treating it with the color spectrum. Even ancient peoples understood the power of color; the temples of ancient Greece and Egypt were deliberately painted with strong colors to induce different psychological states in initiates and worshippers.

A color therapist can diagnose imbalances within the energetic field by assessing which colors draw you most, by asking you your likes and dislikes, and where possible, by sensing what colors are predominant in your aura. If there is an imbalance in the energy field, or it is compromised in any way, that will be directly reflected in the color field of the aura. Color therapy works by restoring the full harmonic resonance of color to the body and redressing this balance.

Working with a color therapist is the best option, since all colors have both positive and negative attributes, and extremes of exposure to different colors can upset the balance. Anxiety and depression respond well to color therapy.

An interesting adjunct to this therapy is the Lüscher Color Test. Developed by Dr. Max Lüscher, this self-administered test can uncover aspects of your psychological makeup that reflect in your personality and your emotions at the time.

Cranial osteopathy

In the 1930s, William Garner Sutherland, an osteopathic student of Dr. Still (see Osteopathy, page 274), discovered that the skull, the dome of bone that protects the brain, is made up of eight separate parts, with an intricate joint system and minute gaps between them. Sutherland found, contrary to the previously held belief that the skull was one complete structure, that these separate parts move very slightly. He felt that if this was true, that the bones of the skull move, then dysfunction could also occur. He experimented by compressing his own skull, which caused grave physical and mental problems, so he decided to find out why.

The brain and the spinal column and nerves are surrounded by cerebrospinal fluid. The fluid has a perceptible rhythm that can be affected by breathing and any disturbance in the cranial bone system. Sutherland's research demonstrated that, by applying a series of gentle manipulations to the skull, the rhythms could be adjusted, thus reducing tension in the tissues.

If the rhythm is imbalanced, this can cause pressure on parts of the brain or affect other parts of the body via nerves originating in the brain. Any injury to the head, or dental work that misplaces the jaw temporarily will affect this delicate system of movement of fluid and displaced bones.

After the practitioner has thoroughly assessed your medical history, treatment will commence, involving movements that include gentle manipulation, tapping, molding, and holding the bones to encourage them into correct alignment.

Craniosacral therapy is a wonderfully relaxing and healing therapy. Although the movements are barely perceptible, they are incredibly powerful and induce a profound sense of healing and balance throughout the entire body and all its systems. Mentally, you can expect to feel calm and peaceful. As with any powerful therapy, issues may come up. Anything that has been held within may resurface. This is part of the redressing and balancing process and will lead to a more relaxed and healthier you.

After treatment, be aware of your needs and, if possible, take time to relax to allow the full effects of the treatment to be instilled within you. You will experience profound benefits to your physical being.

Craniosacral therapy can treat general aches and pains, migraine, neuralgia and headaches, sinusitis, dizziness, stress-related asthma, digestive complaints and irritable bowel syndrome, stomach ulcers, discomfort after blows to the head, including whiplash and dental work, high blood pressure, and breathing problems.

Crystal healing

Precious and semiprecious stones have been appreciated for their beauty and value for thousands of years. They have also long been recognized as possessing healing and balancing properties. In China, jade has been used for centuries to treat bladder and kidney problems. The recent resurgence of power bracelets makes a fashionable use of gemstones and their curative properties.

The therapeutic powers of crystals can form the basis for a complete healing session, or can be used to intensify an alternative modality of healing work. Quartz crystals act as intensifiers for other gemstones and can also be used as a focal point for the dynamic energy of any healing session. Different gemstones resonate with different energy spectra and gems are useful in reflecting single or multiple parts of the energy that we lack back to us.

In a crystal healing session, the therapist will ask questions about your current emotional and physical state, determining what needs to be rebalanced, and then place appropriate stones on different energy centers of the body. The subtle vibrations of the human energy field are balanced through the vibrations of the gemstones, as the stones, in turn, resonate with the energy centers.

After it has been determined what crystals will work best for you at that time, there are many additional ways of linking with that energy during the day. You can carry the stones with you, or place them prominently around your home or work environment. Some crystal therapists may even suggest that you place a stone you are working with in a glass of water, and drink from it: the water will be charged with energy vibrating at the frequency of that particular crystal.

While there are many types of crystals that aid healing, the following is a brief list of the properties of some of the more common gemstones:

Amethyst is excellent for calming the mind and is, therefore, useful in meditation.

Rose quartz, with its dusky pink color, is a gentle but powerful cleanser of the heart.

Citrine is generally a vibrant golden orange in color and is used for energizing the body and stimulating the mind.

Smoky quartz ranges from dark brown to black in color, and is excellent for cleansing and grounding.

Green aventurine is useful for stimulating healing in the heart chakra.

Jasper is generally brick-red in color and works as an all-round grounding and protecting stone.

Tiger's eye, in polished form, is dynamic in appearance and its properties are also dynamic; it is energizing, but, at the same time, stabilizing.

Detoxification

In combination with detoxification, you can use many of the other therapies mentioned in this section to cleanse the system. Looking therapeutically at the wellness of the body as a whole, it is important to treat not just the symptoms, but the root cause of the disorder that creates the imbalance, and to realign that body system accordingly. Since our wellness depends on the proper functioning of the body, it is vital that the waste from the environment around us, as well as the waste products from our organs and body systems, are safely excreted (see more on Detox and Detox Action Plan, pages 85–87).

Fasting

Fasting involves abstaining from solid foods for a period of time and drinking plenty of pure liquids, including water and fruit juices. It allows for the body to focus resources on enhancing the immune system functions, as well as cleansing the body of accumulated environmental and food toxins. The entire physical organism has less stress placed on it by not having to work at digesting foods, thereby allowing the digestive system a well-deserved rest.

Stimulated emotional responses are not uncommon during a fast, as the body now has extra reserves of energy to focus elsewhere. Suppressed emotional states can be brought to the foreground, in which case working with a rebirther or body therapist can help you to clear these states.

As a preventative measure, regular fasting for one or two days a month is often advised by naturopaths. Fasting is also recommended in cases of digestive complaints and during acute cases of rash or skin problems. There are many types of fasts recommended for different conditions, such as juice or saline fasts, all of which should be undertaken with the guidance of a naturopath, nutritionist, or physician.

The initial side-effects of fasting can be extremely unpleasant, and may include diarrhea, headaches, vomiting, dizziness, and bad breath. Fortunately, the frequency of these experiences diminishes as the fast progresses. Extended fasts are best undertaken in a retreat environment or in a residential clinic situation, where you can then avoid the stresses of daily life.

Controlled fasting should be strictly under the supervision of a naturopath. Fasting must never be used for weight loss and should not be practiced if you are pregnant or have diabetes, ulcers, or heart conditions. When starting or finishing a fast, consult your medical doctor or naturopath for advice.

Feldenkrais therapy

Feldenkrais work aims to develop new pathways within the brain, enabling the body to move consistently in ways that do not cause pain or damage. Moshe Feldenkrais, founder of the therapy, was plagued with an old knee injury, which he theorized was compounded by an improper pattern of movement. The ultimate goal of Feldenkrais work is to have the body organized to move with minimum effort and maximum efficiency. This pragmatic approach to movement stems from Feldenkrais's own training as an engineer and applied physicist.

The Feldenkrais method comprises two separate elements: Functional Integration and Awareness through Movement. Functional Integration is a one-on-one therapeutic session in which the practitioner uses manipulation techniques to retrain the body/mind into more efficient pathways of movement. People with strenuous or physically active jobs find that Feldenkrais therapy significantly increases their physical efficiency, and improves performance levels, too.

Awareness through Movement is taught in classes, where students are given apparently minor physical exercises to perform. The goal is to bring as much consciousness as possible to each activity. Recognizing how many extraneous muscles are often involved in simple movements is a fundamental step along the path to relaxing the body and making it more efficient.

Functional Integration and Awareness through Movement work are both useful for patients recuperating from strokes and for those with spinal disorders, chronic pain, arthritis, and muscular injuries.

Flotation therapy

A truly modern-age form of water therapy, flotation therapy allows for the complete relaxation of the body and provides the ultimate way to reduce stress. Flotation therapy effortlessly relaxes the body by floating the client in a dense mineral salt solution. This induces a sensation similar to the weightlessness achieved while bathing in the waters of the Dead Sea. The water in a flotation tank is kept at an even body temperature, and all external stimuli are screened out.

The combination of the water's buoyancy and the lack of external influences allows you to turn your attention completely inward. Once your attention is so directed, you can work powerfully to achieve deep and resonant states of meditative awareness, if desired. In addition, you can work to regulate blood pressure and heartbeat through mental techniques.

Flotation therapy can be used to alleviate problems associated with stress, such as anxiety and insomnia, and can be used to help stop addictive cycles of behavior. Speakers located inside the tank can play hypnosis or meditation tapes to assist you in your journey along the road to complete wellness.

Healing

The aim of healing, or spiritual healing as it is often called, is to restore the physical, spiritual, and emotional bodies back to a peaceful yet dynamic state of balance. Almost every culture in history has acknowledged the power of healing and prayer, and tests have proved that healing works, even in cases where the patient does not believe in a higher power or consciousness.

In a healing session, the therapist actively surrenders his/her will to an energy flow greater than their own. They surrender their perceptions of limitation and ask, while in a meditative state, that the powers of divine mind or universal flow be channeled through them. The healer will act as a receiving vessel and, subsequently, as an instrument for the transmission of this energy to the patient. This process allows for the patient to be reintroduced gently to a state of harmonic balance, restoring them back to their own unique energetic dance with the divine.

Find a healer who resonates with you, and in whose presence you feel comfortable. In a session, the healer will have you either sit or lie down, depending on their particular preference for working. You will remain clothed as the healer either places their hands on your body or simply holds them in your energy field. You may feel warmth or a tingling sensation as the energy being channeled passes through your energy field and into your body.

Although they do sometimes happen, miracle or instant cures are the exception rather than the norm. Most people feel the benefits building up over a period of a few sessions, but you can also feel the effects of balance and a resurgence of energy virtually instantly. How you experience each session is not only individual to you, but also to each time you see the healer.

Some healers will also provide what is

called "absent healing," in which healing thoughts are sent to the person without their actually being present. Some healers choose to do this at certain fixed times, and most will require a full name, as well as some information about the area in which the patient requires healing. Spiritual healing works extremely well with small children and animals, and experiments show that controlled healing has a positive effect on plant and seed growth, as well as a strongly mitigating effect on cancer cells.

Herbalism

Herbal medicine, in its broadest sense, is as old as eating. Throughout history people gradually accumulated a knowledge of the healing power of plants. Those who prepared the food and tended the sick, usually the women, came to know and understand which plants to use when particular problems were encountered. This knowledge of plant remedies was passed on through the generations and has become the basis of herbal medicine.

It is still possible to find communities where people rely heavily on the wild herbs of the countryside for both prevention and healing. Traditionally, the herbs were gathered at specific times of day or on certain days of the lunar months. They were made into soups and drinks or were dried and used in powdered form.

The origins of herbalism are rooted in antiquity. There is evidence of the use of herbs for medicine in every ancient culture, and herbalism still forms the basis for the medicines of most modern-day cultures. Records of the use of herbal medicine date back several millennia before Christ in China, Egypt, and India, to name only a few places. If you could visit an apothecary a few centuries ago, you would find herbal everything—tinctures, creams, poultices, elixirs, syrups, plasters, and cordials.

Herbalism teaches the art and science of using plant remedies to maintain natural optimum strength and wellbeing, in order to prevent degenerative conditions, or to accelerate healing and restore health.

Regular drinking of well-chosen organic herbal teas makes positive use of plants in their most natural state, extracting all their nourishing qualities and medicinal properties to redress and restore bodily balance. (See more on pages 106–108.)

A herb is defined as a plant used for food, medicine, scent or flavor. However, in therapeutic usage, the term "herbs" has developed a broader definition and "herbal medicine" means a form of therapy that involves plant extracts, whether from true herbs or from other plants. In addition to the leaves, herbal remedies are also made from other parts of the plant. Hawthorn berries come from a perennial woody bush, and rose hips, used for treating colds and flu, come from a persistent woody briar. When celery is recommended for the urinary system, the seeds are used; when red clover is the remedy, the flowerhead is used; and when dandelion is given for liver problems, it is the root that is ingested.

Herbs can be used for culinary as well as medicinal purposes, and often are. There are only very fine distinctions between food, nutritional medicine, and herbal medicine. Many times the purposes overlap. Caraway will help to relieve the flatulence that may be caused by cooked cabbage. Cardamom and cumin seeds chewed after a spicy meal help to relieve flatulence and settle the stomach. The same result is achieved with peppermint. Rose hips make a pleasant tea and also add to the intake of vitamin C to help ward off colds; alfalfa tea is refreshing and provides some alkaline minerals for help in acidic conditions, such as arthritis.

Commonly, the term "herbal medicine" covers the use of the active physical ingredients in any part of the plant. This distinguishes herbal medicine from homeopathy and the Bach flower remedies, which make use of the subtly extracted energy of the plant rather than its physical substance. Do not underestimate the efficacy of herbal remedies simply because you may have been used to thinking of herbs as simple

and delicate culinary plants. Some very strong compounds are found in them (as those who use poppy and hemp can tell you), and some very potent drug medicines have been made by extracting, concentrating, and sometimes modifying their active ingredients.

Herbs can be used for treating a variety of simple health problems, ranging from colds and headaches to more serious conditions and illnesses under the guidance of a qualified practitioner. When self-administering, always remember that herbs are powerful substances. Eat or drink them as normal if they come as culinary herbs and spices, or as herbal teas. When you buy and use them in tablet form, or as tinctures or extracts, you must stick to the recommended dosages given with the product. It is all too easy to think that just because it is a herb it can do no harm.

Holistic massage

As discussed in detail on page 223, the benefits of massage go far beyond the simple "feel-good" factor. Holistic massage is a tangent part of therapeutic massage (see page 280), and is more concerned with focusing on the wellness of the whole person, rather than just the physical body. A holistic massage therapist will often incorporate moves from therapeutic massage, but will mainly focus on using effleurage (see page 222), or long connected strokes, that act to soothe the body and emotional states. The aim is to induce a sense of peace and wellbeing within the body.

On your first visit, a holistic massage therapist will ask questions about your medical history. Generally treatments begin with the client lying face-down, and covered. The parts of the body that are not immediately being worked on remain covered and warm, while the therapist works with long connected strokes to soothe away tensions and bring back a state of peace to the physical body. Once induced in the physical body, this is then gently able to affect the emotional state, restoring peace and balance to mind, body, and spirit.

Homeopathy

Homeopathic treatment has been in existence since the 5th century BC, when it was developed by the father of medicine, Hippocrates, the famous Greek physician who proclaimed "like cures like." The word "homeopathy" comes from two Greek words: *homos*, meaning "like," and *pathos*, meaning "suffering."

In the late 18th century, Dr. Samuel Hahnemann, a German physician, rediscovered this highly effective, natural form of medicine after becoming disillusioned with the harsh medical practices of his day. He had been working on a translation of W. Cullen's *Materia Medica* and noticed that the symptoms quinine produced on a healthy body were the same as the symptoms it was used to alleviate. This gave Hahnemann the idea for his theory, "*similia, simillibus curantur,*" "like is healed by like," published in 1796.

Dr. Hahnemann experimented for some years on himself, family, and friends, applying the principles he had discovered, with considerable success. Hahnemann put forward the theory that instead of using drugs that opposed and suppressed the symptoms of an illness, a medicinal substance should be used that, in its undiluted form, would cause the illness. By diluting substances to the point that none of the original substance could be detected, Hahnemann began putting into practice the theory of treating "like with like."

These principles continue to be employed in homeopathic practice to this day. Homeopaths believe that the more the remedy is diluted, the more effective it is. The most commonly available remedies are usually diluted to 1/1,000,000 of the strength of the original active substance. On the label this strength is described as "6x." However, practitioners often prescribe remedies of 30x and sometimes even greater. The numbers and letters refer to the homeopathic potency; the higher the number, the more dilute and the more effective the substance is thought. As can be expected, this theory has caused an enormous amount of controversy in conventional medical circles.

A homeopath will treat the person as a whole, not a list of symptoms. A holistic approach is adhered to, following the belief that all the symptoms, as well as the patient's character, lifestyle, habits, and medical history, must be considered before a remedy can be prescribed. All these aspects to health are thought to be closely interconnected and their relationships and patterns must be traced.

The client may find the questions asked by their homeopath extraordinary, or even bizarre, particularly in the initial consultation. Due to this holistic approach to treatment, two patients presenting with the same illness will often be prescribed entirely different remedies.

Another principle of homeopathy that has caused much consternation and controversy is the belief that the healing process is thought to start inside the body and work toward the outside, with symptoms moving in the same direction. Consequently, as one internal symptom improves, another external symptom may develop. This may mean that a patient feels worse before feeling better.

Many people have responded positively to homeopathic treatment. It continues to grow in popularity, despite no one being absolutely certain how it works. We do know, however, that potentized homeopathic remedies have the power to catalyze a healing response in the patient. It is, without doubt, a gentle approach to helping the body maintain and restore health and balance, and is especially suited to the elderly, the very young, and those with allergies. It is completely safe, nontoxic and free of serious side-effects.

Remedies are made from a variety of sources—animal, vegetable, mineral, and human. They are first dissolved in alcohol and water for a few weeks, during which time they are shaken regularly. This liquid is then strained and becomes the "mother" tincture, which is then diluted to make the various potencies. These are then measured on the decimal (x) or centesimal (c) scale. To make a 1c dilution, one drop of tincture is added to 99 drops of alcohol and water and shaken vigorously. For a common, more diluted, 6c remedy, this would be repeated six times, each time taking a drop from the previous solution.

Dr. Hahnemann was a firm believer in prevention rather than cure, and in the ability of a healthy body with an efficient immune system to fight off infection. He particularly stressed the importance of personal hygiene, in combination with a healthy diet and lifestyle, to help limit the chances of contracting day-to-day viruses like colds, flu, and so on. Furthermore, Dr. Hahnemann argued that the treatment of such minor ailments helps prevent the development of more serious disease. In accordance with this theory, homeopaths will impress upon the patient the importance of dealing with these minor ills, prescribing arnica following an injury to reduce bruising, for example, which in turn limits blood loss and infection of the wound.

You may receive treatment for just one day, or over an extended period of time. A patient can expect to revisit their homeopath about two weeks after first treatment to assess their reaction and progress, at which time continued treatment may be discussed. Homeopathic remedies are widely available from pharmacies, health food stores, and specialty natural medicine outlets, and you and your pets may benefit from many simple homeopathic first-aid remedies. However, always consult a professional homeopath for advice on more serious conditions.

Hydrotherapy

For hundreds of years, wealthy Europeans have retreated to water spas to alleviate and heal numerous illnesses. The civilizations of Ancient Rome and Turkey built spas over natural hot mineral springs, knowing that water in many forms helped restore balance to the body. A renaissance in hydrotherapy occurred in the 19th century, with its great proponent, Father Sebastian

Kneipp, a Roman Catholic priest from Bavaria, at the forefront of the movement.

Hydrotherapy—literally "water therapy"—is often used to alleviate circulatory problems, in addition to chronic pain, through the application of water in its many forms, from liquid to steam and ice treatments, often alternating. Internal hydrotherapy, like colonic irrigation and enemas, is sometimes recommended by practitioners for cleansing, detoxification, and clearing digestive problems, as well as for stimulating the immune system.

Today hydrotherapy is widely accepted by the medical establishment; many hydrotherapy pools are located in hospitals and prescribed by doctors, particularly in cases of recuperation from accidents, for burn patients, and for rehabilitating damaged cartilage and musculature. Various applications of hot and/or cold water treatments can alleviate pain, reduce inflammation, and strengthen muscles after an injury. Controlled immersion in increasingly warm pools of water also acts to stimulate the responses of the sweat glands, in order to more efficiently remove the body's waste products.

Many forms of hydrotherapy can be undertaken at home, including cold compresses and alternating hot and cold showers, which are prescribed to stimulate the circulatory system. Inhalation therapy utilizes the medium of water vapor to allow herbs or oils with medicinal properties to be carried to the particularly receptive respiratory membranes.

Of course, a whirlpool tub at home is a dream for home hydrotherapy, but more rigorous treatments should be undertaken at a clinic's spa, with a trained therapist. With home treatments, please consult a physician before starting if you have diabetes, arteriosclerosis, or are pregnant.

Hypnotherapy

We all have access to a naturally-occurring trance state in which the consciousness is equally balanced between sleeping and waking. This state of equilibrium provides the working space for clinical hypnotherapy, a widely recognized and medically established complementary therapy.

In a hypnotherapy session, the client reaches this state through guided imagery techniques. Clear vocal modulations help the client relax deeper into this natural trance, where the consciousness is simultaneously alert and deeply relaxed.

In the trance state, both halves of the brain are equally receptive and both process suggestions that are made. The client remains fully aware of all that is being suggested and, because of this state of equipoise, the subconscious easily receives these suggestions, which are generally therapeutic choices the client and practitioner have discussed before the treatment begins. The hypnotherapy trance state can easily be left, either through the simple suggestions made by the therapist or by the client, if they should choose to end the session at any time.

Hypnotherapy can be successfully used for a number of beneficial outcomes—from stopping addictive patterns to reprogramming emotional states of imbalance. A good therapist will help you navigate the waters of the subconscious and allow for new and more life-affirming values to replace old negative and limiting beliefs. The root cause of the imbalance can also be examined and addressed while in the trance state.

Hypnotherapy helps to guide the choices of the subconscious and assists the client with automatically making the right life-supporting future choices. It is particularly effective in treating the causes of panic and anxiety, depression, and low self-esteem, in addition to assisting the body in coping with stress factors in positive and dynamic ways. (See also Self-hypnosis, page 279.)

Iridology

To an iridologist, a map of the imbalances within the physical body can be found by studying the markings on the iris of the eye, as well as tracking how these markings change and evolve. Iridology can, therefore, act as a diagnostic tool as well as an easily accessible method of monitoring the progress that a course of healing treatments has on rebalancing the internal organs.

In 1881, the father of iridology, the Hungarian Dr. Ignatz von Peczely, published his findings, claiming that illnesses in the body can be linked to abnormal flecks, white lines, spots, or dark streaks in the iris. In the 1950s, Dr. Bernard Jansen, leading American iridologist, published an eye map, precisely pinpointing the exact location linked to each of the organs in the body, which revolutionized the use of iridology as a diagnostic tool.

The left iris reflects the left side of the body; the right reflects the right side. The eye is then divided into six zones or rings around the pupil, each of which link to systems within the body. The zone or ring closest to the pupil links with the stomach; the health of the intestines can be studied by examining the second zone or ring; the third reflects the lymphatic system; the fourth ring relates to the state of the internal organs and glands; the fifth to the muscular and skeletal system; and finally, the outer ring links to the elimination of waste and the skin. In general, top parts of the body are reflected in the upper half of the iris, and the lower organs in the lower part of the iris. In addition there are ten physical constitutional types within the framework of iridology, corresponding to the ten fiber pattern types found in the iris.

Because iridology is such an effective diagnostic tool, it can be used to identify early signs of imbalance or illness, and a skilled iridologist can recommend a course of treatment to prevent problems before they occur.

Kinesiology

Kinesiology takes its name from the Greek word *kinesis*, which means "motion." Kinesiologists believe that each group of muscles is related energetically to other parts of the body, such as the organs, glands, circulatory system, bones, and digestive system. Kinesiologists diagnose by muscle testing; that is, applying light pressure to muscles to ascertain whether or not there are imbalances in the areas of the body.

For example, the pectoral muscle relates to the stomach meridian and reveals the condition of digestive health. Another example is the hamstring muscles, which relate to the large intestine. If a muscle is strong (it does not give way when pressure is applied), then health is good. If a muscle is weak (it gives way under pressure), then this indicates an imbalance. Rather than diagnosing for illness, kinesiologists look for imbalances or deficiencies in nutrition and energy.

This system was developed in 1964 by an American chiropractor, George Goodheart. While working on a patient who had severe leg pains, massaging a muscle called the fascia lata (which runs from the outside of the leg from the hip to just below the knee), Goodheart discovered that the patient experienced pain relief. Through this treatment, the muscle had been strengthened, whereas massage of other muscles did not produce similar results. Goodheart remembered research undertaken by osteopath Dr. Frank Chapman at the turn of the 20th century, which showed that massaging pressure points could improve the flow of lymph fluid throughout the body.

Light therapy

Light therapy makes use of natural and artificial light to create a state of balance and wellness within the patient. In a naturally balanced state, our bodies are exposed to all the wavelengths in the spectrum of sunlight, from ultraviolet to infrared. While taking in the right amount of full-spectrum light is important for balance, consistently taking in the wrong kinds of light can create hyperactivity in children and stress in adults.

Full-spectrum light therapy will activate the pineal gland via light entering the eyes. This, in turn, induces a healing within the parasympathetic system.

Serotonin levels are raised, which in turn increases calcitonin, thyroid and growth hormones, in the bloodstream. In addition, because the patient is in a meditative state while receiving light therapy, the intake of oxygen is automatically increased.

Light therapy is widely known as an effective treatment for cases of seasonal affective disorder (SAD). In addition, it is used successfully in treating high blood pressure, depression, sleep disorders, skin problems, premenstrual syndrome (PMS), jaundice in infants, and even migraines.

Sunlight is like food, and a minimum adequate amount of light is necessary for the complete functioning of the human body. For example, not only does artificial full-spectrum light increase the absorption of calcium in the body, but the circadian rhythms that regulate the body's sleep patterns are also directly affected by the amount of light we absorb.

One of the benefits of light therapy is that it can be self-administered, once you have purchased the equipment. Getting a full spectrum of light indoors can be as simple as replacing fluorescent lightbulbs (which only emit a small portion of the light spectrum) with full-spectrum lightbulbs.

Bright light therapy boxes can also be purchased, and these require that you sit in front of them every morning for about 30 minutes. Colored light therapy can be used to bathe the body in filtered floodlights, or through beams of light specifically directed over the area of the body that needs healing.

The biological rhythm of the body is affected by light, and various forms of light therapy aim to keep these rhythms in a normal flow, and in doing so, maintaining both physical and mental wellbeing. Light therapy can easily be used in conjunction with other forms of therapy. However, if you have any eye problems, consult your optometrist first to be safe.

Magnetic therapy

Our entire physical organism is dependent for life on the constant influences of magnetic energy. Most organs in the

human body have a magnetic functional vibratory rate of approximately 7.96 cycles per second. Working with either the static or electronically pulsed energies of magnets can increase the efficiency of all internal organs, as well as stimulate the blood flow.

Magnetic or oxygen deficiencies in an internal organ can precipitate the degeneration of cell structures, eventually leading to a lack of operational efficiency within that organ. The application of negative magnetic fields allows the oxygenation of tissues by creating a high-energy field, directly leading to an increased number of electrons within that organ.

Research currently being carried out suggests that negative magnetic energy is a primary-force healer. Treatments involving positive and negative magnetic force therapy are useful in the rehabilitation of physical injuries. In addition, magnetic forces can act as a controlling agent against the formation of free radical cells—precursors to many known illnesses. Magnetic therapy is also useful in the treatment of pain and injury, and with such conditions as tendonitis, fibrositis, rheumatism, neuralgia, sciatica, carpal tunnel syndrome, and migraine.

Treatment with magnets takes place by means of either static or pulsed techniques. Working with static magnetic energy simply involves positioning magnets over various parts of the body, wearing belts or bandages with magnets sewn into them, or magnetic jewelry, or sleeping on a pillow or mattress that has magnets already placed inside. With pulsed magnetic therapy, an electronic device directs alternating positive and negative magnetic fields at the affected area.

Magnetic and electromagnetic therapy are also useful in prolonging the beneficial effects of many other alternative and complementary therapies, and work well as an adjunct to many holistic therapies.

Manual lymphatic drainage

Manual lymphatic drainage (MLD) is a gentle form of massage that actively works to stimulate the lymphatic system of the body. Movements are deep, rhythmic, and methodical, and stretch the tissues in the direction of the lymphatic flow.

Because the lymphatic system has a directly regulatory effect on the immune system, MLD can assist in protecting the body against the development of serious illnesses and infections. In addition to stimulating these vital immune defenses, manual lymphatic drainage is useful in the detoxification of the body. The lymphatic system is responsible for the production of antibodies and the transportation of fats, hormones, and proteins. If the body is overloaded with toxins, the lymphatic receptors are tender to touch. This acts as an alarm for the body, signaling that a detoxification is in order.

As a beauty treatment, MLD is a successful adjunct to a weight-loss regime, since it helps eliminate excess fluid. Facial appearance can also be dramatically altered because MLD improves the quality of the skin and reduces swelling and puffiness. (See more on pages 223–24.)

Naturopathy

The history of naturopathy, a collage of natural therapies, is long and rich. Botany, the study of plants, and herbalism, the application of plants and herbs for medicinal purposes, reaches back to the beginning of time. The great Chinese herbal, the *Pentsao*, dates from around 3000 BC and presents a detailed analysis of herbal treatments. Until the birth of "modern medicine" in the last hundred years, doctors prescribed herbal and natural remedies as a matter of course. Indeed, the orthodox drugs of today are often synthetic versions of the natural medicines of the past—from those of the early Greeks, Egyptians, Chinese, Native Americans, or many other cultures. Each has some sort of natural herbal tradition, often passed down as part of oral teachings, through medicine men and wise women.

Hippocrates, who was born in 460 BC, created one of the very early written herbal pharmacopoeias. There are, however, much

earlier ones, such as the Chinese *Pentsao* mentioned earlier and the Ebers Papyrus, dated about 1500 BC, which lists about 900 herbal remedies/treatments.

Hippocrates is not only considered the "father of medicine," but the father of naturopathic medicine as well. His was a holistic school, which taught how to prevent and cure disease by releasing inner vitality and allowing the body to heal itself. In the Hippocratic school, preventative medicine was practiced and diseases treated by means of diet, herbs, fasting, exercise, spinal manipulations, cleansing, and relaxing with hydrotherapy. They believed in the body's ability to heal itself and their basic philosophy is summed up in the language of their time: *medicatrix naturae*, or "only nature heals."

In his book, *Better Health Through Natural Healing*, internationally renowned naturopath Ross Trattler describes the philosophy of naturopathic medicine: "The natural therapeutic approach maintains that the constant effort of the body's life-force is always in the direction of self-cleansing, self-repairing, and positive health. The philosophy maintains that even acute disease is a manifestation of the body's efforts in the direction of self-cure. Disease, or downgraded health, may be eliminated only by removing the real cause and by raising the body's general vitality so that its natural and inherent ability to sustain health is allowed to dominate. Natural therapeutic philosophy also maintains that chronic diseases are frequently the result of mistaken efforts to cure or attempted suppression of the physiological efforts of the body to cleanse itself."

Negative ion therapy

The atmosphere contains both positive and negative electrical emissions, known as positive and negatively charged ions. An excess of positive ions can drain the body of energetic reserves, while negatively charged ions are energizing. These negative ions act beneficially to improve a person's health and mental wellbeing.

Negatively charged ions are mainly the direct result of cosmic radiation from space and electromagnetic radiation from the sun. Air near waterfalls or by ocean waves, as well as high up in the mountains and around lightning, is also highly negatively charged. We can all feel the charge that is released directly following a thunderstorm, when the air is dynamic and electrically charged with negative ions. Being in such places has a direct beneficial effect on the metabolism, the central nervous system, and the respiratory system. Simply standing in a shower can act to charge the electrical current around us with negatively charged ions, enabling us to feel more spontaneously alert and uplifted.

For the most part, air particles are electrically neutral. Other particles acquire either a positive or negative electrical charge. Unfortunately, aspects of modern living directly contribute to the positive charging of particles: pollution and central heating each contribute to removing the negative charge from the air. Electronic devices, such as televisions and computers, favor positive ions. In places where there are too few negative ions, people may experience headaches, depression, lethargy, and general irritability.

Ion machines are available that negatively charge the ions in the air. These machines can be used in the home or office and directly act to reduce such problems as hay fever, allergies, and headaches, as well as increase wellness within the respiratory system. Such machines are often used in conjunction with light therapy in treating cases of seasonal affective disorder.

Nutritional therapy

Food is the most natural medicine there is; it has powerful restorative and healing powers. By understanding the nature of food, we can use it to treat specific deficiencies which lead to an underfunctioning body or, more seriously, illness. More importantly, by being aware of what you eat and paying attention to breaking bad habits, while implementing good new eating habits, you can prevent many health problems that are the result of poor nutrition.

Discovering your own optimum diet makes good health sense. It is not the same for everyone. Many people have food sensitivities or more serious allergic reactions or natural dislikes to certain foods. There are a few ways you can determine food intolerances. You could take a food intolerance test, but you can also find some obvious sensitivities by reducing to the simplest diet and then starting to add foods, one by one, and noting how you feel after each one. Food sensitivity increases if you are run down, stressed, or ingesting toxins like pesticides in your food.

Regardless of your individual preferences and sensitivities, there are certain basic guidelines you can follow to achieve a healthier level of nutrition. Most of these are covered in the chapter on Healthy Eating (see pages 36–87).

Diet is the most direct way to treat all kinds of common ailments and illnesses. For example, few people realize that such conditions as allergy, asthma, alcoholism, arthritis, dry skin, eczema, inflammatory conditions, learning difficulties, poor memory, schizophrenia, and many others relate to deficiencies or imbalances of fatty acids (see pages 41–42). The huge changes to diet during the past century mean that almost everyone has a deficiency of these essential nutrients, or an unbalanced consumption of them, which can also cause chaos in the body's chemistry.

Understanding how to correct these imbalances could be life saving. It could also help to heal long-standing symptoms and delay the progress of degenerative disease. Mothers-to-be need to know the facts before conception because brain growth, intelligence, eyesight, and many other functions need the correct supply of fatty acids for optimum development.

Discover the best possible diet for you by consulting a qualified nutritionist, who will help you create an eating plan that offers you the greatest benefit and may even cure an ailment or two. A detailed consultation with a nutrition consultant could help put your health on a better course for life.

You will be asked to fill in a detailed health questionnaire before your first consultation, and depending on your answers, you may be advised to have food intolerance tests. The nutritionist will adjust your diet to your body ailments and symptoms: one person may need more raw food; another more warm, cooked food.

Even if you are highly disciplined and eat a diet of fresh, healthy foods every day, you may still need a good vitamin/mineral supplement. There are many reasons for taking supplements. Very few people eat a diet with maximum nutrients every day, and most people compromise along the way. Often there seems no choice; many foods are now grown in soils that are depleted in some trace minerals and are picked before they have ripened and are able to develop their full vitamin content. Or foods lose freshness and some nutrients because they have been transported and stored for varying lengths of time before they are purchased. Experts agree that a healthy, balanced diet has to be your priority, since pills do not contain the fiber, protein, and carbohydrates, as well as the wide range of phytochemicals (see pages 27 and 93), that are essential for a healthy body. However, many experts now agree that supplements are not only a good thing, but are essential to health and wellbeing. (For more advice, see Supplements, pages 90–105.)

Osteopathy

Osteopathy was founded in 1874 by Andrew Taylor Still, an American doctor who had become dissatisfied with orthodox medicine. In addition to being a doctor, he was an accomplished engineer, and this combined knowledge gave him an interesting slant on the human body, viewing it like a machine.

His disillusionment with the methods of orthodox medicine, including the overprescribing of sometimes dangerous drugs with side-effects, fostered his desire and research into other methods of healing. He became certain that much illness is caused by misalignment in the body and he devised a system of manipulation which could bring the body back into balance. Osteopathy rapidly became accepted by the orthodox world and is now a highly regarded and established medicine.

Osteopathy treats the body's large framework of bones, joints, muscles, and ligaments. The body is meant to have a full range of motion, allowing it to run, walk, jump, twist, dance, speak, write, play sports, drive, and perform any task that requires even the slightest movement. Problems in the musculoskeletal system, which may have evolved through habitual poor posture, injury or accident, repetitive strain, disease, and abuse or misuse, can be successfully treated with osteopathy.

Stress alone can cause problems in the framework of the body, when muscles tighten and restrict blood supply to the muscle tissues and surrounding areas, causing defects in the bones which the muscles surround or to which they are attached. Dr. Still believed that the body should run like a well-tuned engine, with the minimum of wear and tear. Like an engine, a body may require maintenance, and certainly taking care of yourself and adopting a healthy lifestyle helps keep the engine running smoothly.

Treatment will begin with detailed questions about your symptoms, for example to establish whether the problem is worse in the morning, the evening, after walking, or when sitting. The osteopath will take your medical history, along with details of any other treatments you are receiving, and will undertake a thorough physical examination. You will be observed performing a normal range of movements and adopting various positions, including sitting, lying down, standing, and bending forward, backward, and sideways.

Particular joints will be assessed and the osteopath will apply pressure to various areas of soft tissue to ascertain whether they are overly tired, tense, or stressed. Reflexes may be tested with a small hammer and, in some cases, an X-ray may be necessary, especially if your visit to the osteopath follows an accident or serious injury. An assessment will then be made as to the appropriate treatment. In acute and long-term conditions, treatment may continue for several months; however, some other problems can be cleared up with only a few sessions.

Each session will last about half an hour and most people find the release of tension and the following relaxation in the surrounding muscles a very soothing and enjoyable experience. The osteopath may use a variety of techniques, including massage, soft tissue manipulation, and gentle repetitive movement of certain joints to aid mobility. In the case where fixed joints are a problem, the joint may be released by guiding it rapidly through its normal range of movement. This will produce the clicking sound that is often associated with osteopathic treatment. An immediate release of tension will be experienced, almost like a drug-induced high, with instant relief of pain.

The osteopath will advise you on postural correction. In order for the condition not to recur or become permanent, it is important that you continue to practice postural correction and take care of yourself in accordance with any advice given.

Osteopathy can be used to treat arthritis, asthma, athletic injuries, back problems, bronchitis, bursitis, carpal tunnel syndrome, constipation, earache, headache, flu, endometriosis, hearing problems, heartburn, hemorrhoids, menstrual problems, muscle cramps, chronic and acute pain, prostate problems, sinusitis, and varicose veins.

Polarity therapy

Polarity therapy draws from a wide range of Eastern and Western healing techniques. The main belief of this system is that all illness is caused by blockages of the body's vital energy. By freeing up the blockages

and allowing energy to flow naturally, illness can be alleviated, prevented, or stopped from recurring.

This therapy was developed by Austrian-born Dr. Randolph Stone, who lived from 1890 to 1983. Over a period of fifty years, Dr. Stone utilized knowledge he had gained from a vast range of training, which included chiropractic, osteopathy, and naturopathy, in addition to Eastern systems, such as acupuncture, yoga, and Ayurvedic medicine. His main training, in which he used manipulation, often brought good results and relief from symptoms, but he discovered that illness sometimes recurred and that there was often an underlying, residual condition that had been hidden by the acute symptoms.

His therapy draws deeply from the Chinese belief in *chi* (vital energy), also called *prana* in India. He found that good health is wholly dependent on "polarity relationship"; that is, between the positive, the negative, and the neutral. Achieving balance between these polarities is essential to good health and wellbeing, including spiritual wellbeing, and so the aim of polarity therapy is to bring about balance in all areas. The techniques used include manipulation and touch, stretching postures, correct diet, and healthy mental attitude through counseling. Negative thoughts and attitudes can bring about illness in the body as reliably as a poor diet.

Polarity therapy does not generally deal with specific symptoms, but instead concentrates on achieving and creating balance throughout. Anyone who suffers from any kind of illness will benefit from taking responsibility for their body through addressing diet, correcting their posture, and stretching regularly, as well as addressing any issues through counseling. With the help of a polarity therapist to see the process through, the benefits can be all-encompassing. It is important that the patient is able to commit fully to their own health care and is not simply wanting someone else to "do it for them," handing over responsibility.

The polarity therapist will take a full medical history. Your energy patterns will then be assessed and any blocks within your system will be found by testing the pressure points and reflexes. You will be encouraged to be aware of the body's own healing processes throughout; for example, if you have an unrelenting headache, you will be asked to focus your attention and to concentrate on the affected area, and then to note any thoughts, mental images, and emotions that come to you. This process will then be repeated so that a complete picture of your physical, emotional, and mental health can be drawn up.

You may be asked to make changes to your diet at this point, and, if there are valid reasons, you may be given a cleansing diet, devised by Dr. Stone himself, for an appointed period. If necessary, counseling may also be advised in cases where there are significant issues that require more focused attention and you need support in dealing with them.

The benefits of this form of therapy cannot be overstated. Anyone who is willing to incorporate regular attendance at a polarity practitioner's, and to take responsibility for themselves, can only grow enormously in self-awareness. With the therapist's support throughout, this process is hugely enhanced.

Psychological therapies

While most of the therapies in this section take a holistic, mind/body approach, it is important to remember that the mind is very complex and, as such, deserves a section of its own. Therapy has become an increasingly popular form of self-discovery and new theories are emerging all the time. Descriptions of some of the most important therapies in the field of psychology follow.

Behavioral therapy

This form of psychotherapy seeks to predict and control behavior in a scientific way. Based on learning theories, it began in the early years of the 20th century. During the 1960s, cognitive therapy developed; this form is concerned with belief systems and perception, helping the client change the way they view situations and, therefore, change the outcome.

Analytical therapy

This form of therapy began toward the end of the 19th century and includes many variations, such as psychoanalytical and psychodynamic psychotherapies and psychoanalysis. The theory behind analysis considers an individual's mindset as the outcome of conflict between internal forces, and looks for answers within the individual's unconscious. The aim is to analyze the effects of early experience and to discover how they may be causing difficulties in the present.

Freudian psychoanalysis

Freudian psychoanalysis is based on the theory that unconscious factors play a large part in determining behavior. Its founder, Sigmund Freud, worked extensively with patients suffering from mental problems in the late 19th century. While his theories were ridiculed at the time, they still endure today, and are the foundation for many other types of therapy.

The relationship between therapist and patient is paramount in psychoanalysis, as it is important to the process of recovery that the patient is able to trust and confide in their therapist. By analyzing physical manifestations of the workings of the unconscious—dreams, emotions, and thoughts—and re-experiencing key events with the therapist, repetitive patterns of behavior and emotional blocks are revealed, which over time provide clues as to the source of the patient's problems.

Typically, psychoanalysis is a long-term process; patients will often have several sessions a week over a period of six months or more in order to work through their problems. Psychoanalysis is thought to work particularly well for people who are physically strong, and may have achieved a lot, but who tend to be plagued by problems like depression and low self-esteem.

Jungian psychoanalysis

Psychiatrist Carl Jung built on Freudian psychoanalytic theory by extending the definition of the unconscious mind to include the "collective unconscious." This part of the mind contains elements that, unlike Freud's unconscious, are not dependent on personal experience, but are a result of the collective unconscious, made up of archetypes based on primitive images that shape our perception of the world and are universally present, regardless of race, gender, etc.

Because of the close connection with Freudian theory, a typical Jungian psychoanalysis session provides a very similar experience. Dream analysis and the open discussion of feelings and emotions are tools common to both disciplines; however, the methods of interpretation differ between the two. A Jungian therapist will analyze a dream, for instance, with reference to the symbolic imagery of the collective unconscious—ancient motifs that mirror and describe our external experiences. The therapist aims to help the patient become aware of patterns of behavior and recurring themes in such dreams that highlight areas of difficulty in their life. Again, this is a long-term process and is suitable for people with specific problems, such as introversion or low self-esteem, or those who simply want to increase their self-awareness.

Gestalt therapy

The aim of this type of therapy is to achieve self-realization through here-and-now experiments in awareness. The feelings and emotions of the patient in the present moment are paramount, in contrast to psychoanalysis, which emphasizes the importance of past experiences and repressed desires in determining behavior. Because extensive discussion of emotions tends to result in a "theorizing" of those feelings, emotional honesty is hard to achieve in traditional psychoanalysis.

Patients are encouraged to bring their feelings into the present using role-play

and other methods of improvization to reenact important situations in their lives. In this way, the patient feels spontaneous and genuine emotions about that particular situation, and can recall past experiences with clarity rather than playing out learned responses tainted by hindsight. The aim of gestalt therapy is to help the patient develop new reactions to stressful and emotional situations based on genuine, in-the-moment feelings.

Group therapy

There are many kinds of "therapeutic groups" which have many dynamics in common: group therapy, group counseling, encounter groups, awareness groups, support groups, T (training) groups, self-help groups, and personal awareness or sensitivity-training groups. Individuals in "therapeutic" or "growth" groups give themselves and the other participants an opportunity to explore feelings in a safe and confidential atmosphere (even if all the participants do not feel equally safe or up to the risk). Things you never discuss regarding your personal or professional life may find an outlet in the context of a group, which gives you permission—and, indeed, encourages you—to explore and share your individual agendas and the feedback it provokes.

Group therapy and group counseling evolved during the World War II, when there was a shortage of trained therapists available to provide individual therapy. At first, the group therapist assumed a traditional, therapeutic role, frequently working with a small number of clients with a common problem. However, leaders gradually began to experiment with different roles. Many discovered that a group setting offered unique therapeutic possibilities, and began to take advantage of these. The dynamics of a group offered support, caring, confrontation, and other qualities not found in the framework of individual therapy. Within the group context, members could practice social skills and apply some of their new knowledge.

Group counseling is not aimed at stimulating major personality changes and is not concerned with treating neurotic and psychotic disorders in the way that group or individual therapy is. The counseling group seeks to resolve specific, usually short-term, issues and deals with more conscious problems than the "therapy" group.

Integrative therapy

This form of therapy is holistic and many therapists working in this way have a humanistic background. Integrative therapy considers the whole person—mind, body, and spirit—and seeks to achieve integration between the three aspects.

Transactional analysis

Transactional analysis (TA) focuses on external behavior patterns, rather than internal psychological processes, by looking at our interpersonal interactions and how these reveal toxic patterns of behavior that prevent us from dealing honestly and openly with others.

The TA theory of the ego provides an easily understandable way of describing our relationships. The interplay of the three ego states, and the degree to which one dominates, determines the types of "games" —devious strategies used to manipulate others into doing what we want—the individual plays. In theory, the "child" is emotional and seeks approval and attention; the "adult" is rational and logical; and the "parent" is disciplinary and moralistic. This translates into real life; for example, a dominating partner may act out the "parent" role in a relationship in order to get what they want. The "games" we play make up the damaging patterns of behavior or "life scripts" that the individual follows, and the aim of the TA therapist is to expose these toxic games. In doing so, the therapist tries to encourage the individual to throw away dysfunctional life scripts and replace them with honest and direct interactions.

Transpersonal therapy

See page 257.

Psychosynthesis

The purpose of psychosynthesis is to unite the separate and sometimes conflicting elements of the mind to form a complete and comprehensive whole, including, for example, those parts that determine personality, desires, impulses, and values and morals. The aim of this integration is to increase self-awareness and to aid the mental and emotional growth process, in order to fulfill the massive human potential we all possess and which too often goes unrecognized.

Psychosynthesis is based on the premise that life has meaning and purpose, which is to further the universal evolution of consciousness. Therefore, it represents a strongly holistic approach to psychology, with the emphasis on the spiritual.

Radionics

As in so many other areas of natural medicine, every aspect of physical existence is seen to vibrate on multiple levels. Radionics is a method of working with the interface between the energetic realm and the psychical. Radionic practitioners recognize that all aspects of existence, including states of illness and wellness, vibrate at specific rates that are directly reflected through sound in the calibrated dials of radionic instruments, which look a little like sophisticated radio sets.

Someone seeking radionic treatment will send in a sample of hair or blood, which the practitioner uses to tune into their frequency. Harnessing the energetic interface between the psychic realm and the physical, the treatment takes place in the more subtle realms of energy fields. The patient doesn't need to be present at the time diagnosis takes place.

A radionics practitioner uses the equipment to tune into the patient's energetic imbalances simply through the medium of the sample of the patient's hair or blood. In addition to the use of the radionic instrument, the practitioner uses what is a type of ESP or radiesthetic faculty to obtain answers to questions posed in the

therapist's mind about the patient's health. The vibratory rate of the illness is subsequently reflected on the frequencies received through the radionic instrument.

Using the hair or blood spot as a direct link back to the patient, the radionic practitioner then finds the right frequency to counteract directly the frequency of the imbalance or illness of the patient. A supplementary healing effect can be added by placing a homeopathic remedy, flower remedy, or vitamin or mineral sample near the hair or blood sample, while the practitioner is broadcasting the radionic treatment back to the patient.

Since radionics is such an effective diagnostic tool, other forms of alternative healing or dietary changes can be suggested once the nature of the imbalance has been determined. Radionic divining can help find other methods that would additionally facilitate wellness for the patient. Like many forms of alternative medicine, radionics can be used as an adjunct to other healing modalities.

Rebirthing

Mention the word "rebirthing" and images spring to mind of reliving your own birth. But why, since your mother was likely to have been in extreme discomfort at the time, call a beneficial healing therapy after that moment?

The name "rebirthing" is taken because some therapists have felt that the strength of "life-denying" and limiting choices can trail all the way back to the choices made at the moment of birth. In the rebirthing therapy, the process of "conscious connected breathing" allows you to go back in time and "choose again" at the moment of birth—or, indeed, any other moment since. This time, you can choose thoughts that support the highest and most loving experience for the self. The activity of breathing safely in a conscious, connected fashion means that you are able, spontaneously and gently, to confront whatever choices are blocking the experience of joy that is your birthright.

This transformational breath work allows deep memories and repressions to be gently accessed. The opportunity for forgiveness is then offered to you by your rebirther, thereby facilitating the highest possible emotional healing at that moment. Rebirthers often work with bodywork and/or affirmations to support the client in making the most loving and valuable choices in any session. However, it is not always necessary to relive the moment of birth in order to reap numerous benefits.

Often people experiencing a series of sessions (initially twelve sessions are the usual recommended amount) find their lives improving dramatically as their previous choices to hold back their life force are renegotiated. The individual may be consciously aware of making the choice to live differently/more joyously/more peacefully, but these realizations can also happen subtly. People sometimes simply feel their life force and capacity for joy expanding, without consciously having to access the memories or the stuck patterns that have held them back.

Making the highest choices possible in life is the most supportive dynamic tool you can have, and can create a more loving space for your relationship with yourself, your family, and your friends. Rebirthing work is profoundly life-altering, and working in a series of sessions can dynamically improve the quality of your life. Rebirthing allows for the expansive beauty of the soul to be experienced in healing breath work and loving choices made in the present moment.

Reflexology

Reflexology is a popular natural therapy that treats health problems or potential problems by massaging the feet and sometimes the hands. This is an ancient healing art practiced by the Chinese more than 5,000 years ago and by the ancient Egyptians, Greeks, and native North Americans, such as the Hopi.

Reflexology is based on the idea that the whole body and its systems are reflected in specific areas of the feet. These areas are called reflex zones and there are particular spots that link to a specific organ or function, which are called reflex points. The use of pressure therapies to clear blocks along the paths of energy is commonplace in the East. Acupuncture, acupressure, and shiatsu are other well-respected Oriental energy therapies.

A reflexologist gently and firmly massages the feet, pressing various reflex points to clear blockages and toxic build-up in the organs and various internal body systems that can lead to something more serious if unchecked. Although it does not hurt, you may experience a certain sensitivity and tenderness to pressure on certain points on the feet, ankles, and the hands. Not all reflexologists use the hands in their treatment—but the feet are always treated. Precisely where you feel the most tenderness or sensitivity reflects the point in the body where you may be experiencing congestion or imbalance.

According to practitioners, reflexology stimulates the body's immune system and recharges your personal powers for self-healing. It divides the body into ten zones, each of which corresponds to an area on the foot. The left side of the body is linked to the left foot and the right side to the right foot. Perhaps this is why it was known as "zone therapy" before it was called reflexology.

The heel relates to the lower back; the ball of the foot to the lungs; and the big toes to the head and brain. For example, if you are treated for migraine, the reflexologist will massage and press the corresponding zone and point on your feet, in this case the top of your big toes. It is a simple principle—for every important organ or body system, there is a tiny area that corresponds to it on one or both feet.

Reflexology seems to have many beneficial effects and is gaining recognition as more and more testimony comes to light. Reflexology is an excellent complementary therapy to any orthodox treatment because it doesn't use drugs or devices and has a wonderful, soothing, relaxing benefit, which seems to help eliminate stress after even just one session. Increasingly, the medical establishment is integrating reflexology into its hospital wellness programs, with nurses training in reflexology and using the treatment in hospitals nationwide.

Reflexology can help protect your health and prevent illness. An area of pain on a particular point may indicate a problem in the corresponding organ or body system—or it may just mean there is a potential weakness in that area that may lead to a more serious problem later if not addressed. In this way, reflexology can be a very useful tool in your prevention program. Always consult your doctor for any persistent or serious symptoms.

Reflexology can be used to treat arthritis, asthma, bronchitis, constipation, depression, digestive disorders, irritable bowel syndrome, insomnia, migraine, muscular tension, PMS, sciatica, sinus problems, and stress.

Reiki

Reiki, pronounced "ray-kee," is Japanese for "universal life energy." This ancient healing art is believed to have originated thousands of years ago in Tibet via Tibetan Buddhism. It was rediscovered in the 19th century by Mikao Usui, a Japanese minister, at a Christian seminary in Kyoto, Japan.

Dr. Usui spent fourteen years seeking the ability to heal, and it was his belief that he might achieve this by studying Buddhism and learning both Chinese and Sanskrit to promote his research. According to tradition, Usui spent 21 days fasting on a sacred mountain outside Kyoto, and it is there that he received a vision incorporating four symbols that could be used to aid healing to pass onto others. His vision revealed how the universal life energy, described in ancient Sanskrit writings, Indian *sutra* or sacred texts, could be accessed and utilized to provide hands-on healing.

Tuning into the symbols creates the ability to channel healing power. Dr. Usui died in the 1930s, having initiated sixteen other people into the secret of reiki, teaching them the master attunement. Thanks to Dr. Chujiro Hayashi, one of Usui's students, reiki has remained with us. He established a reiki clinic in Tokyo after noting all the sequences of hand movements in a reiki session and the results of healing sessions.

Now reiki is flourishing worldwide and is available to everyone. Reiki practitioners hold the belief that the body becomes ill only when the universal life energy is imbalanced. The treatments therefore aim to bring balance and harmony to the physical, and treat any emotional or spiritual disorders at the same time. Anyone can train to be a reiki practitioner through a series of courses, although it is not actually taught but "transferred" from teacher to pupil.

A reiki treatment promotes emotional, spiritual, and physical wellbeing. Clients usually lie down, clothed, while the practitioner gently lays his or her hands over the energy centers of the body, thus allowing healing energy to flow into the body. The treatment usually begins with the head and ends with the feet, to promote grounding of energy. There are some reiki practitioners who do not make contact with the body, but instead send healing energy into the aura, the energy field that surrounds the earthly body.

Reiki can be used successfully as a self-treatment, and for those in training this is actively encouraged to promote their own wellness. Reiki energy can even be directed into the future or faraway places. Animals and plants also respond well to reiki healing.

Courses are a series of "degrees," the first usually lasting a weekend and then four more initiations by a reiki master. By the end of the first degree, trainees will be able to send healing energy to themselves and others. After completion of the second degree, the trainees will be able to give distant healing. Those wanting to train others take the third degree, based around "teaching" transferral.

The results of reiki treatment are often quite dramatic and sudden, but just as often, they are gradual. The recipient of reiki must seek to take on responsibility for themselves as well as receive treatments from a practitioner. The results of reiki can be long-lasting and can effect cures if the recipient makes the decision to foster a self-loving and self-caring attitude.

Reiki practitioners believe that daily self-treatment, together with taking active preventative measures in terms of physical health, provides spiritual growth and emotional support. They make a huge effort to work on themselves to ensure their efficacy in treating others. Treatments normally last from 30 to 60 minutes, and the format is usually four sessions over four consecutive days. Depending on the individual, sessions may be spread out over two months, once a week or more.

Reiki can treat absolutely anything and has no contraindications. Anyone who feels they are experiencing serious illness of any type will benefit from reiki, but should always take the precaution of at least having a diagnosis from an orthodox doctor. Minor illnesses, including emotional disturbances, can be treated with this peaceful, loving therapy as successfully as more chronic or acute conditions.

The ever-growing popularity of this particular form of healing worldwide indicates that vast numbers of people have benefited from the treatment. Perhaps it is the disciplined "education" that this healing therapy employs that adds to its appeal among Western populations, who are increasingly looking to Eastern forms of healing and health.

Relaxation therapy
See page 252.

Self-hypnosis
Self-hypnosis, incorporating visualization techniques (see page 211), can be used in conjunction with a course of hypnotherapy. It is especially useful in cases where the patient requires on-the-spot treatment and the therapist can't be around, such as when suffering from insomnia or asthma. Self-hypnosis makes use of the mind's own unconscious healing powers to help alleviate pain, speed recovery, and lessen depression, anxiety, phobias, and addictions.

An excellent time to practice self-hypnosis is at night, just before falling asleep, and in the morning, just after waking up. The countdown to trance can be provided for you on a tape by the hypnotherapist with whom you are working. Otherwise, you can make use of the natural trance-like state between sleeping and waking.

Self-hypnosis is particularly valuable in the alleviation of pain. One technique for this is called "glove anesthesia." The person puts themselves into a trance or uses a tape to provide the countdown to trance. Their hand is placed over the painful area and the suggestion is made to feel the hand as heavy, numb, and completely relaxed. The sensation is then transferred into the body part in pain, allowing the pain to decrease and a comforting sensation of peace to follow.

Shiatsu
Shiatsu is a Japanese holistic bodywork system that aims to achieve wellbeing through an efficient flow of energy around the body. The shiatsu system is similar to acupuncture in that it involves stimulation of the body's meridians or energy paths, but uses a rhythmic series of massage techniques instead of needles—shiatsu literally means "finger pressure." These techniques aim to reduce muscle tension, release toxins, such as lactic acid and carbon monoxide, from the joints, and relieve any general stiffness that can impair the body's energy flows.

Although largely preventative, aimed at maintaining the quality and quantity of the body's *chi,* and its flow around the body, shiatsu is also believed to treat specific complaints, including stress, fatigue, back pain, migraine, irritable bowel syndrome, constipation, diarrhea, menstrual problems, circulatory problems, arthritis, allergies, asthma, insomnia, and sexual problems.

A shiatsu practitioner will diagnose your state of health by asking about your medical history and how you feel physically and emotionally. He or she may also use traditional Oriental methods of diagnosis, such as a pulse- or face-reading, to look for signs of fatigue, bloating, and so on.

The shiatsu session takes place lying down, since correct body positioning and gravity play a large part in achieving effective results. The session may begin with stretching and breathing exercises aimed at relaxing the muscles and creating a quiet and meditative atmosphere. After the initial general energy-balancing moves, the practitioner concentrates on specific problem areas, holding each point for three to five seconds to release blocked energy. The session ends with calming techniques, aimed at pacifying disturbed energy and restoring an efficient flow.

Sound therapy

The use of sound and music for healing and therapeutic purposes is now accepted in many academic circles (as well as artistic ones). Most of us have some first-hand experience of the depth of feeling evoked by a particular sound or song, but the concept of the healing power of sound is finally gaining recognition and respect.

More and more people have awakened to their own natural voice and the power that comes from giving themselves permission to use it. Our real natural voice is a gift, and everyone has the right to treasure, explore, and share the gift of their true voice to express themselves, whether by sounding the meditative "om" or singing a favorite song.

Music is one of the most ancient forms of expression, and the recent rediscovery of sound healing is the "hot" alternative therapy. More complementary therapists are using chanting and singing to heal the body. Many believe that we made music before we made words, and when we reclaim or discover our voice and give ourselves permission to use it, we are rewarded with increased vitality and self-esteem.

Qualified music therapists now work at numerous hospitals and health care facilities. In addition to professional therapists, choir leaders, and music teachers, there are other ways to tap into the benefits of sound, such as simple chanting or just plain singing in the shower. The journey through sound is so individual—what really moves you or stimulates a "peak" experience may irritate or grate on your partner. Unless you live on an isolated mountain top, it's an idea not to try to join the "dawn chorus"! Nevertheless, while respecting that what makes your heart sing may make another weep, remember that your natural voice is beautiful and that you have the right to use it when and how it feels natural for you.

Thai massage

Like many Oriental systems of medicine, Thai massage aims to disperse energy blockages that are believed to be the cause of illness. Traditional Thai medicine takes a particularly holistic approach to wellbeing, seeking to restore equilibrium to the mind/body/spirit relationship. Drawing on Buddhist philosophy, it has a strong tradition of practice within the family. Massage is only one component of the total Thai medicine system; the others being nutrition, herbal remedies, and spiritual counseling, especially meditation.

Thai massage is strongly influenced by yoga, which is evident in the passive stretching techniques that are its trademark, and also by traditional Chinese medicine, in the stimulation of the body's meridians. At first Thai massage may seem too vigorous to be relaxing, but it has the power to calm disturbed energies and emotions while simultaneously energizing the body. Other benefits include improved circulation, increased flexibility, pain relief, release of muscle tension, realignment of the spine and bones, and stimulation of the internal organs and nervous system.

The typical Thai massage session lasts one to two hours and is performed on a mat on the floor. It is important to wear loose,

comfortable clothing that you can move around in easily. The masseur/masseuse applies gentle pressure to various points of the body, depending on the individual's needs, using fingers, thumbs, palms, elbows, knees, and feet.

A key part of Thai massage is the passive stretching of the torso and limbs— the practitioner will support your body in various poses that encourage the opening up of joints without straining the muscles, in order to release toxins and relieve stiffness. A Thai massage should leave you feeling balanced and energized.

Therapeutic massage

Sometimes called Swedish massage, therapeutic massage is a medically respected therapy, based on the oldest healing modality in the world. Hippocrates suggested a daily massage was the way to maintain optimum health, and therapeutic massage treatments are certainly one of the nicest ways to take your medicine.

Using a basis of five different moves, pressure is applied to the body either in small rhythmic motions, long connected strokes, deep kneading, or cupping moves, all which stimulate the circulatory system and allow the efficient removal of waste from the lymphatic and muscular systems.

The therapeutic massage therapist will first ask you questions about your medical history, making sure that you do not have any contraindications to the treatment. Once this has been established, you lie down on the massage table, and the therapist usually starts the treatment on the back, using either talcum powder or oil as the massage medium. Pressure is firm, but gentle, and the overall effect is both stimulating and soothing. (See more on pages 220–29.)

Tissue (cell) salts

Biochemical remedies are the result of the life's work of a German doctor, Wilhelm H. Schuessler, who lived from 1821 to 1898. Our bodies are made up of millions of cells, and in order to function properly, they require a constant supply of chemical substances, including natural substances like mineral salts. Dr. Schuessler believed an imbalance or deficiency of certain mineral substances in the cells could cause a disturbance of function and health. He isolated twelve mineral salts as essential cell nutrients and called them "tissue salts," although they are commonly referred to as "cell salts." Dr. Schuessler's form of treatment became known as nutritional biochemistry, and to support his findings, he put forward five main principles:

1 Disease does not occur if cell activity is normal.

2 Cell activity is normal if cell nutrition is normal.

3 The human body requires both the complex organic compounds and inorganic (mineral) substances as cell nutrients.

4 A mineral salt deficiency will impair the ability of cells to assimilate and utilize the organic compounds.

5 Cell nutrition and metabolism can be revitalized by supplying the deficient mineral salts in a readily assimilated form.

Even with a balanced diet, it is still possible to have a localized deficiency because of fatigue or injury, but which will respond well to cell salts. The principle of assimilation is fundamental to Dr. Schuessler's theory of biochemistry. Assimilation into the body can be achieved by the administration of a micro-dose of the cell salts, which pass quickly into the bloodstream through the mucus lining of the mouth and throat.

The homeopathic principle of trituration—a controlled, slow mixing and grinding process to break down the active ingredients—is used to incorporate the mineral salts in micro-dose amounts into a milk-sugar base. Small molded tablets are prepared from the mixture. When these are placed on the tongue, assimilation immediately begins.

Cell salt therapy is suitable as a first-aid treatment for many minor, simple, and easily recognized conditions. All cell salts are totally safe and free from side-effects.

Tui na

Tui na is a Chinese form of bodywork similar to physiotherapy in Western medicine and to shiatsu in Japanese medicine. By means of vigorous massage and bone manipulation, using a wide variety of hand movements, Tui na stimulates the body's meridians—or paths of energy flow—and disperses the energy blockages that lead to illness and disease.

After a general question-and-answer session, covering illnesses, allergies, and other health problems, the practitioner will identify the important energy trigger points for your condition, or surrounding the affected area for more specific complaints. Tui na is very much a collaborative effort its effectiveness depends to some degree on the practitioner's ability to harness their own energy and redirect it into their hands, encouraging a revitalizing flow of energy between the two of you.

Tui na translates literally into "push grasp," a good indication of the hand movements used. Typical techniques include pressing and dragging, rolling, vibrating, twisting, shaking, patting, and beating the skin and muscles, to stimulate blood flow and flexibility and relieve stiffness in the muscles and joints.

Tui na is believed to be effective for a wide range of conditions, including bone misalignment, migraines and neck pain, digestive disorders, and viral illnesses, as well as various pediatric complaints. You should, however, avoid Tui na if you are pregnant, or have heart disease or cancer (particularly of the skin or lymphatic systems), if you suffer from brittle bones (osteoporosis), or if you have particularly sensitive skin.

Yoga therapy

Yoga therapy involves the patient working with specifically directed yoga asanas (see page 168) in conjunction with a yoga therapist. The yogic asanas work directly on toning the muscles, but they also have a profound effect on revitalizing the internal organs, since working yogically helps to realign the body. The life force of the body becomes more readily available, thereby allowing the complete healing process to speed up in cases where there has been an injury or illness.

Yoga therapy has successfully helped millions of people with cases of chronic and acute pain, anxiety, menstrual problems or disorders, asthma, and bronchitis. If you are considering directed yoga therapy for an injury or illness, make sure that your condition is first diagnosed by your doctor.

Zero balancing

Zero balancing is a hands-on type of bodywork that works directly at the interface points between the muscular and skeletal systems. Points where these structures meet are used as vital energetic pathways to access and rebalance the vibrational and physical bodies. In this respect, zero balancing works with both the physical and energetic structures of the body to give a full body-mind attunement.

Created in the 1970s by Dr. Fritz Smith, zero balancing combines both Western and Eastern healing modalities. Applied specific finger pressures are combined with held stretches called "fulcrums." The work allows a still point through which old energetic and physical patterns that no longer serve the client can be released. The resulting effect is the release of deeply accumulated tensions that have been held in the physical body.

Zero balancing is so called because the work enables the client to reach a "zero point," an energetically balanced state that feels clear and neutral. This integrated state allows a deep and profound sense of peace and relaxation, akin to that of intensive meditation.

The evaluation of the body by the therapist is performed by testing the range of motion around a joint. This work is a very effective and safe way of treating physical pain, as well as for integrating emotional stress. The experience is one in which the client's overall sense of wellbeing is ultimately enhanced.

index

bibliography

Alexander, Jane. *Spirit of the Home.* Thorsons, 1998.

American Heart Association. *2001 Heart and Stroke Statistical Update.* Dallas, Texas: American Heart Association, 2000.

Anderson, Dr Norman B., *Emotional Longevity* (Penguin Books Ltd., 2003).

Appleton, Nancy. *Healthy Bones: What You Should Know About Osteoporosis.* Avery, 1997.

Atkins, Dr. Robert. *Dr. Atkins' Age-Defying Diet Revolution.* Vermilion, 2000.

Baker, Dr. Sidney MacDonald, and Karen Baar. *The Body Clock Diet.* Vermilion, 2001.

Balch, Dr. James F. *10 Natural Remedies That Can Save Your Life.* Doubleday, 1999.

Beeken, Jenny. *Yoga of the Heart.* White Eagle, 2000.

Borysenko, Joan. *Guilt is the Teacher and Love is the Lesson.* Warner, 1991.

Brownstein, Dr. Art, and Joan Borysenko. *Healing Back Pain Naturally.* Harbor Press, 1999.

Cameron, Julia. *The Artist's Way.* Pan, 1995.

Campion, Kitty. *Holistic Family Herbal.* Bloomsbury, 1997.

Challem, Jack. *The Inflammation Syndrome.* John Wiley & Sons, Inc., 2003.

Cherewatenko, Dr Vern S. and Perry, Paul. *The Stress Cure.* Harper Resource, 2003.

Cochrane, Amanda. *Perfect Skin.* Piatkus, 2000.

Cochrane, Amanda. *Treat Your Child the Natural Way.* Thorsons, 2001.

Consadine, Mike, ed. *Whole Person Catalogue.* Brainwave, 1992; mail order only.

Chopra, Deepak. *Ageless Body, Timeless Mind.* Rider, 1999.

Chrystyn, Julie. *Lifeforce.* Blake, 1998.

Clark, Susan. *The Sunday Times Vitality Cookbook.* HarperCollins, 2000.

Cousin, Pierre Jean. *Facelift at Your Fingertips.* Quadrille, 2001.

Crawford, Dr. Michael, and David Marsh. *Nutrition and Evolution.* Keats, 1995.

D'Adamo, Dr. Peter, and Catherine Whitney. *The Eat Right Diet.* Century, 1997.

Dean, Dr. Ward, and John Morgenthaler. *Smart Drugs and Nutrients.* B&J, 1990.

Dossey, Dr. Larry. *Meaning and Medicine: A Doctor's Tales of Breakthrough and Healing.* Bantam, 1992.

Edwards, Betty. *Drawing on the Right Side of the Brain.* HarperCollins, 1993.

Farris, Russell and Marin, Dr. Per, *The Potbelly Syndrome.* Basic Health Publications, Inc., 2006.

Firshein, Dr. Richard. *The Nutraceutical Revolution.* Vermilion, 1998.

Geffen, Dr. Jeremy. *The Journey Through Cancer.* Vermilion, 2000.

Goodrich, Janet. *Natural Vision Improvement.* Celestial Arts, 1987.

Harris, Gail. *Body & Soul.* Kensington, 1999.

Heller, Dr. Raechel F. and Dr. Richard F. *The Carbohydrate Addict's Diet.* Vermilion, 2000.

Herbert, Victor, and Genell J. Subak-Sharpe, eds. *Total Nutrition: The Only Guide You'll Ever Need, from the Mount Sinai School of Medicine.* St. Martin's Press,1995.

Hoffman, David. *The New Holistic Herbal.* Element, 1983.

Holford, Patrick. *100% Health.* Piatkus, 1999.

Holford, Patrick. *The Optimum Nutrition Bible.* Piatkus, 1998.

Holford, Patrick, and Judy Ridgway. *The Optimum Nutrition Cookbook.* Piatkus, 1999.

Ivker, Robert S.; Robert A. Anderson; and Larry Trivieri. *The Complete Self-care Guide to Holistic Medicine.* Jeremy P. Tarcher, 1999.

Keating, Kathleen. *The Little Book of Hugs.* Doubleday, 1998.

Kenton, Leslie. *The Raw Energy Bible.* Vermilion, 1998.

Lee, Dr. John R. *Natural Progesterone.* John Carpenter, 1999.

Mellor, Constance. *Natural Remedies for Common Ailments.* Beekman, 1981.

Peirce, Andrea. *The American Pharmaceutical Association Practical Guide to Natural Medicines.* William Morrow, 1999.

Plant, Jane. *Your Life in Your Hands.* Virgin, 2000.

Powell, Trevor. *Free Yourself from Harmful Stress.* Dorling Kindersley, 1997.

Reavley, Nicola. *New Encyclopedia of Vitamins, Minerals, Supplements, and Herbs.* M. Evans and Company Inc., 1998.

Reid, Daniel. *The Tao of Health, Sex and Longevity.* Simon & Schuster, 2000.

Richardson, Rosamond. *Natural Superwoman.* Kyle Cathie, 1999.

Robinson, Lynne. and Gordon Thomas. *Pilates: The Way Forward.* Pan, 1999.

Shapiro, Debbie. *Your Body Speaks Your Mind.* Piatkus, 1996; Sounds True, 2006.

Shapiro, Eddie and Debbie. *A Time for Healing.* Piatkus, 1994.

Shapiro, Eddie and Debbie. *Ultimate Relaxation.* Quadrille, 1999.

Spillane, Mary, and Victoria McKee. *Ultra Age.* Pan, 2000.

Sun, Howard and Dorothy. *Colour Your Life.* Piatkus, 1998.

Tisserand, Maggie. *Aromatherapy for Women.* Thorsons, 1985.

Trattler, Ross. *Better Health Through Natural Healing.* Thorsons, 1987.

Van Straten, Michael, and Barbara Griggs. *Superfoods.* Dorling Kindersley, 1990.

Washnis, George J. *Discovery of Magnetic Health.* Nova, 1993.

Weil, Dr Andrew *8 Weeks to Optimum Health.* Warner, 1998.

Wellings, Nigel, and Elizabeth Wilde McCormack. *Transpersonal Psychology.* Continuum, 2000.

Williams, Xandria. *Fatigue.* Ebury, 1996.

Williams, Xandria. *From Stress to Success.* Thorsons, 2000.

Williams, Xandria. *The Liver Detox Plan.* Ebury, 1998.

Wills, Judith. *The Food Bible.* Quadrille, 2000.

Yesudian, Selvarajan. *Yoga Week by Week.* Translated by D. Stephenson. Allen & Unwin, 1976.

addresses

SUPPLIERS

Circle of Health
PMB 399
2852 Willamette Street
Eugene, OR 97405–8200
541 349 8680
www.ayurveda-herbs.com
Ayurvedic supplements and
more; online store.

Dr. Hauschka Skin Care, Inc.
359C North Street
Hatfield, MA 01038
1 800 247 9907
www.drhauschka.com
Supplements, cosmetics,
treatments, and information on a
store or salon near you.

Flower Essence Society
P.O. Box 459
Nevada City
CA 95959
916 263 9163
1 800 736 9222
www.floweressence.com
Distributors of California
flower essences and Healing
Herbs, research information;
online store carrying FES
products and Tisserand oils,
and store locator.

General Nutrition Centers (GNC)
300 Sixth Avenue
Pittsburgh, PA 15222
1 888 462 2548
www.gnc.com
Store locator for Canada and
U.S.A., or www.drugstore.com
for online store.

GNLD Golden Neo-Life
orders: 773 721 5968
www.gnldusa.com
Quality nutrients, herbs, and
supplements; online ordering.

Herbal Remedies U.S.A.
225 North Wolcott
Casper, WY 82601
1 866 467 6444
www.herbalremedies.com
Vitamins, minerals, herbs,
homeopathic and Ayurvedic
remedies, teas and tinctures,
aromatherapy oils and products,
and magnetics; online store.

Herbs First
501 West 965 North
Suite 3
Orem, UT 84057
801 437 3538 (fax)
www.herbsfirst.com
Vitamins, minerals, teas, aminos,
tinctures, traditional Chinese
medicines, Ayurvedic remedies,
aromatherapy, magnetics, and Dr.
Christopher and Dr. Schulze
formulas; online store.

Nature's Answer
75 Commerce Drive
Hauppauge, NY 11788
1 800 439 2324
www.naturesanswer.com
Homeopathic extracts, herbs,
supplements, and creams; online
store and store locator.

Nelson Bach
100 Research Drive
Wilmington MA 01887
978 988 3833
1 800 319 9151
www.nelsonbach.com
Information on training, research,
products, treatments, and
seminars on Bach flower
remedies; online store.

Solgar Vitamins and Herbs
500 Willow Tree Road
Leonia, NJ 07605
1 877 765 4274
www.solgar.com
Wide range of the famous-brand
vitamin and herbal supplements;
online store and store locator.

Vitamin World
4320 Veterans' Memorial
Highway, Holbrook, NY 11741
1 800 228 4533
www.vitaminworld.com
Wide range of herbal remedies
and supplements; online store
and store locator.

Weleda Apothecary
6 Red Schoolhouse Road
Chestnut Ridge, NY 10977
845 352 6165
http://usa.weleda.com
Homeopathic tonics, supplements,
creams, and essential oils; online
store and store locator.

Winds of Change Health Products
300–2339 Hwy 97 North
Dilworth Shopping Centre
Kelowna, British Columbia
V1X 4H9 Canada
250 861 3699
www.vitaminscanada.com
Wide range of supplements; online
store and links.

USEFUL ADDRESSES

The following organizations can
be contacted for information on
treatments, education and
training, and referrals to certified
practitioners in your area.

Acupuncture
American Association of Oriental Medicine
433 Front Street
Catasauqua, PA 18032
610 266 1433
www.aaom.org

Chinese Medicine and Acupuncture Association of Canada
154 Wellington Street
London, Ontario N6B 2K8
519 642 1870
www.cmaac.ca
Education and clinic for
treatment at the institute.

Alexander Technique
Alexander Technique International
1692 Massachusetts Avenue
3rd Floor, Cambridge, MA 02138
1 888 668 8996
www.ati-net.com

American Society for the Alexander Technique
P.O. Box 60008
Florence, MA 01062
1 800 473 0620
www.alexandertechnique.org

Canadian Society of Teachers of the Alexander Technique
465 Wilson Avenue, Toronto,
Ontario, M3H 1T9, Canada
877 598 8879
www.canstat.ca

Aromatherapy
Pacific Institute of Aromatherapy
P.O. Box 6842
San Rafael, CA 94903
415 479 9121
Information on courses, and
locating products or practitioners.

The National Association for Holistic Aromatherapy
4509 Interlake Ave N., 233
Seattle, WA 98103-6773
888-ASK-NAHA
www.naha.org
Information on courses, and
locating products or practitioners.

Ayurvedic
Maharishi Ayur-Veda Health Center
RR # 2, Huntsville, Ontario
POA 1KO, Canada
705 635 2234
Ayurvedic treatment center.

American Academy of Ayurvedic Medicine
100 Jersey Avenue
Building B, Suite 300
New Brunswick, NJ 08901
732 2247 3301
www.ayurvedicacademy.com

National Institute of Ayurvedic Medicine
584 Milltown Road
Brewster, NY 10509
845 278 87004
http://niam.com
Workshops, retreats, courses, and
online products imported directly
from India.

also: Dr. Scott Gerson (founder)
5th Floor, 375 Fifth Avenue
New York, NY 10016
212 685 8600

Chelation therapy
American College for Advancement in Medicine
23121 Verdugo Drive, Suite 204
Laguna Hills, CA 92653
949 455 9679 (fax)
www.acam.org

Chiropractic
American Chiropractic Association
1701 Clarendon Boulevard
Arlington, VA 22209
703 276 8800

Canadian Chiropractic Association
1396 Eglinton Avenue West
Toronto, Ontario M6C 2E4, Canada
1 800 668 2076
www.ccachiro.org

Guided Imagery
Academy for Guided Imagery
P.O. Box 2070
Mill Valley, CA 94942
1 800 726 2070

Health Associates, Inc.
P.O. Box 220
Big Sur, CA 93920
408 667 0248 (fax)

Holistic Dentistry
Holistic Dental Association
P.O. Box 5007
Durango, CO 81301
www.holisticdental.org

Homeopathy
National Center for Homeopathy
801 North Fairfax St., Suite 306
Alexandria, VA 22314
703 548 7790

North American Society of Homeopaths
1122 East Pike Street
Seattle, WA 98122
206 720 7000
www.homeopathy.org

Hypnotherapy
American Institute of Hypnotherapy
1805 East Garry Avenue
Suite 100, Santa Ana, CA 92705
714 261 6400

American Society of Clinical Hypnosis
2200 East Devon Avenue
Suite 291
Des Plaines, IL 60018
708 297 3317
Register for M.D.s and dentists trained in hypnosis for treating health conditions.

International Medical and Dental Hypnotherapy Association
4110 Edgeland, Suite 800
Royal Oak, MI 48073
313 549 5594
1 800 257 5467

Massage
National Certification Board for Massage and Bodywork
8201 Greensboro Drive, Suite 300
McLean, VA 22102
800 296 0664
Referrals to NCTMB therapists in Swedish massage, shiatsu, rolfing, reflexology, and more.
www.ncbtmb.com

American Massage Therapy Association
820 Davis Street, Suite 100
Evanston, IL 60201-4444
847 864 0123
www.amtamassage.org

Meditation
Mind-Body Clinic
New Deaconess Hospital
Harvard Medical School
185 Pilgrim Road
Cambridge, MA 02215
617 632 9530
Treatments and training.

Stress-Reduction Clinic
University of Massachusetts
Medical Center
55 Lake Avenue
North Worcester,
MA 01655
508 856 2656
Training programs teaching meditation techniques.

Institute of Transpersonal Psychotherapy
P.O. Box 4437
Stanford, CA 94305
415 327 2066
Information on activities, research, and teachers

Naturopathy
American Association of Naturopathic Physicians
3201 New Mexico Avenue,
NW Suite 350
Washington, DC, 20016
866 538 2267
www.naturopathic.org

Homeopathic Academy of Naturopathic Physicians
12132 SE Foster Place
Portland, OR 97266
503 761 3298
www.hanp.net

Canadian Naturopathic Association
4174 Dundas St. W,
Suite 303
Etobicoke, Ontario,
M8X 1X3 Canada
416 233 2924

Nutrition
Society of Certified Nutritionists
2111 Bridgeport Way West 2
University Place,
WA 98466
1 800 342 8037

International and American Association of Clinical Nutritionists
16775 Addison Road
Suite 100
Addison, TX 75001
972 407 4089

Organics
Organic Trade Association
74 Fairview Street
P.O. Box 547
Greenfield, MA 01302
413 774 7511
www.ota.com
Information on all organic business in the U.S.A. and Canada, research, and news.

Osteopathy
American Academy of Osteopathy and the Cranial Academy
3500 DePauw Boulevard, Suite 1080, Indianapolis, IN 46268
317 879 1881

American Osteopathic Association
142 East Ontario Street
Chicago, IL 60611
800 621 1773
312 202 800
www.aoa-net.org

Pilates
The Pilates Studio
www.pilates-studio.com
Searchable online listing for certified Pilates guild members and course locations.

Pilates Physical Mind Institute
1807 Second Street, Suite 40
Sante Fe, NM 87505
505 988 1990
1 800 505 1990
www.the-method.com
Courses and studios.

Reflexology
International Institute of Reflexology, Inc.
P.O. Box 12642
5650 First Avenue North
St. Petersburg, FL 33733–2642
727 343 4811
www.reflexology-usa.net
Worldwide referral service for practitioners of the Ingham method of reflexology.

Reflexology Association of America
4012 Rainbow Ste. K-PmB 585
Las Vegas, NV 89103–2059
www.reflexology-usa.org

Reflexology Association of Canada
L201–17930 105th Avenue
Edmonton, Alberta T5S 2H5
Canada
780 484 2097
1 877 722 3338
www.reflexologycanada.ca

Shiatsu
Boston Shiatsu School
East-West Institute of
Alternative Medicine
1972 Massachusetts Avenue
Cambridge, MA 02140
617 876 4048
Classes and courses in shiatsu, traditional Chinese medicine, meditation, and yoga.

Sound Therapy
American Association of Music Therapy
P.O. Box 80012
Valley Forge, PA 19484
215 265 4006
Offers treatment for music healing, stress reduction, psychological counseling, and referrals to music therapists.

Yoga
American Yoga Association
P.O. Box 19986
Sarasota, FL 34276
941 927 4977
www.americanyogaassociation.org

Himalayan Institute of Yoga, Science, and Philosophy
RRI Box 400
Honesdale, PA 18431
717 253 5551
1 800 822 4547
Nationwide yoga centers.

Sivananda Yoga
5178 South Lawrence Boulevard
Montreal, Quebec H2T 1R8
Canada
514 279 3545
Centers worldwide; in North America.
  Chicago: 312 878 7771
  New York: 212 255 4560
  San Francisco: 415 681 2731
  Los Angeles: 310 478 0202
  Toronto: 416 966 9642

International Association of Yoga Therapists
P.O. Box 1386
Lower Lake, CA 95457
707 928 9898
Information on yoga centers, therapists, news and journals.

288

acknowledgments

1 Images Colour Library; 9 Gettyone Stone/Mark Davison; 10–11 Telegraph Colour Library/Antony Nagelmann; 12 Gettyone Stone/Bill Pogue; 16 Gettyone Stone/Steve Ragland; 18–19 Images Colour Library; 24 Image Bank/M Regine; 27 Images Colour Library; 28 Gettyone Stone/Mark Davison; 31 Gettyone Stone/D Young Riess MD; 33–36 Images Colour Library; 38 Lorry Eason; 39 Anthony Blake Photo Library/ Martin Brigdale; 40 Anthony Blake Photo Library/ Matthew May; 42 above Photonica/ CSA Plastock; 42 center Anthony Blake Photo Library /Maximilian Stock Ltd; 42 below Photonica/CSA Plastock; 43 Images Colour Library; 44 Gettyone Stone/Z & B Baran; 46 Marie Claire Maison /Manfred Seelow/stylists Jacqueline Saulnier & Eric Solal; 48–49 Images Colour Library; 51 Insight Picture Library/Michelle Garrett; 52 Stockbyte; 54 Special Photographers Library /Barbara & Zafer Baran; 56–59 Images Colour Library; 61 Anthony Blake Photo Library/Paola Zucchi; 62 Gettyone Stone/D Young Riess MD; 64–65 Images Colour Library; 67 Telegraph Colour Library/Stuart Hunter; 69 Gettyone Stone/Sheena Land; 70–71 Gettyone Stone; 72–73 Gettyone Stone /Sheena Land; 74–75 Stockbyte; 76 Telegraph Colour Library/Francesca Yorke; 78 Gettyone Stone/Deborah Davis; 79 Stockbyte; 80 Telegraph Colour Library/Andy Eaves; 82–83 Gus Filgate; 84 Stockbyte; 85–86 Images Colour Library; 87 Stockbyte; 88 Gettyone Stone/Moggy; 90 Gettyone Stone/Ray Massey; 92 Hémisphères /Stéphane Frances; 93–95 Images Colour Library; 96 Gettyone Stone/Spike Walker; 97 Images Colour Library; 98–99 Collections/John Wender; 99 Images Colour Library; 100 Photonica/CSA Plastock; 101 Martin Brigdale; 102 Gettyone Stone/Chris Craymer; 102–3 Telegraph Colour Library/Hugh Jones; 104 Gettyone Stone/Tony Stone Imaging; 104–5 Images Colour Library; 106 Gettyone Stone/Z & B Baran; 107 Images Colour Library; 108 robertharding.com/Lee Frost; 110 Gettyone Stone/Amy Nennsinger; 110–11 Gettyone Stone /Steve Taylor; 112–14 Images Colour Library; 115 Gettyone Stone/Anwell; 116 Food Features; 116–17 Images Colour Library; 118 Photonica/Patricia McDonough; 120 Gettyone Stone/Nick Vedros & Associates; 121 Gettyone Stone/Darryl Torckler; 122 left Stockbyte; 122 right Photonica/CSA Plastock; 124 Stockbyte; 126 Images Colour Library; 128 Gettyone Stone /Darryl Torckler; 129 Gettyone Stone/David Epperson; 130 Images Colour Library; 131 Gettyone Stone/Claudia Kunin; 132 Gettyone Stone/Stuart Miclymont; 134 Gettyone Stone/Sheena Land; 136–37 Gettyone Stone/Jack Ambrose; 138 Gettyone Stone/David Roth; 140 Gettyone Stone /Nicholas Devore; 141 Gettyone Stone/Gary Faye; 142–43 Gettyone Stone/Christopher Thomas; 143 Gettyone Stone/Paul Edmondson; 144–57 Vic Paris; 156 Gettyone Stone/David Ash; 158–59 Gettyone Stone /Aldo Torelli; 160–61 Gettyone Stone/A & L Sinbaldi; 162 Gettyone Stone/Gary Nolton; 162–63 Gettyone Stone/Sheena Land; 164–65 Photonica/Richard Seagraves; 166–67 Gettyone Stone/Bill Pogue; 169 Gettyone Stone/Michelangelo Gratton; 170–81 Vic Paris; 182 Gettyone Stone/Eric Larrayadien; 183 Gettyone Stone/Martin Barrand; 185 Contact Images/Michael Cole; 186 Image Bank/Juan Silva; 187 Photonica/Ann Cutting; 188 Encore; 190–91 Gettyone Stone/Hulton Getty; 192–93 Encore; 194 Gettyone Stone/Laurence Monneret; 196–99 Encore; 200 Gettyone Stone/Hulton Getty; 202 Gettyone Stone /David Chambers; 203 Gettyone Stone /Shaun Egan; 204–5 Encore; 206 Gettyone Stone/Ross Anania; 207 Gettyone Stone/Bob Torrez; 208 Image Bank/Rob van Petten; 211–13 Images Colour Library; 214–15 Encore; 216 Image Bank/Paolo Curto; 218 Gettyone Stone/Keren Su; 220 Image Bank/Marc Romanelli; 221 Gettyone Stone/Nina Rizzo; 223–25 Encore; 225 Gettyone Stone/Jack Ambrose; 226 Image Bank/Nino Mascardi; 228–29 Images Colour Library; 230 Gettyone Stone/Claire Hayden; 231 Gettyone Stone/Donna Day; 232 Powerstockzefa; 235 Gettyone Stone/Don Bousey; 238–39 Gettyone Stone/Chip Porter; 240–41 Gettyone Stone/Natalie Fobes; 242–43 Images Colour Library; 243 Gettyone Stone/Hulton Getty; 246 Gettyone Stone/Ebby May; 247 Gettyone Stone/Reza Estakhrian; 248 left Gettyone Stone/Stanley Brown; 248 right Gettyone Stone/Brandtner & Staedeli; 251 Impact/Mike McQueen; 253 Gettyone Stone/Giantstep; 254–55 Gettyone Stone/Giantstep; 256 Encore; 257 Gettyone Stone/Eric Larrayadien

Author Acknowledgments
My heartfelt thanks and deepest gratitude to Jennifer Dodd and Catharine Christof, whose continual support has made this project possible. I am also grateful to Anne Furniss, Mary Evans, Françoise Dietrich, Rachel Gibson, Jane O'Shea, and all the team at Quadrille, and to freelance editor Anne McDowall, for their excellence and perseverance. Thank you also to Caroline Turner, Vic Paris, Amanda Clarke, Paul Bailey, Paul Walker, Carole Diplock, Michael Skipwith, Sue Beechey, Anne Harling, Michael Phillips, Joanne Sawicki, Alannah Tandy, Graham Wilson, Bridget Bodoano, Nick Parsons, and Sophie Bracken. I am especially grateful to the generous contributions and support of many people who have inspired me and taught me much of the information that is included in this book.

Love and thanks to my family and friends, especially Eleanor and Philip Schwartz; Jane Silk and Alan Nathan; Zoe, Sean, Aron, Charlotte, Thea and Evie Wellband; Peter and Ruth Schwartz; Sandy and Millie Schwartz; Paul and Marion Dattelbaum; Kim and Jim Corbett; Alex and Amanda Lowson; Tina Fletcher, Pleasure John Riley; Nancy Howard; Barbara Freije; Mani Morice; Jennifer and Mark Sprackling; Catherine Christof; Helena Coghlan; Jane and Tony Weldon; Susie Allfrey; Andrew Homewood; Prue Faull; John Prudhoe; Toni Liberthson Hunter; Nancy and John Franco; Eileen Ahearn; Georgina Hale; and Toni and Peter Sturtevant.

The author is grateful to these people for their permission to use extracts, as follows: Pierre Jean Cousin; Patrick Holford and Judy Ridgway; Eddie and Debbie Shapiro; Mary Spillane and Victoria McKee; Xandria Williams; and Celia Wright.

Thank you to the following people for their permission to use their text:
Alison Belcourt; Sarah Bridgland; Jerome Burne; Catharine Christof; Pierre Jean Cousin; Jennifer Dodd; Lewis Esson; Emma Noble; Susie Perry; and Caroline Turner.

We are grateful to the consultants listed at the front of this book for their valuable expert advice and recommendations.